Leadership and Management in Nursing

Mary Ellen Grohar-Murray, RN, PhD
Associate Professor of Nursing
Saint Louis University School of Nursing

Helen R. DiCroce, RN, MSN
Emeritus Associate Professor of Nursing
Saint Louis University School of Nursing

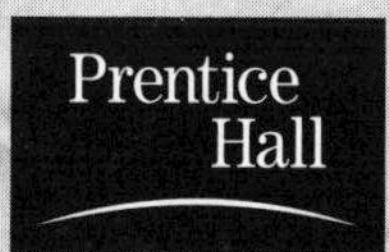

Upper Saddle River, New Jersey

Library of Congress Cataloging-in-Publication Data

Grohar-Murray, Mary Ellen.
Leadership and management in nursing / Mary Ellen Grohar-Murray, Helen R. DiCroce.— 3rd ed.
p.cm.
Includes index.
ISBN 0-13-061777-6
1. Nursing services—Administration. 2. Leadership. 3. Nurse administrators I. DiCroce, Helen R. II. Title.
RT89 .G76 2003
362.1'73'068—dc21 2002016921

Notice: Care has been taken to confirm the accuracy of information presented in this book. The authors, editors, and the publisher, however, cannot accept any responsibility for errors or omissions or for consequences from application of the information in this book and make no warranty, express or implied, with respect to its contents.

The authors and publisher have exerted every effort to ensure that drug selections and dosages set forth in this text are in accord with current recommendations and practice at time of publication. However, in view of ongoing research, changes in government regulations, and the constant flow of information relating to drug therapy and drug reactions, the reader is urged to check the package inserts of all drugs for any change in indications of dosage and for added warnings and precautions. This is particularly important when the recommended agent is a new and/or infrequently employed drug.

Publisher: Julie Levin Alexander
Executive Assistant and Supervisor: Regina Bruno
Executive Editor: Maura Connor
Assistant Editor: Yesenia Kopperman
Editorial Assistant: Sladjana Repic
Marketing Manager: Nicole Benson
Product Information Manager: Rachele Strober
Director of Manufacturing and Production: Bruce Johnson
Managing Production Editor: Patrick Walsh
Production Editor: Amy Hackett/Carlisle Publisher Services
Manufacturing Manager: Ilene Sanford
Manufacturing Buyer: Pat Brown
Media Managing Editor: Amy Peltier
Media Project Manager: Stephen Hartner
Design Director: Cheryl Asherman
Design Coordinator: Maria Guglielmo
Cover Design: Gary J. Sella
Composition: Carlisle Communications, Ltd.
Cover Printer: Phoenix Color Corporation
Text Printer: RR Donnelley & Sons, Harrisonburg, VA

Pearson Education LTD.
Pearson Education Australia PTY, Limited
Pearson Education Singapore, Pte. Ltd
Pearson Education North Asia Ltd
Pearson Education Canada, Ltd.
Pearson Educatión de Mexico, S.A. de C.V.
Pearson Education – Japan
Pearson Education Malaysia, Pte. Ltd

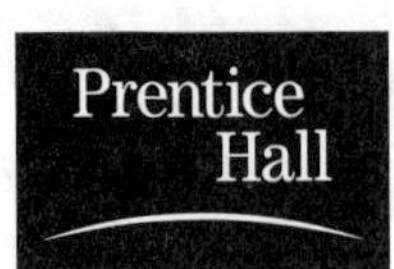

10 9 8 7 6 5 4 3 2
ISBN: 0-13-061777-6

Contents

UNIT 2: An Overview of Organizations and Management 121

7 Overview of Nursing Management 149

13 Managing Change 251

Preface

The third edition of this text offers students updated content that reflects the major changes in health care delivery that have occurred over the past several years. Many have impacted nursing as a profession in a profound way. One of the most striking changes is the number of professional nurses who have been displaced in acute-care settings in favor of ever-increasing nonprofessional care providers. In order to ensure safe care to patients, nurses who did survive the cuts became responsible for supervising nonprofessional personnel in practice settings. Along with the changed configuration of caregivers in care settings, nurses experienced a loss of professional autonomy in decision making relative to care delivery. Physicians found themselves in a similar bind. In their stead, business and health insurance considerations dominated decisions about the types and length of services patients were entitled to. At no other time in the history of health care in the United States have changes in the system resulted in such unprecedented turmoil. Administrative decisions failed to take into account the vital role nursing has historically played in health restoration and preservation over the decades. Nursing titles came to resemble those of the business world as the differences between business and professional standards were blurred. Over time, problems that emerged from such changes forced administrators to recognize the important role that only nursing can fill in the delivery of comprehensive health care. As a result, administrators are rethinking many of their cost-cutting strategies. On the plus side of the unprecedented changes, many physicians have a new appreciation for professional nurses as colleagues in the delivery of care. The time is right for nursing to reclaim its autonomy within the practice of nursing, and renew its role as an equal collaborator with other health professionals in the planning, delivery, and evaluation of health care. All of these factors influenced our approach to the updating of content for the third edition of this text. Several references to problems that came from the new system, along with ideas for resolution, are made throughout the chapters.

The content and concepts presented in this edition remain the same as in previous editions, reflecting their timeless nature. The latest literature from management, leadership, and nursing have been added to the references used in the text. Examples illustrating the concepts are updated to reflect current practice and new case studies, and learner exercises are provided at the end of each chapter. We were pleased to learn that the second edition of the text was recognized in the 1998 Brandon/Hill Selected List of Nursing Books and Journals under the heading "Administration and Managed Care." Books included in the list represent contemporary concepts, theories, and trends in nursing and set forth sound clinical methods. This recognition reinforces our belief about the value of the book's contribution to the nursing literature for both generic students and registered nurse students returning to universities to complete a baccalaureate degree in nursing.

The content in this edition is divided into four units — Unit 1: Leadership; Unit 2: An Overview of Organizations and Management; Unit 3: Special Responsibilities of the Manager; and Unit 4: Managing Resources. In Unit 1 there are five chapters — The New Health Care System, Leadership Theory, Interactive Processes of Leadership, Decision Making and Conflict Management, and the Ethical Responsibilities of the Nurse Leader. There are three chapters in Unit 2 — Organization and Management Theory, Overview of Nursing Management, and Delegation. Unit 3 focuses on nursing managers and divides their responsibilities into five chapters — Maintaining Standards, Motivation in the Work Setting, Monitoring and Improving Performance, Legal Issues in the Workplace, and Managing Change. Unit 4 has four chapters devoted to managing resources — Managing Resources: The Staff, Managing Resources: Time, Managing Resources: The Budget, and Informatics in Nursing.

We continue to believe the flow of content in this text is logical and lends itself well to study by beginners. This belief is reinforced by reports of students relative to its readability. Using exercises in the book as a basis for written reports about their practice, students continue to provide us with contemporary evidence that this book is useful to beginners in the profession. Incorporating those reports into classroom discussions adds significantly to the value of a leadership course because their personal experiences replace sterile textbook content and they feel some ownership in the presentations. Student reports continue to provide us with some insight into the world of the beginner. It is an invaluable source of material for the classroom. We believe this edition will be helpful to students' understanding of the place nursing occupies in the overall health care system.

Additional exercises and activities to complement the third edition can be found on the Companion Website and Distance Learning Courses. Some of the features included are:

- Objectives
- Key Concepts
- Outline Review
- Critical Thinking
- NCLEX Review
- Message Board
- And more!

To access these features, visit the homepage for *Leadership and Management* in Nursing, 3rd Edition at www.prenhall.com/grohar-murray

Acknowledgments

We are indebted once again to several individuals for their assistance and support during the writing of revisions for the third edition. We are grateful to the publishers for showing an interest in a new edition, and for the assistance they provided us through sending reviewers' comments along with all the other materials needed to meet their publishing requirements. We are most grateful for the expertise of the contributing authors who add so much to selected chapters. Their dedication to nursing and knowledge in their respective fields are highly valued. The revisions by Judith A. Roos (Chapter 12 on legal issues), Dr. Carol Quinn (Chapter 5 on ethics), and Dr. Joan Carter (Chapters 9 and 16 on standards and the budget, respectively) would not be as valuable without them. Dr. Carter was very ably assisted by Lee Stoll, retired administrator of Saint Louis University Hospital, in revising her chapters. We feel very fortunate that the contributing authors were willing to share their backgrounds for the benefit of future nurses.

We would be remiss in not acknowledging the support of our families for their forebearance during the many hours the writing of revisions took from family activities. Their patience and understanding are very much appreciated.

Lastly, we wish to acknowledge the influence that promising, bright students continue to have on us. It is through their eyes that we have a glimpse of their world as new practitioners of nursing. From them we continue to learn and to marvel at their dedication to nursing in turbulent times of unprecedented change. They sustain the deep-seated belief we have that the profession of nursing is an undying service to society.

Mary Ellen Grohar-Murray
Helen R. DiCroce

Contributors

Joan H. Carter, RN, PhD
Associate Dean and Associate Professor
Saint Louis University School of Nursing
St. Louis, Missouri

Carrol Quinn, RN, DNS
Vice President of Quality Improvement
Mercy Franciscan Partnership
Cincinnati, Ohio

Judith A. Roos, RN, MSN
Doctoral Candidate
University of Illinois
Chicago, Illinois

Lee Stoll, RN, MSN
Consultant
Ioverus Consultants
Clayton, Missouri

Cherill I. Stockmann, RN, MSN(R)
Doctoral Candidate
Saint Louis University School of Nursing
St. Louis, Missouri

Reviewers

Julie K. Baylor, MSN, RN
Assistant Professor, Nursing
Bradley University
Peoria, Illinois

Debby Brown, RN, BS, MS, MS, PhD(c)
Assistant Professor
University of Rhode Island
Kingston, Rhode Island

Dawna Martich, RN, BSN, MSN
Clinical Trainer
American Healthways
Pittsburgh, Pennsylvania

Mary Carol Galichia Pomatto, EdD
Professor and Assistant to the President
Pittsburg State University
Pittsburg, Kansas

Patricia A. Thomas, PhD, RNC
Professor, Department of Nursing
Rhode Island College
Providence, Rhode Island

Maureen Tremel, MSN, ARNP
Nursing Instructor
Seminole Community College
Sanford, Florida

UNIT 1

Leadership

1

The New Health Care System; Challenge to Nursing Leadership

"I studied the lives of great men and famous women, and I found that the men and women who got to the top were those who did the jobs they had in hand with everything they had of energy and enthusiasm."

Harry S. Truman

INTRODUCTION

The time is right for nursing to take charge of the profession's place in health care delivery. A serious nursing shortage has firmly placed the spotlight of attention on nurses and what they do. This is an opportunity to form alliances with powerful and influential people in the government and media to generate public support for nursing's unique contribution to the nation's health. In order to formulate a framework in which the nursing role will be used appropriately, leadership skills will be needed. The goal of this textbook is to introduce the student to a comprehensive leadership and management theory and to give suggestions for the acquisition of these skills.

The health care industry has been in the midst of revolutionary changes for almost three decades. Health care priorities, services rendered, structures, and personnel have all been radically affected. Dynamic forces, among them 43.4 million uninsured Americans,[1] continue to influence health care delivery. Consequently, the nursing profession has been expected to meet the new challenges. These challenges include taking on more responsibility in the management of patient care, redesigning systems of nursing care delivery, incorporating new technologies into practice, and struggling with the inherent conflicts between the nursing professions' values and the demands of the new health care system.

Because of the dramatic changes, opportunities for nurses willing to accept the challenges abound. In particular, nursing leaders are needed to ensure that values held by the nursing profession continue to define the nursing role in health care delivery. The current health care system and foreseeable future will be dominanted by managed care, professional issues (especially the shrinking and aging workforce of nurses), and society's demand for accessible, quality, and cost-conscious health care. This chapter will discuss the health care environment, the basis for nursing leadership, and challenges for the future.

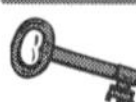

KEY CONCEPTS

Ambulatory Care refers to the health care services provided on an outpatient basis; no overnight stay is required. The services provided by ambulatory care centers, hospital outpatient services, physician's offices, and home health care fall under this category.

Ambulatory Payment Classification (APC) refers to The Health Care Financing Administration (HCFA) new outpatient prospective payment system for outpatient health care (Primary care and ambulatory settings).

Behavioral/Situational Framework is a theoretical foundation that suggests appropriate behavior results from a detailed framework analysis of a situation. The variables that define the situation include the greater society, the organization, a particular event, and leader and follower characteristics. The appropriate behavior refers to leader/manager behavior that provides guidance, inspiration, or direction toward accomplishing an end.

Capitation refers to a preset amount of money allocated to provide a set of services for a population over a stated period of time, regardless of the services used.

Diagnosis-Related Groups (DRGs) are one of the first systems that categorized patient and disease information based on averages leading to uniform cost for each category. The following variables determine the category: primary and secondary diagnosis, primary and secondary procedures, age, and length of stay.

Fee-for-Service refers to the traditional payment method whereby patients pay doctors and hospitals.

For-Profit Organizations are organizations with stated financial structures that include profit goals and tax liabilities.

Health Maintenance Organization (HMO) is an alternative health care delivery agency and financing mechanism (prepaid comprehensive health coverage for hospital and physician services), which provides primary care services and refers specialty needs to appropriate sources (contracted partners).

Leadership is a concept and process that is capable, through interactional phenomena, of influencing a group toward goal achievement.

Managed Care refers to the assumption of responsibility and accountability for the health of a defined population and the simultaneous acceptance of financial risk.

Managed Competition refers to the future goal of health care delivery to allow patients and payers to choose among available integrated systems that would best meet their needs. Service, price, quality, and availability would be among the issues to consider.

Management is a concept and a process that uses resources (human, technical, financial, time, and so on) to meet specific goals efficiently and effectively.

Medical Industrial Complex is a term given to the network of clinics, hospitals, and practices that comprise a unit to deliver health care in a managed care environment and capable of engaging in managed competition.

Not-for-Profit Organizations are organizations with financial structures that project financial goals with particular tax and legislative protections or shelters.

Preferred Provider Organization (PPO) is a term used to describe an arrangement between purchasers of care (employers and insurance companies) and a group of practitioners who provide services to patients for a designated network at a discounted rate to encourage the use of available services.

Primary Care is a term used to describe the basic health care all persons require. It is also the entry point of care in the managed care environment.

MANAGED CARE

The United States does not have a unified vision of how health care should be delivered. Thus, providing health care to the U.S. population has increasingly become a major economic, political, and social issue. The growing number of medically uninsured continues to be a serious ethical problem. The tension between delivering care that is high quality, cost conscious, and accessible has led to the development of managed care. **Managed care** is intended to provide health care to patients through one seamless system as they move from wellness to sickness and back to wellness. Continuity of care, prevention, and early intervention are the goals of the system. It provides the kind of primary health care that nurses do best.[2] While managed care continues to dominate the health care delivery system, problems and criticism have also increased. Reports of poor quality of care, depersonalized care, poor comunication, and confusion over roles are some of the problems cited. In response to these public and professional concerns, a variety of managed care models were developed and a serious study of managed care has been instituted by the Center for Health Systems Change.[3] Analysis and discussion by experts has begun the evaluation process. Concerns and issues are being reviewed in a slow and methodological process.

HEALTH CARE REFORM

Events leading to the development of managed care began in the mid-1950s. Up to this time, care was provided on a **fee-for-service** basis. In addition, at that time, there was a vast expansion of the health care system in terms of volume, intensity, dollars, and personnel.

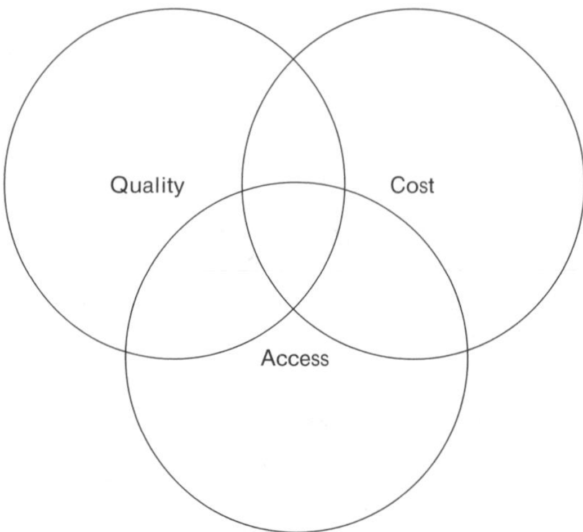

FIGURE 1-1. The dominant elements of nursing's values for health care reform.

This unrestrained investment in the health care industry led to a rapid escalation of health care costs. All payers (those who reimburse care), especially the federal government, were greatly affected. As a result, in 1983, Congress deliberately enacted what has become known as the Social Security Amendments of 1983 Law HR-1900 (PL 98-21). This legislation included the establishment of a prospective payment system based on 467 **diagnosis-related groups (DRGs)** that allowed pretreatment diagnosis billing categories for almost all U.S. hospitals reimbursed by Medicare. This amounted to a set of maximum fees that would be paid for Medicare patients. Hospitals would make a profit only if the cost of hospitalization was less than agreed upon by the corresponding DRG category. For the first time there was an incentive to keep costs down. This was the major event that started a revolution within the entire medical care industry, which dramatically altered the nature of health care delivery. Soon major insurance companies followed suit by establishing price ceilings as reimbursement for hospital care received. Because health care was accountable for cost containment, nursing departments were also expected to account for the cost of direct and indirect care. In the process, nursing service departments reorganized the delivery of nursing care, and in some cases nurses were laid off and several hospitals were no longer operative. In addition, major hospital reorganization efforts ensued by the formation of networks, consolidation of services, and development of partnerships (see Figure 1-1).

These activities, while substantial, were not sufficient to harness the increasing rise of health care costs. In response, the Clinton administration actively attempted to overhaul the health care system and stop the rate of growth. A task force, led by Hillary Clinton, (the First Lady) was controversial from its inception. Nevertheless, in September 1993, amid considerable public interest and continuing political controversy, the task force proposed a program for health care reform. This government initiative was rejected; however, it pressured the marketplace and insurance company financing to continue their efforts toward change.

The changes translated into managed care. Initially, the shift of working (and insured) Americans into managed care plans held health care costs down, but health care costs eventually began to rise. Each year health care costs increased, and estimates suggest the health care costs will exceed 2.1 trillion dollars by the year 2007.[4] Again, the problem of how to harness the growth of costly care is before policymakers. High health care costs in the United States is attributable to a variety of reasons. People are living longer, often with a greater risk of chronic disease; technology innovations; prescription drugs; innovative and expensive interventions for the treatment of illness (transplantation, stem cell therapy, and reproductive technologies also have ethical implications); and more contribute to the cost factor. Since the financing of health care continues to plague health care delivery, concerns and questions have been posed. Among them:

Is the quality of care better?
Can cost be controlled?
Where are cost-cutting strategies being realized?
How have these changes affected the nursing profession? Other health care professions?
Where is care being delivered?
Who is receiving care? Who is deprived of care?
What effect does the vast number of medically uninsured have on the health care system?

MANAGED CARE CHARACTERISTICS

Consequences of these questions are being felt in the current health care system. Managed care continues to be the dominant financing mechanism moving from fee-for-service that proposes effective, responsible, and cost-efficient care for an individual within a given population. The care is intended to be a cooperative process between the managed care organization and the patient. Managed care is a system that integrates the financing and delivery of appropriate medical care by means of the following mechanisms:

- **Care is population based.**
  Population-based care encompasses the concepts and methods of epidemiology and public health. It is comprehensive care that recognizes not only the individual but also the community and environment with special emphasis on healthy practices that promote health. Thus, the health care professional's role of delivering care to the individual has expanded to consider other factors that impact that care. The overarching goal is to improve the health status of the population.

- **All participants are held accountable.**
  Joint accountability is expected on the part of all parties involved for the cost and quality of health care. This includes the patient, practitioner, and administrators of the managed care system (the insurance provider). This may be accomplished through coinsurance or a cost-sharing requirement under a health care policy, which provides the insured (patient) will assume a portion of the cost (usually 20 percent)

of covered services. The cost, quality, and value of care are evaluated to ensure quality of care and efficient use of resources through monitoring, controlling cost, and judiciously using medical services.

- **Information to assess value is necessary.**
All relevant information is collected about the delivery of care, including patient data, population information, cost data, and technological information, in order to ensure that patients receive the most appropriate care. Evidence-based care, critical paths, and quality controls are used to ensure, as well as evaluate, care. Reliance on information management is mandatory as a methodology to ensure the most appropriate and cost-effective care.[5]

- **Primary care is of central importance.**
Primary care is considered the chief mechanism by which preventive, therapeutic, and restorative care is provided in the least expensive cost center. **Primary care** is the entry point to access care, serves as a partner for a long-term caregiving relationship, and provides coordination of specialty care as well as all other services needed. Typically, this care is provided in **ambulatory care** settings.

Because of the growth and central importance of ambulatory care, the Health Care Financing Administration (HCFA) instituted a Medicare outpatient prospective payment system known as the **Ambulatory Payment Classification (APC)** System. The new system was authorized by the Balanced Budget Act of 1997.[6] Preset fees are established for ambulatory care services. It is predicted that the APC will be as important as the DRG system was to inpatient financing. The APC system was inevitable because of the effectiveness of the DRG system in substantially reducing expenditures in the hospital. Similar financial incentives will be in place for the APC; efficiency in delivery of care will have financial rewards. The APC system will not facilitate high-cost providers with cost-based Medicare payments. This particular activity has allowed primary care practitioners to be reimbursed for services on the basis of specified criteria. Nurse practitioners (NPs), as well as primary care practitioners, are eligible for reimbursement based on specified codes and regulations. Payment for services will be capped on the basis of care delivered. This was an extremely important event for NPs who now have statutory authority for the reimbursement of Medicare and Medicaid patients.[7] As was suspected, the private insurance companies and independent **HMOs** are following suit, and reimbursing primary care at a similar rate.[8]

- **Interdependence is a necessary component for health care delivery.**
The complexity of today's care requires numerous caregivers and specialists. This demands coordinated care that is not fragmented. Interdisciplinary care has long been used with specific populations (psychiatric and elderly, to mention two). The concept of the interdisciplinary team takes on more importance in managed care. The ultimate aim is to provide a mechanism for a seamless health care delivery system through a variety of interconnected services.

- **Contracts are used to detail finances and delivery of care.**
Currently, managed care organizations have a variety of ways of providing and financing health care. To support the specifics of the caregiving process, explicit contracts are provided. This informs all involved parties exactly what they will receive and what financial risk each party will assume. This means all participants—patient,

practitioner, and provider—have a responsibility for financing care and incentives to keep costs down.

The actual contract process is complex and evolving as more information and strategies for negotiation are developed. The integral components of the contract are the following:

- Contracted health plans are the basic set of agreements that an organization is willing to provide to its employees.
- Contracted providers represent the health care providers and the services they offer. In addition, the terms under which the providers will provide service must be stated.
- The membership characteristics refer to information about the individuals/employees covered by a plan, which may include a particular age demographic with known problems (health, language barriers, working hours). These descriptors of the membership allow the ability to target resources and services.
- Employer groups are the actual companies/organizations who provide health care benefits to employees. Their particular ability to provide health care benefits must coincide with the cost and services provided by the contracted health care organization. [9]

As the contract process becomes more sophisticated, the ability to compete among health care systems is becoming more intense,[10] leading to managed competition.

Managed Care Organizations

The formation of the **medical industrial complex**, a result of merging and reorganization of free-standing institutions, was an early step toward a competitive market-dominated system known as managed competition. Managed competition occurs when providers and insurers compete to provide services to defined capitated groups. Because these systems are integrally involved with finances, the language used is that of business and the insurance industry. For instance, **capitation** is a term that refers to a given amount of money allocated for a set of services for a particular population over a stated period of time. Prepaid medical groups are given a monthly fee regardless of the services used. With total capitation, the integrated health system is responsible for its enrollees. Patients who are paid enrollees are called covered lives. The system receives payment based on a negotiated single price per covered life, and it is paid upfront. The objective of this system then becomes to keep people healthy and out of the hospital by delivering quality care at affordable prices (ideally in primary care settings).

A wide variety of organizational arrangements provide managed care. Complicated legal and financial imperatives dictate whether the organization be a **for-profit** or **not-for-profit organization**. Some of the more common arrangements are referred to as health maintenance organizations (HMOs), **preferred provider organizations (PPOs)**, or exclusive provider organizations (EPOs). These organizations provide a wide range of services from prevention to designated acute care. A more detailed discussion of each follows:

Health Maintenance Organizations (HMOs)

A typical HMO is an entity that ensures health care services in a specific geographic area and provides basic and optional benefits to those who choose to enroll. This model is the original prototype of managed care, and existed long before the onset of managed care. It became an extremely useful organized system when managed care essentially became a mandate. There are different types of HMOs which contract and provide services, including the staff model HMO, group model HMO, network model HMO, and independent practice association model HMO.

A *staff model* HMO is a somewhat self-contained organization. Physicians, nurse practitioners, and other providers are hired as employees of the HMO and deliver care to those patients who are members (by virtue of employment or choice) as needed. Services may be limited to primary care or be more comprehensive. A limiting factor is that patients do not choose a provider, but rather are seen by any available practitioner.

A group model HMO represents a contractual agreement with a multispecialty group(s) of providers to deliver care for their membership. Reimbursement is by capitation (a preset fee is available for all members of the HMO whether they exceed or underuse the allocated amount), which means depending on the population's health needs, the HMO has a profit or a loss. Provider choice (while greater) is limited and recognized as a negative aspect.

A network model HMO represents contractual agreements with small medical practice groups or even solo practitioners who serve patients (members of HMOs) from their own office space. Capitation is the reimbursement method. The advantage is individual members have a choice of providers.

Independent practice association HMOs represent contractual agreements with a wide variety of providers, allowing members a great choice in providers. The limitation is the increased expense of this plan and less ability of the HMO to coordinate the patient record. [11]

A preferred provider organization (PPO) is an entire network of providers and organizations which coordinate and manage the managed care contracts. Because of the large volume of patients and providers, discounts are available for services rendered. Typically the members pay a co-payment. This model offers a great deal of choice for the members.

Exclusive practice associations represent a form of PPO where members must use the available list of providers or pay the entire cost of health care. [12]

There are other models, and more are being developed, that attempt to eliminate problems and yet maximize the objectives of cost consciousness and quality care. In a managed care system, the hospital is no longer the center of care. Rather, primary care (ambulatory care service) is the focus. Managed care places more emphasis on education, self-help, preventive services, and limits access to tertiary care or hospitals. Because the patient or enrollee is treated in the lowest cost setting, it is not desirable or cost effective to keep every hospital bed filled. In this system, the primary care practitioner is the central figure in controlling and managing health care delivery. The term "panel" is used to describe the group of providers. Panels serve to provide policy direction and control the configuration of practicioners within the managed care organization.

CHARACTERISTICS OF THE HEALTH CARE SYSTEM

Characteristics of the current health care system were first detailed by the Professional Education Workforce report,[13] and for the most part continue. However, the growing nursing shortage is a serious and ominous problem that dominates professional issues in nursing and will influence the delivery and quality of health care in the near future.

Professional Issues: The Nursing Shortage

The United States will be facing a critical nursing shortage of nearly 500,000 nurses by the year 2020, and by the year 2010 more than 40 percent of the nurses will be 50 years of age and over. [14] Implications of the declining and aging workforce are devastating for the nation's health. The health care system reorganization (low staffing ratios, reduced wages), opportunities in other fields, and misunderstandings about the nursing profession are among the conditions contributing to the nursing shortage. Unfortunately, if this trend continues, the nursing shortage will coincide with the aging baby boomer generation's health care needs. While every institution is not currently experiencing a lack of registered nurses, the prediction is the problem will worsen over time. [15]

In a study conducted by Buerhaus et al., the researchers examined the reasons for, and consequences of, an aging registered nurse workforce. There was a declining propensity for those born after 1960 to enter the nursing profession. Shortly thereafter, in the 1970s, women, who still composed the greatest percentage of nurses, were offered an expansion of career options. This further narrowed the number of candidates for the nursing profession. The net effect of these forces reduced the pool of young registered nurses in the 1980s and the 1990s who traditionally would have replaced those who were retiring or leaving the field.

From 1983 to 1998, the average age for registered nurses rose from 37 to 42 years of age, and approximately 60 percent of the workforce is now over 40 years of age. The decline in nurses has become noticeable in the specialty areas such as critical care and perioperative care. Traditionally, intensive care units have attracted young nurses, and operating and post-anesthesia recovery rooms have attracted older nurses. The number of nurses under 30 years of age is decreasing and older nurses are retiring. The shortage of nurses in these areas is predictive of things to come. The registered nurse workforce will be shrinking after 2010, and the supply of working RNs will be 20 percent below requirements by the year 2020. [16]

The implications for a nursing shortage are overwhelming and threaten the health of the nation. The shortage is expected to impact the quality of care, hospital staffing, and health care in general. Potential problems include reduced access to care, increased waiting times for patients from emergency care to primary care, and reduced positive patient outcomes. Patient outcomes, in particular, are sensitive to nursing input.

In response to the nursing shortage, the U.S. senate initiated hearings through the Subcommittee on Aging. Senator Barbara A. Mikulski of Maryland issued a statement describing the impact of the shrinking and aging nursing workforce and her commitment to finding a solution.[17] Long-term workforce planning is required and a variety of experts are suggesting efforts to address the problem. Buerhaus, a researcher and expert in nursing staffing, offered the following suggestions:

- Improve the image of nursing.
- Remove barriers and stigmas to men and minorities to induce their participation in the profession.
- Consider ways to keep older nurses in the workforce.
- Allow internationally educated nurses to practice in the United States, as well as offering admission to U.S. nursing programs.
- Take the message (shortage of nurses) to physicians, hospital administrators, policymakers, the general public, and the media. [18]

Leaders in nursing also recognize the magnitude and momentum of the powerful demographic and social forces driving this problem. The Tri-Council of Nursing (composed of four powerful autonomous organizations), the American Association of Colleges of Nursing, the American Nurses Association, the American Organization of Nurse Executives, and the National League for Nursing proposed strategies to reverse the new nursing shortage with long-term implications for the nursing profession. The recommendations include plans/programs in education, work environment, legislation, and regulation, as well as technology, research, and data collection. [19] The initiatives in education include developing career progression activities such as moving new nursing graduates through graduate school more rapidly, identifying alternative roles for nursing (innovative roles), instituting a more equitable compensation plan for different levels of nursing education, supporting staff development programs, and stimulating a more diverse group of youth to consider nursing as a career.

Initiatives in the work environment include implementing specific strategies to retain experienced nurses who provide direct care through flexible scheduling, rewarding preceptor and mentoring activities, implementing appropriate salary and benefit programs, establishing a more acceptable work environment by ensuring autonomy and appropriate management structures, and redesigning work to enable an aging workforce to remain active.

Advocating legislative and regulatory bodies to increase funding for nursing education, as well as providing support for the reimbursement of nursing activities, were suggested. The last set of suggestions included investigating technologies to accommodate a reduced nursing staff and support initiatives for workforce planning, while promoting data collection to account for variations that might affect workforce planning.[20] These suggestions, while worthwhile, require collaboration with policymakers to adequately address this threatening problem.

HEALTH CARE PRIORITIES

Participation by government officials, insurers, health care leaders, and input from the greater society have identified those aspects of health care that are most important. The following set of priorities represent their combined views. Each will be discussed independently, and the implications for professional nursing will be discussed. [21]

1. **An emphasis from treatment of disease to health promotion and disease prevention.** The managed care environment is part of a profound change in the culture of health care whose emphasis is moving away from the treatment of illness and toward wellness and health. Health promotion and disease prevention are long-held values of the nursing profession. Nursing organizations and the nursing press advocate preventive health services, quality of care, and accountability for health care outcomes. Underlying this precept is a major cultural transformation, with patients expecting a very different response from practitioners. Today, an information-rich middle class culture, and a population no longer content with an emphasis on illness, dominates society. In essence, these attitudes provide a positive environment for nurses, who are uniquely suited to provide this desired style of health care.

2. **A continuing need for primary care providers.**
   Primary care is the routine care needed by most people. It includes an annual physical, treatment for minor illness, periodic immunizations, and health screening. Within the managed care environment, primary care is the entry point to receive more complex medical treatment.

   Because of the need for primary care practitioners, advanced practice nurses (APNs) or nurse practitioners (NPs) provide primary care. APNs are registered nurses whose formal education (a master's degree) and clinical preparation extend beyond the basic requirements for licensure, resulting in a certificate, or second license. Specialties of APNs include: (1) certified nurse midwives (CNMs), (2) certified registered nurse anesthetists (CRNAs), (3) clinical nurse specialists (CNSs), and (4) nurse practitioners (NPs). Within these specialties are subspecialties for which APNs assume high levels of responsibility.

   In particular, NPs are educationally prepared to perform a wide range of professional nursing functions, including obtaining a medical history; performing a physical examination; providing prenatal care and family planning; providing well-child care (screening and immunizations); providing health maintenance care for adults; and collaborating with other health professionals as needed. In addition, NPs are prepared to perform some functions traditionally performed by MDs, such as diagnosing and treating common acute and chronic health problems and prescribing medications. NPs have a proven ability to offer quality, cost-effective primary care. Three decades of research give clear evidence that APNs provide care of comparable quality and at a lower cost than do doctors. Yet, many legislative barriers frustrate their potential. The extent to which NPs are able to perform traditional physician functions [for example, prescriptive license (the right to prescribe some medications)] is limited by individual state regulations, although nearly all states have acknowledged in varying degrees the expanded role of the APN. The issue of legislative approval, which changes and expands the scope of APN practice, involves complex public policy, specific legislative actions, and overcoming political obstacles with other health practitioners.

   The current system is demonstrating a growing support and acceptance of the variety of health care professionals, who deliver care in accord with their education. In this system, nurses are used to improve access to affordable health care. This is particularly true of patients who are at high risk for serious problems that might have been prevented. In particular, the elderly are served by gerontologic nurse practitioners (GNPs), while mothers and children are served by family nurse practitioners (FNPs). Minorities, immigrants, and children living in single-parent families are at risk for health care problems. They are traditionally underserved and exhibit problems that would benefit from preventive care such as immunizations and prenatal care. Opportunities for nursing to provide care to these groups is worthwhile and meaningful.

3. **More than half the nursing care will be provided outside the hospital, while the hospital will provide only critical care.**
   The acute care hospital provides care and interventions that cannot be offered in an outpatient setting. There has been a steady increase in hospital admissions since the

major reorganization effort following the institution of DRGs. Most hospitals are part of medical industrial complexes associated with specific managed care models. Despite consolidation efforts, urban and rural hospitals are reporting difficulty in hiring nurses, and longer recruitment times for management roles.

Nursing employment has a history of being erratic. However, as emphasis continues to grow regarding ambulatory and home health care, as well as an expansion of preventive and primary care services, more nurses will be required, and there is a looming nursing shortage. New and expanded practice sites, other than the hospital, have emerged. These sites include parishes, schools, ambulatory and day surgery centers, clinics, holistic care centers, and group practices. Some practice sites are integrated with an acute care system and some are stand-alone. Patient care depends on nurses, and strategies to retain and recruit nurses have never been more urgent.

4. **Clinical nursing knowledge will be challenged to include new skills.**
The practice environment requires evidence-based clinical knowledge from nurses. Nurses with specialty skills and experience are in demand. Nurses are in particular demand if they can lead multidisciplinary teams, serve as patient educators, and perfom as managers of care across the continuum or demonstrate a high level of skill in the operating room, recovery room, emergency room, intensive care unit, critical care areas, pediatric units, and labor and delivery. [21] In addition, nurses need to be prepared to share decision making with patients and evaluate treatment effectiveness. The ability to understand the total organizational perspective in the delivery of care will require leadership/management knowledge. Lifelong learning is a responsibility of the workforce.

5. **Scientific knowledge and technology will continue to increase.**
Modern times have given us computers and advanced technology whose full capability is yet to be determined. This can only be viewed as a positive step forward for the science of health care. However, modern technology challenges the profession to incorporate these advancements into the holistic philosophy of nursing, which is concerned with the total patient. The expense of modern technology makes cost containment a challenge.

6. **Ethical issues will continue to grow in complexity.**
Ethical problems will continue to exist on two levels: (1) those problems that have direct bearing on a patient's life and (2) policies that impact the health care system. Access to health care continues to be a major ethical and political issue for the health care system. The problem of the medically uninsured persists. The ability to provide access to all individuals is organized around two major issues. The first concerns the available mechanisms to finance health care, and the second concerns the allocation of scarce resources.[22]

FORECAST FOR HEALTH CARE

The nursing profession is a vital participant in health care delivery and is both affected by, and capable of, influencing the system. If the current trend continues (the shrinking

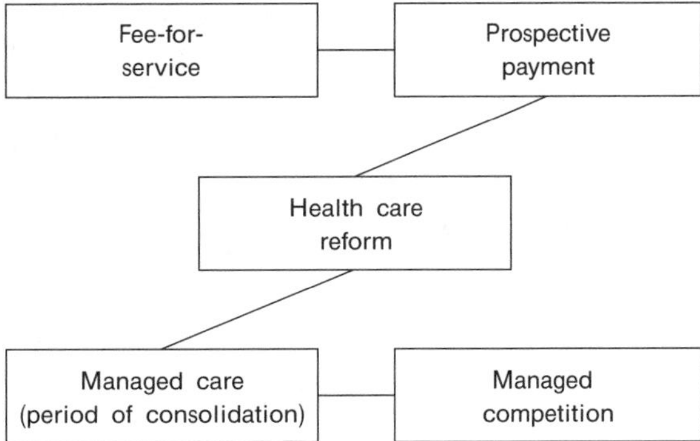

FIGURE 1-2. A depiction of the evolution of health care from the traditional fee-for-service to the future of managed competition.

nursing workforce), then major changes will be needed in the recruitment, education, and retention of professional nurses. The Bureau of Labor Statistics reports jobs for RNs will grow by 23 percent by 2008. Nurses will be required in literally every area of health care. This includes specialty areas and outpatient areas, in both rural and urban settings.

Just as there is a growing demand for nursing services, nursing school enrollments are down, older nurses are retiring, and serious concern is building. Thus, being a leader/manager in an unsettled environment demands that the nurse be prepared with the appropriate knowledge and skills. The nurse manager's preparation should include the analytical ability to identify problems and the skills to effectively lead and manage people through difficult and changing times. This makes the need for nursing leadership even more important to provide creative solutions to facilitate quality nursing and health care. The innovative nurse leader/manager of the future will be expected to use creative problem solving and interpersonal techniques, such as collaboration and negotiation. The future environment for health care delivery for which the nurse leader and manager must be prepared includes recognizing the values held by the nursing profession, supporting and empowering nurses, and marketing the work of nursing not only in the delivery of health care, but also health promotion, disease and accident prevention, research, and education (see Figure 1-2).

NURSING LEADERSHIP'S HERITAGE

Throughout history, there have been great nurse leaders. Their accomplishments have been studied through case study analysis, revealing personal characteristics of greatness. Several studies by Christy[23] reviewed the characteristics and contributions of Lavina Dock, Annie Warbuton Goodrich, M. Adelaide Nutting, Sophia F. Palmer, Isabel Hampton Robb, Isabel Maitland Stewart, and Lillian Wald. These nurse leaders became effective change agents and influenced legislation, nursing practice, and nursing education. Through their efforts, valuable contributions were made in areas of nursing education, nursing literature, and professional organizations, all of which proved to be substantial aids in the development of the profession. Today, outspoken nursing leaders (especially leaders in the American Nurse's Association and state chapters) continue to voice the values of nursing, share the accomplishments, and inform the nation of professional concerns and issues.

Challenge to Nursing

While changes are required to meet the demands of the managed care environment, some essential elements of the past must be retained to preserve the nature of holistic care, which is central to the very philosophy of nursing. Specific changes in nursing education were implemented as advocated by the National League for Nursing (NLN).[24] Reform of nursing education realigned programs to be more congruent with the changing direction of health care. Specifically, NLN directed "in a consumer-driven, community-based, primary care–focused based system, nursing education will have to concentrate on increasing the number of primary and tertiary care practitioners." While curriculum changes reflected the appropriate changes and clinical learning experiences continue to prepare practitioners with the skills needed for quality patient care in a variety of settings, there is an inadequate number of enrolled nursing students.

Serious changes, however, are needed in the practices that have led to the nursing shortage. Nursing salaries, change in working conditions, and recognition of the value of nursing care have to be addressed. Nursing education is sophisticated, scientific, and challenging. The workplace must change policies and financial incentives to reflect the knowledge and skills of professional nursing. The nursing profession has the unique power to influence both health care delivery and health care policy. This demands leadership skills at the national and local policymaking levels. The introduction of health-related policymaking and implementation concepts in nursing curricula, combined with that of leadership, management, and research theory, maximize nursing's efforts to society and the profession (see Figure 1-3).

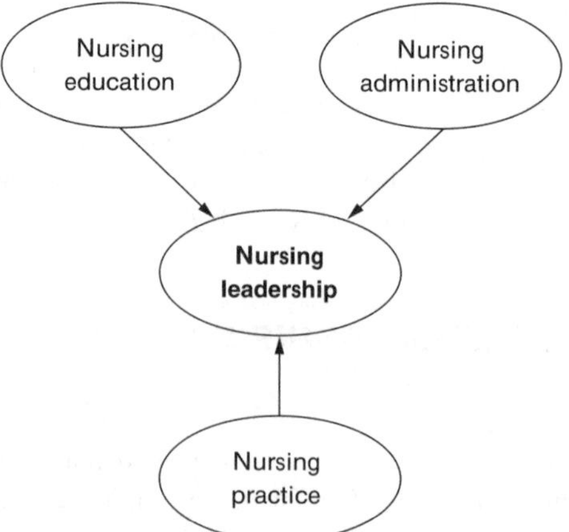

FIGURE 1-3. Factions of the nursing profession that define and guide the nursing profession and nursing leadership.

Leadership Framework

This is one of the most challenging and potentially rewarding times to be involved in the nursing profession. Never before has leadership been a more important concept to the practice and the profession of nursing. The ability to analyze situations, create objectives, and move others in the appropriate direction will be called upon by every practicing nurse. The transition from student to leader and manager is a process that involves knowledge, skill, experience, and time. What is common to the leadership and management process is that appropriate leader/manager behavior depends on the situation and available resources. Leadership and management skills are essentially cognitive. By reviewing the essential forces that affect a situation, appropriate decisions can be made. For this text the leadership/management process will be based on a **behavioral/situational framework**, which refers to the necessary behavior the nurse leader should use to achieve a goal. Appropriate leader behavior depends on conditions found in the situation and those affected by the situation. Consistently, the future nursing leader will be exposed to a way of analyzing situations from a broad base. From this perspective, decisions may be formulated from critical factors found in the environment, in a situation, within the leader, and within the group.

New leaders are going to be challenged to develop new and efficient methods of nursing care using older and fewer nurses, influence the working conditions for professional nurses, be outspoken advocates for professional nursing, and allow nurses to assume appropriate roles in new structures. A theoretical basis for leadership and management, as well as work experience, provides a good foundation for the nurse leader during these dynamic times. The importance of experience in the development of leaders has been well described in the experiences of executives from the public domain. Successful leaders provide evidence for the need of both knowledge and seasoning. This is particularly important in times of organizational and professional stress similar to the current health care system. The conclusion suggests preparation and mentoring are mandatory for those willing to assume leadership responsibility. Identifying potential leadership and management capabilities of individuals is critical in the selection of candidates for important roles. Stress in the workplace, staff morale, and general upheaval in the work setting prove to be quite costly when poor leaders and managers are in place. Identifying valuable traditions and practices through the efforts of nurse managers, nurse researchers, nurse educators, and nurse clinicians who work in concert with each other is sensible and brings unity to the profession.

Differentiating Leadership and Management

The terms **leadership** and **management** have been used several times throughout this chapter. It is appropriate to point out the way in which these key terms will be used in this textbook. Leadership and management are viewed as separate entities. Leadership is viewed as being a more fundamental and creative coordinating process than management, which selects actions that use resources effectively and efficiently. The authority of leadership is derived from the ability of the leader to influence others to accomplish goals, whereas the authority of management is derived from the manager's position in the organization. Anyone in a setting can serve as a leader by generating and proposing creative, innovative ideas and by applying predictive principles to problems. To be a leader, one does not have to occupy a formal managerial position. Managers, however, occupy formal positions in an organization and are accountable for the effective use of available resources. The chief executive officer (CEO) expects managers to "make the place run" according to a design. Skills of both managers and leaders are needed for successful operation of any organization. The skills of both might be embodied in one individual, but this is not necessarily true. Some who excel as leaders are poor managers, whereas others excel at managing an established situation while seldom generating ideas for needed redesign. Bennis,[25] a management scientist whose views were reiterated by Fred Manske,[26] points out the differences between a manager and a leader. He says a leader inspires and a manager administrates; a leader develops and a manager maintains; a leader relies on people and a manager relies on the system; and, lastly, a leader requires trust, while a manager requires control.

CASE STUDY

New Graduate Employment in an Emergency Room

Kim Jones just graduated from college with a baccalaureate degree in nursing. Kim entered the profession because she had an interest in serving people. Kim had planned to work on a general medical surgical area for a year to gain experience and then move to the Emergency Department. Since Kim had her senior year practicuum in the ED, she understood the depth and variety of knowledge needed to practice safely and effectively. In addition, the ED had a policy of only hiring nurses with at least two years of experience, which eliminated new graduates. As Kim was finishing her clinical experience as a student in the ED, the nurse manager approached her and said, "Kim, I have something I would like to talk to you about." The nurse manager explained that, since the nursing shortage, she had staff positions that needed to be filled. While it had never been the ED's policy in the past, they were reconsidering their hiring practices and wanted to hire Kim as a new employee of the ED. She also added that a special preceptor program would be developed. She inquired if Kim would like to participate in the planning of this program to prepare new nurses for positions in the ED. Kim was overwhelmed and felt she had some thinking to do.

- How would you go about advising Kim whether or not to accept this position?
- Is the establishment of a preceptor program sufficient for a new graduate?
- What should be the components of an ED preceptor program?
- What skills are necessary for working in an Emergency Department?
- What should Kim negotiate with the nurse manager in order to feel comfortable with this opportunity?

NOTE: It is believed to take at least a year of intense education and experience for a new employee to achieve competence in the ED. Studies are being conducted to determine the necessary aptitudes and critical thinking skills of potential candidates. Preceptor programs have proven effective coupled with education. New ways of enticing and retaining nurses in these highly skilled areas is challenging.

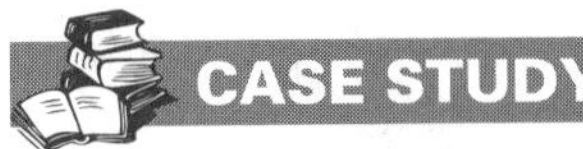

CASE STUDY

Leadership or Management?

In the managed care environment, St. Joseph's Hospital joined a network of other not-for-profit hospitals. Major reorganization efforts had consolidated surgical services to St. Joseph's. The nurses on 4 South, a general surgery division, were becoming increasingly angry about the short length of stay of patients, the high acuity level of the patients, and inadequate nursing staffing to this increasingly more complex patient census. The nurses began complaining. Were patients receiving quality care? The nurses felt there was too much emphasis on cost containment and most of the nurses felt they had no control over the situation. Mr. Smith, the nurse manager, recognized the turmoil and called a staff meeting to discuss the issues.

- Is Mr. Smith practicing leadership or management? What is the difference?
- What value is there in calling a meeting among the staff?
- Aren't the nurses powerless in this situation?
- What potential strategies might address the nurses' issues?

NOTE: The beginning of a meaningful solution to a problem starts with analysis. Individuals who share their perceptions and concerns may also develop meaningful solutions. Nurses in similar situations have instituted policies that insure quality through follow-up phone calls, referral to home care, hotlines for patients and families, data collection instruments (patient satisfaction surveys, quality improvement instruments), establishing services such as sitters (for patients who need constant surveillance), liberal visiting hours for families, and informing administration of the current situation.

SUMMARY

This chapter has described the evolution of events that have led to the current conditions in health care. These characteristics represent the role of managed care, professional nursing issues with emphasis on the looming nursing shortage, and the priorities of health care delivery. Future nurse leaders/managers will practice in a managed care environment where emphasis will be on health promotion, prevention, and primary care. Sick people will be cared for everywhere, not just at the hospital; thus, nurses must have new professional skills that deal with the assessment of individuals and families in a complex integrated health care system. Because cost containment continues to dominate health care delivery, most patients will be provided care in managed care organizations. Technology and scientific advancements will continue. The ethical issue of access to health care continues to be debated. These characteristics represent the forces that will influence the work environment serving, and ultimately the decisions about, patient care. The challenge and opportunities available to nursing have never been greater. Fortunately, there is a heritage of past leaders to inspire present efforts. The value of leadership theory is an important tool to influence health care and policy as well as the future role of professional nursing. The transition from students to leaders and managers is a process that requires knowledge, skills, experience, and time. Throughout this textbook, the process will be emphasized and structured according to models. Practice takes place in a dynamic environment in which varying degrees of control and structure are possible. It is in a behavioral and situational context that students are challenged to contribute to nursing early in their careers by thinking and acting like leaders.

LEARNER EXERCISES

1. What are the dominant forces in the current health care system? Discuss both the positive and negative effects of these forces on the nursing profession.
2. Define managed care. What implications does it have for professional nursing? What would you tell someone interested in entering the nursing profession today?
3. A patient enters the community HMO with a serious respiratory problem. The patient needs immediate medical attention. What will be the likely process of care the patient will receive? How many types of managed care organizations are there? How do they differ?
4. What strategies would you consider to address the shortage of nurses in the workforce?
5. As a student in a nursing program, what skills do you believe will be helpful to you in your professional career?
6. Evaluate the health care environment in your current organization or complex using this checklist:

The Health Care Environmental Checklist

Directions: Check "yes" or "no" to the list of attributes to determine to what extent your organization/complex is consistent with the stated priorities for today's health care.

Attribute	Yes	No
• Wellness and prevention programs are offered to the public.	❑	❑
• Patients are discharged in a timely manner.	❑	❑
• Case management is the system of nursing care delivered	❑	❑
for inpatient and outpatient care.	❑	❑
• Home care services are provided.	❑	❑
• Ambulatory or outpatient surgery services are offered.	❑	❑
• Opportunities exist for Advanced Practice Nurses.	❑	❑
• Standardization of medical and nursing care plans are in effect using critical paths and evidence-based care.	❑	❑
• Skilled nursing units are available.	❑	❑

	Yes	No
• Staffing requirements are based on acuity levels and optimum staffing models.	❑	❑
• Supervision of non-licensed personnel is by professional nurses.	❑	❑
• Information systems are in place.	❑	❑
• Efficiency methods are sought in departments.	❑	❑
• Opportunities exist for nurses.	❑	❑
• Nursing leadership and management roles are prominent.	❑	❑

The extent to which your current work environment reflects these elements is the degree to which it is congruent with current health care delivery systems. Your desire for continued participation in an organization depends on your personal priorities in the practice of nursing, and how well your priorities fit within the organization.

REFERENCES

1. Kilborn, P. (1998, October 5). Reality of the HMO system doesn't live up to the dream. *New York Times*, A1, A16.
2. Himalu, U. (1996, October). Managed care: Does the promise meet the potential. *American Nurse*, 1–14.
3. Finkelman, A. (2001). *Managed care: A nursing perspective*. Englewood Cliffs, NJ: Prentice Hall, p. 10.
4. Broder, D. (1997). The problems persist. *Washington Post*, A1.
5. Diers, D., & Bozzo, J. (1999). Using administrative data for practice and management. *Nursing Economics, 17*(4), 233–237.
6. *Federal Register*. (1998 September). Washington, DC: Washington DC Press.
7. Balanced Budget Act. (1997).
8. Duncan, D. G. (1999, July). Preparing for Medicare's APC System. *Health Care Financial Management*, 43.
9. Golden, S. (2001, Fall). When it's tailor-made it fits better. *Health Associates 2001 PIAN Contracting*, 6.
10. Golden, S. (2001, Fall). When it's tailor-made it fits better. *Health Associates 2001 PIAN Contracting*, 7.
11. Finkelman, A. (2001). *Managed care: A nursing perspective*. Englewood Cliffs, New Jersey: Prentice Hall, pp. 56–67.
12. Finkelman, A. (2001). *Managed care: A nursing perspective*. Englewood Cliffs, New Jersey: Prentice Hall, pp. 56–67.
13. PEW Health Professions Commission. (1995, August). *Health professions education and managed care: Challenges and necessary responses*, 1st ed. PEW Health Profession Commission, p. 6.
14. Buerhaus, P., Staiger, D., & Auerback, D. (2000). Part one: Implications of a rapidly aging RN workforce. *Journal of the American Medical Association, 283*(22), 2248–2954.
15. Sigma Theta Tau. (2001). Facts about the nursing shortage: Resource info: Nurses for a healthier tomorrow. Retrieved March 22, 2001, from the World Wide Web: *http://www.nursingsociety.org*.

16. Buerhaus, P., Staiger, D., & Auerback, D. (2000). Part one. Implications of a rapidly aging RN workforce. *Journal of the American Medical Association, 283*(22), 56–67.
17. Mikulski, B. (2001, February 13). Opening statement, Subcommittee on Aging. Washington, DC.
18. Buerhaus, P., Staiger, D., & Auerback, D. (2000). Part one: Implications of a rapidly aging RN workforce. *Journal of the American Medical Association, 283*(22), 29–53.
19. AACN (2001). Strategies to reverse the new nursing shortage. Retrieved from the World Wide Web: *http://aacnnche.edu/publications/positions/trieshortage.htm.*
20. AACN (2001). Strategies to reverse the new nursing shortage. Retrieved from the World Wide Web: *http://aacnnche.edu/publications/positions/trieshortage.htm.*
21. PEW Health Professions Commission. (1995, August). *Health professions education and managed care: Challenges and necessary responses*, 1st ed. PEW Health Profession Commission, 10.
22. Executive Summary. (2000). Nursing values challenged by manager care. *Nursing Trends and Issues*. Retrieved September 22, 2001 from the World Wide Web: *http//www.nursingworld.org/readroom/nti/980/nti.htm.*
23. Christy, T.E. (1987). Leadership in nursing. In J.C. McCloskey & M.T. Molen (Eds.), *Research on the profession of nursing*, 8(230). New York: Springer Publishing.
24. AACN. (2001). Nursing educations' agenda for the 21st century. Retrieved from the World Wide Web: *http://www.aacnnche.edu/publications/positions/nrsgedag.htm.*
25. Bennis, W., & Nanus, B, (1985). *Leaders. The Strategies for Taking Charge*, New York: Harper & Row, pp. 218–222.
26. Manske, F. (1999). *Secrets of Effective Leadership*, 3rd ed. Columbia, TN: Leadership Education and Development, Inc.

2

Leadership Theory

"Leadership is the capacity to translate vision into reality."

Warren Bennis

INTRODUCTION

In the nonstop pace of managed care, all nursing roles are evolving. Nursing leaders at every level have seen their positions and scope of responsibilities change. Leaders are faced with multiple priorities[1] and increased demands. The current health care system requires nurses at all levels of the organization to possess and exercise leadership skills. Nurses both individually and collectively are struggling with new issues and questions posed by this new system.[2] To address these concerns, the profession has been challenged to change its education and practice. Nurses must be prepared as leaders who are competent, flexible, and able to energize others to adapt to change. This book will lead the reader to the realization that leadership involves a process that encourages each individual in the work setting to contribute to effectively meeting organizational goals. In addition, it will become evident that the usefulness of a leadership position is in relation to situational factors. The objective of this chapter is to describe leadership theory as it progresses from a simple concept to a complex process.

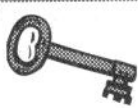

KEY CONCEPTS

Autocratic is a decision-making style used by a leader in which the leader does not consider the group's input.

Behavioral School is a way of explaining leadership by virtue of the decision-making style used by the individual, ranging from autocratic to laissez-faire.

Connective Leadership is a process that connects individuals with their tasks and visions to one another, to the group, and to the larger network.

Contingency Model is a way of explaining leadership on the basis of specific contingencies or variables. They include leader-member relationships, the structure of the task, and the position, or role, of power.

Democratic is a decision-making style used by the leader that equally considers the group's input as well as the leader's.

Great Man Theory defines leaders as those who are born with abilities to lead others.

Laissez-Faire is a decision-making style used by a leader that is group centered.

Leadership Behavior refers to the actual choice of the decision-making style the leader uses toward meeting a specific goal. These behaviors are commonly thought to be telling, selling, testing, consulting, and joining.

Leadership Style refers to the underlying motivation of a leader who directs goal-oriented behavior. These styles are commonly referred to as autocratic, democratic, laissez-faire, or eclectic.

Life-Cycle Theory of leadership is a way of explaining leadership based on the following assumptions: (1) the follower's readiness for task completion is based on his or her motivation and competence, and (2) leadership behavior is adaptable based on the follower's task maturity.

New Theory of Leadership is a way of explaining leadership, as offered by Warren Bennis and Burt Nanus, through four human handling skills that suggest that leaders are those who have vision, can communicate, are steadfast, and demonstrate a positive self-regard.

Process Model of Leadership is a conceptualization of the essential factors and activities that comprise appropriate leadership decisions and behaviors.

Situational Theory is a way of explaining leadership through taking into account forces that occur in the situation, the leader, and the followers. Leaders are determined by the situation.

Trait Approach is a way of explaining leadership in light of a set of traits an individual possesses. These traits include instrumental and interactional characteristics.

Transactional Leadership is the traditional leadership process that emphasizes leaders influencing a process over followers.

Transformational Leadership is a process of influencing followers through creating relationships that focus on vision and values. This method relies on a climate of trust and mutuality.

DEFINITION OF LEADERSHIP

Leadership continues to be debated among members of the nursing profession. Does nursing have a real ability to change the system through the exercise of leadership behaviors? Will the policymakers address nursing's concerns? Is it accurate to imply that nursing can stand shoulder-to-shoulder with those who determine the direction of health care delivery? Does nursing have the power to determine its destiny? Until the members of the nursing profession are prepared to stand behind nursing leaders with a unified voice, these questions will continue to be debated. Leadership theory offers a framework to understand how to meet goals and objectives even with diverse views among the group members. Leadership as a concept addresses collective action.

However, leadership continues to be the subject of study, as there is no one agreed-upon definition. Leadership has been examined by many disciplines who add insights, dimensions, and meanings. Most definitions reflect the discipline's perspective. Thus, the following comprehensive definition, compatible with nursing's values, is offered.

Leadership may be considered as:

> A collective function in the sense that it is the integrated synergized expression of a group's efforts; it is not the sum of individual dominance and contributions, it is their interrelationships. Ultimate authority and true sanction for leadership, where it is exercised, resides not in the individual, however dominant, but in the total situation and in the demands of the situation. It is the situation that creates the imperative, whereas the leader is able to make others aware of it, is able to make them willing to serve it, and is able to release collective capacities and emotional attitudes that may be related fruitfully to the solution of the group's problems; to that extent one is exercising leadership.[3]

Leadership Theory

Leadership is a complex and multidimensional concept. It includes intrapersonal, interpersonal, intergroup, and situational variables. As a result, it is not easily defined or measured. However, leadership may be analyzed as a process that includes social, ethical, and theoretical components. The social nature of leadership entails the interpersonal skills necessary to be effective in a variety of situations. The ethical nature of leadership involves the inherent power of a leadership position that, when exercised, should benefit the common good. All components of the leadership process will be discussed throughout the text. The following discussion focuses on the theoretical nature of leadership. This review includes tradition, theory, and research.

Great Man Theory of Leadership

At one time leadership was considered a birthright. Kings and queens ascended to thrones because of custom. Individuals in formal leadership roles were accepted without question. This is similar to the **great man theory**, which states that great leaders are born with the ability to lead, influence, and direct others. As such, only those possessing these qualities are leaders. Under this perspective, leaders may not be developed. Fortunately, the study of leadership was pursued.

Trait Theory

The serious study of leadership began when the following question was asked: Who is a leader? Early theorists recognized that leadership was by nature elusive, but might be explained by virtue of a leader's traits. The **trait approach** states that leadership exists as an attribute of a personality. If certain traits are exhibited, an individual is a leader. However, because the traits necessary for successful leadership varied from situation to situation, no exhaustive list of traits was offered.

Even though no one leader type was described, certain personality traits have been identified through early psychological studies to correspond to effective leadership behavior. Among these are intelligence, social sensitivity, social participation, and communication skills.[4] This particular group of traits identifies the leader as the one who has the capability to influence a group through innate intelligence and well-developed interpersonal skills.

Nurse researchers have also conducted studies to determine the characteristics of nursing leaders. Two different studies were conducted independently by Dunham and Fisher, as well as Murphy and DeBack, who sought the characteristics and behaviors of hospital nurse executives.[5,6] Both studies reached comparable conclusions. Nurse executives display similar characteristics, such as being visionary, credible, enabling, willing to serve as role models, and having the ability to master change. Interestingly, Meighan, another nurse researcher, conducted a similar study, only this time using staff nurses with the same leadership characteristics identified.[7] Findings from these studies reveal characteristics that facilitate effective leadership behavior. However, common agreement about strength and priority of the suggested traits, as well as conformity to a single personality profile, is lacking.[8] Nonetheless, identified leadership traits serve as adjunct knowledge to explain what makes an effective leader.

Behavioral School of Leadership

Because traits were insufficient to explain leadership, the study of what leaders do was a predictable next step. This change in perspective examined specific leadership behaviors in the workplace.[9] The early work of Lewin and colleagues explained leadership in terms of decision-making behaviors.[10] Their classic work and terminology is foundational to the study of leadership style.

Leadership Style

Leaders have been described in terms of their decision-making styles in one or more of the following ways. **Autocratic**, or dictatorial, means that the leader makes all decisions and allows subordinates no influence in the decision-making process. Such supervisors are often indifferent to subordinates' personal needs. The second system of decision making is entitled participative, or **democratic**. In this case, the supervisor consults with the subordinates on appropriate matters, giving them some influence in the decision-making process. This type of supervisor is not punitive and treats subordinates with fairness and dignity. The third system is called **laissez-faire**, or free reign, which means that supervisors allow their group to have complete autonomy. Because they rarely supervise the group directly, the group makes its own decisions. These decision-making styles have become synonymous with the concept of leadership styles, which by definition refers to the underlying needs of the leader that motivate behavior. There exists more agreement among authorities on the classification of leadership styles than on a definition of leadership. The **behavioral school** (because of its emphasis on style) has led other authors to expand on its usefulness. For example, styles of leadership can be depicted on a continuum developed by Schmitt and Tannenbaum, ranging from autocratic, or

Leader Centered					Group Centered
		Use of Authority by Leader			
					Freedom of the group
Autocrat ______	______		Democrat		Laissez-Faire
______ Tells	Sells	Tests		Consults	Joins

FIGURE 2-1. The relationship between leadership style and leadership behavior. Leadership styles exist on a continuum and are characterized by particular behaviors. *(Adapted from Schmitt, W and Tannenbaum, R.)*

TABLE 2-1. Comparison of Leadership Style and Limiting Conditions

	Autocratic	Democratic	Laissez-Faire
Leader			
Holds:	Absolute power	Limited power	No power
Knowledge:	Unique	Shared	Same or less
Behavior:	Dominates	Participates	Joins
Position:	Inflexible	Flexible	Neutral
Followers			
Relates:	Dependent	Expects involvement	Independent
Knowledge:	Less	Different	More
Behavior:	Submissive	Involved	Independent
Situation			
Appropriate:	Crisis, emergency, or great skill required of leader only	General goals, controls, and time pressure understood	No clear purpose, control, or time pressure
Inappropriate:	Misuse of employees talents	Cannot influence	Need answer

leader-centered, to abdicate, or group-centered, supervision.[11] This continuum is depicted in Figure 2-1.

To make a decision regarding a leader's placement on the continuum, it is necessary to analyze what constitutes a **leadership style.** This examination includes considering one's personality and intelligence, the characteristics of the task to be performed, the roles of the leader and group members who will complete the task, and the characteristics of the group. In essence, this comprehensive analysis will help the leader to understand what is necessary to complete the task and will ultimately lead to the appropriate leadership behavior in a given situation. For a comparison of leadership styles and their relationships with the leader, follower, and situation, see Table 2-1.

Leadership Behaviors

Leadership behavior refers to a variety of behaviors a leader may enact to meet a goal or to complete a task. These behaviors range from being highly leader-centered to highly group-centered. The leadership behaviors are telling, selling, testing, consulting, and joining (Figure 2-1); these correspond with the different leadership styles. When a leader identifies a problem, considers alternative solutions, decides on the best course of action without consulting the group, and then informs the group of what is to be done, the leader is using *telling* as a mode of behavior. The group members clearly do not participate in the decision-making process. This is a most appropriate behavior in an emergency or crisis situation, such as a cardiac arrest. Certainly it would be an inappropriate leadership behavior for decisions affecting professional responsibilities.

Selling, or persuading, is another behavior the leader may use. It involves, as in telling, a leader making a decision without consulting the group. For example, rather than just informing the group members, the leader tries to appeal to the group's sense of logic by identifying the positive aspects of the decision. This might involve pointing out the decision's benefit because of its congruence with organizational goals or the fact that the group's interests have been considered in the decision. An appropriate use of this behavior is when the leader conveys a new policy to the staff, a policy that could otherwise be interpreted in a negative way, by giving the reason for the policy. An inappropriate use of this behavior will occur if the leader only deals with the positive side of a new policy without sharing all relevant reasons for its necessity. The group may resent the leader's positive explanation of a policy or decision that will be very difficult for the staff to follow.

Business Plans: A Tool for Selling Ideas

Today, nurse leaders need to learn the art of selling. The changes that will benefit nursing require the cooperation of chief executive officers (CEOs), policymakers, and the public. Some of the elements of selling an idea include:

- **Understanding the power of numbers.**
  How many individuals are involved in the initiative? In the case of nursing, how many nurses are involved? Does the number include the entire workforce of nursing or a substantial percentage of individuals? The power of change is proportional to the number of individuals who are in favor of the new plan, particularly if it is positive for a majority.

- **Allowing collaboration among the staff.**
  When an interesting and controversial idea is suggested, allow the group to generate solutions or ideas that would be worthwhile.

- **Create a business plan.**
  When trying to promote an interesting idea, a serious business plan would be helpful. Suggest a pilot project for the initiative to minimize disruption to the organization. Focus the plan on results. Minimize the amount of work the decision makers will have to do. A business plan includes the objectives of the project, a time frame for evaluation, and projections of cost and personnel. Information to write a business plan is available from a variety of sources. (see Figure 2-2)

- **Ask yourself "Would you approve of this plan?"**
  Finally, ask yourself if this idea were presented to you, would the logic sway you to agree or would you have serious reservations about the plan?. The extent to which the plan is organized, logical, and has implications for many will determine its inception.[12]

A template for a business plan

To and From line: This is the objective of the plan to go from one place to a proposed other.

Cash Outlay: This would estimate the amount of money necessary to implement the plan.

Purpose: This would address why this is an important service.

Benefit: Why is this a valuable project?

Need: This would discuss the reasons why such a program is required.

Alternatives: A discussion of alternate approaches.

Best Alternative: The plan that you believe to be the best.

Staple supportive documents to the plan.

Executive Summary : A short, and to the point, summary of what you are proposing, while encompassing all of the major issues.

FIGURE 2-2. A business plan.

Testing is a behavior available to the leader that begins to involve the group members. In this case, the leader identifies a problem and proposes a tentative solution, but before finalizing the decision, the group is consulted for helpful information and input. For example, the leader will discuss the problem with the group and say, "I'd like to have an honest reaction to this proposal." After hearing what the group has to say, the leader will then—and only then—make a decision. It is possible that the leader may change what had been proposed as a solution and follow the recommendations from the group. The proper use of this behavior occurs when the group has the legitimate right to be involved in decision making about policies that they will implement. There is no reason to involve the group if they cannot influence the decision. Indeed, using testing might be harmful to leader-member relationships if the position of the group is ignored.

Consulting is a leader behavior that allows the group to be involved with the decision from the very beginning. The leader presents a problem to the group with its relevant background and asks the group to propose a solution. In effect, the group increases the number of alternative actions to be considered. The leader then selects the decision that best meets the needs of the problem and the group. This is an excellent behavior to use in an interdisciplinary team conference. Another case may be the leader who has a very important yet complicated problem to present to the staff, requiring their input to achieve more commitment to the solution, since they will implement the decision. It would be inappropriate to use this behavior in a highly structured situation in which there is simply only one course of action.

Joining is a leadership behavior that also allows the group to be involved from the very beginning. The leader functions more like a member than a formal leader and agrees in advance to carry out whatever decision the group chooses. The leader does, however, provide the limits within which the decision may be made. This leadership behavior is applicable under special circumstances, such as a problem that requires a solution from a group of people who have comparable positions with equal authority. An example might be the vice president of nursing meeting with other administrators to determine a policy that will influence expansion of the hospital services. An inappropriate use of this behavior would be relinquishing decision-making authority to a group that does not have adequate experience or knowledge to solve the problem.

The aim of leadership development is to produce an effective leader capable of using the proper leadership behavior according to the situation, no matter what the leader's personal inclinations. Leadership style and behaviors are the means by which leadership is exercised. Learning to use these behaviors in the right set of circumstances determines one's personal success as a leader.

Following the classic work of decision-making styles, others in the behavioral school studied leadership effectiveness. For instance, the Ohio State studies in the late 1940s attempted to: (1) develop instruments to measure leadership, such as the Leader Behavior Description Questionnaire (LBDQ) and (2) evaluate factors that influence group effectiveness. Two of the major characteristics that define group effectiveness discovered by these studies were: (1) *consideration*—the extent to which the leader is likely to have a group relationship characterized by mutual trust, respect for subordinates' ideas, and consideration of their feelings, and (2) *initiating structure*—the extent to which a leader is likely to define and structure the roles of subordinates toward goal attainment.[13] The most effective leaders scored high on both of these measures. This kind of research marked the beginning of empirical work to demonstrate the complex interactional nature of leadership.

Later, another study, conducted at the University of Michigan, concluded that there were four major leader behaviors: (1) *supportive behavior*—behavior that enhances someone else's feelings of personal worth and importance, (2) *interaction facilitation*—behavior that encourages members of the group to develop close, mutually satisfying relationships, (3) *goal emphasis*—behavior that stimulates an enthusiasm for meeting the group's goals or achieving excellent performance, and (4) *work facilitation*—behavior that helps achieve goal attainment through such activities as scheduling, coordinating, and planning and by providing resources such as tools, materials, and knowledge. To a great extent, the Michigan studies can be credited with being foundational to the situational theories of leadership by expanding the notion of effective leadership action.[14]

Situational Theory

The next stage of leadership theory development was **situational theory**. Researchers suggested that traits required of a leader differ according to varying situations. In 1948, Stogdill conducted a comprehensive review of the literature and concluded that leadership traits differ in varying situations.[15] No single personality typifies a leader; rather, leadership is a relationship that exists among people in a social situation. Thus, a person may be a leader in one situation and not in another. There are three main factors to consider for the leadership process: (1) a leader, (2) a situation, and (3) followers. The group of factors that determine leadership effectiveness are referred to as forces within the managers, subordinates, and situations.

Forces in the supervisor include: (1) the supervisor's view of people, performance, and status, (2) the degree of confidence held for the subordinates, (3) leadership inclinations, and (4) feelings of security in an uncertain situation. Forces in subordinates include their: (1) need for independence, (2) readiness to assume responsibility, (3) expectations to share in decision making, (4) tolerance for ambiguity, and (5) level of knowledge and experience to deal with situations. Forces in the situation include: (1) the organization's values and traditions, (2) the organization's reaction to change (e.g., is it slow to change or volatile?), (3) whether the organization is dominated by physicians, administrators, or nurses, and (4) to what extent the group is effective, cohesive, and able to assume responsibility in different situations.[16]

Situational theories suggest that, based on an analysis of all these critical forces, an individual may be a leader in one situation and a follower in another. Some of the more recent developments in leadership theory are strongly based on the assumptions represented by situational theory.

Contingency Model

One example of leadership effectiveness based on situational theory is Fiedler et al.'s **contingency model** developed in 1965 (see Table 2-2).[17] This very complex theory consists of a three-dimensional model of a given situation. Components of the model are: (1) leader-member relations, (2) a task structure, and (3) a position of power. Leader-member relations represent the amount of confidence and loyalty followers have in their leader. Task structure refers to the number of correct solutions to a given situational dilemma. Position of power means the amount of organizational support available to the leader. Based on this theory, it is possible to predict the most productive leadership style through a complicated analysis of these components and their relationship to a critical situation. For example, if a nurse manager who is well-liked has an ambiguous task to

TABLE 2-2. Fiedlers's Contingency Theory

Group Situation			
Leader-Member Relations	*Task Structure*	*Leader's Position of Power*	*Leadership Style of the Leader*
Good — Moderately poor — Poor	Structured — Unstructured	Strong — Weak	Directive — Permissive

Note: Different sets of conditions predict proper leadership behavior.

request of the staff, a considerate, accepting leadership style is most appropriate. If the nurse manager is disliked and asks the same ambiguous task to be completed, a very direct leadership style would be considered best. This theory requires a great deal of study and creates a matrix for the user so that a person can change his or her leadership approach after an appropriate analysis of a situation.

Situational Leadership Model

One of the most interesting and useful theoretical perspectives of leadership is the **life-cycle theory** of Hersey.[18] This practical theory suggests that leadership behavior may be predicted on the basis of the follower's readiness. The illustration of the model in Figure 2-3 shows four quadrants, each representing the degree of emphasis on relationship behavior and task behavior. The leader will alter the style of leadership based on an analysis of the follower's readiness. Readiness refers to the level of motivation and competence an individual has for an assigned task. The leader assesses the follower's capacity to complete the assigned task and provides the appropriate leadership behavior that best meets the needs of the follower in the given situation. The leader behaviors are telling, selling, participating, and delegating. The leader behavior conforms to the followers' requirements of needing (1) guidance and (2) relationship or emotional support. This is a tool that may be used with individuals or groups.

This model's original categories have been refined, and published work demonstrates its success in a variety of arenas besides leadership. The underlying assumptions, however, remain the same:

1. The followers' ability and willingness for task completion based on their task readiness is assessed by the leader.
2. The leader adapts behavior to best guide and/or support the followers to meet the specified objectives.[19]

A New Concept of Leadership

Modern theorists are continuing to struggle with the elusive quality of leadership. One of the most dynamic approaches to leadership is that offered by Bennis and Nanus, published in 1985.[20] These authors stated that leadership is the most studied and least understood of the social sciences, and these changing and turbulent times require uniquely effective leaders. They suggest a **new theory of leadership** based on an extensive study of 90 leaders who participated in interviews for the purpose of discovering what is common to leadership and leaders.

The findings of this study concluded that there are four types of "human handling skills" common to leaders. The authors elaborate in great detail the specifics of these skills and refer to them as strategies:

- Strategy I—attention through vision.
- Strategy II—meaning through communication.
- Strategy III—trust through positioning.
- Strategy IV—the deployment of self through positive self-regard and the Wallenda factor.

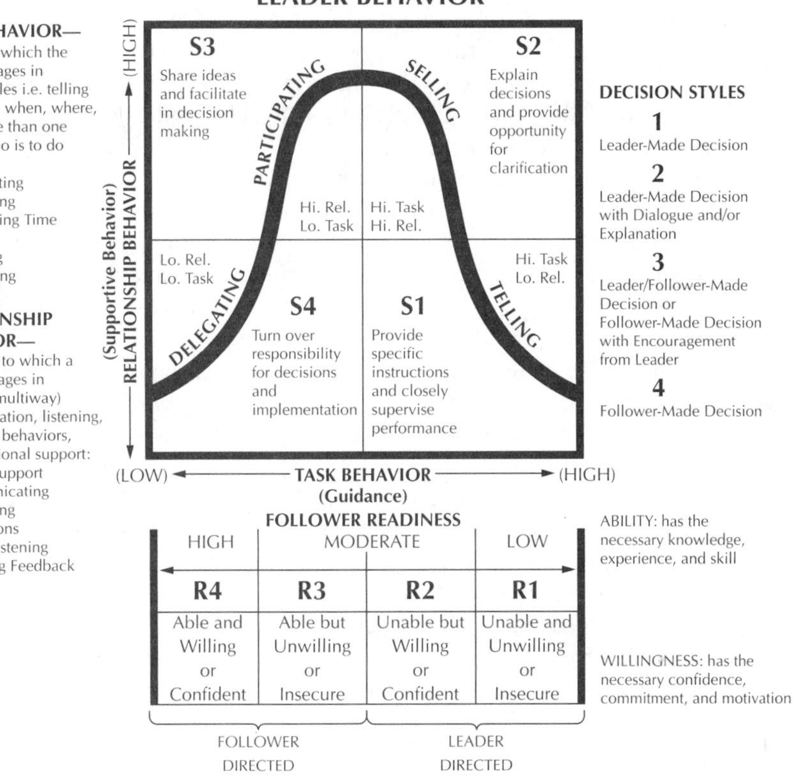

When a Leader Behavior is used appropriately with its corresponding level of readiness, it is termed a High Probability Match. The following are descriptors that can be useful when using Situational Leadership for specific applications:

S1	S2	S3	S4
Telling	Selling	Participating	Delegating
Guiding	Explaining	Encouraging	Observing
Directing	Clarifying	Collaborating	Monitoring
Establishing	Persuading	Committing	Fulfilling

FIGURE 2-3. Leader behavior.
Source: Management of Organizational Behavior. 6th ed. 1993, p. 197. Copyrighted material. Reprinted with permission of Center for Leadership Studies, Escondido, CA 92025. All rights reserved.

Strategy I, or the management of attention through vision, refers to the leader's ability to create a focus or a clear picture of an outcome. The leaders who were interviewed were all results oriented. The ideas they held were very clear in their own minds, making it easy for people to see where they were going.

Strategy II, or the meaning through communication, means that this group of leaders was able to turn its vision into images that others could understand. These leaders had the ability to translate their ideas into symbols with real meaning. From this ability, referred to as the management of meaning and the mastery of communication, leaders are able to inspire by capturing the imagination of others.

Strategy III, or trust through positioning, refers to the leaders' ability to inspire trust in others by contributing to the organization's integrity. This means the leader never loses sight of why the organization exists. The leader knows what the organization stands for and what it has to do. A second component of a leader's contribution to the management of trust is the facilitation of constancy, or staying the course. Like a pilot and an airplane, the leader takes the organization in the right direction. In this way a leader, through positioning, maintains the organization's harmony and purpose but also recognizes the need for change and incongruities and provides for innovations. In essence, the leader provides stability for the organization but also allows for the necessary changes that provide for organizational growth.

Strategy IV, or the deployment of self through positive self-regard, means that the leader leads in a very personal way. The leader will display a positive self-image, and especially self-respect. This is achieved by the leader recognizing his or her strengths and compensating for weaknesses while nurturing the talents and skills that he or she possesses.

Another aspect of the management of self is the deployment of self through the Wallenda factor. This is best explained through a story about Karl Wallenda, a tightrope aerialist. For three months prior to his fatal fall, Wallenda talked about falling and not succeeding, rather than walking the tightrope. It was as though he were destined to fail. The conclusion is: attitudes influence outcome. Positive attitudes that concentrate on success are what this special group of leaders shared. The groundbreaking work of Bennis and Nanus provides much that can be applied to beginning students of leadership.

Transformational Leadership

Leadership theorists began to recognize that for leaders to really be effective, the organizational culture needed to be changed. **Transformational leadership** proposes just that. Burns, an early formulator of transformational leadership, proposes there are two kinds of leadership, transactional and transformational. Traditional or **transactional leadership** occurs when one person takes the initiative for the exchange. Both leader and follower have separate but related purposes, and their differences are the focus of the system. In transformational leadership, both the leader and followers have the same purpose, and they raise one another to higher levels of performance. This new expression of leadership relies on mutuality, affiliation, acknowledgement of complexity, ambiguity, cooperation versus competition, an emphasis on human relations, process versus task, acceptance of feelings, networking versus hierarchy, valuing intuition, and empowerment of all employees.[21]

The transformational leader mobilizes others and grows and develops with the followers. Emphasis is on the outcome because the process of achieving the outcome changes. The right actions may change from day to day because the focus remains on the goals and end product. The result is that both leader and follower develop a love of the work. The central task of the transformational leader is to create a vision and build a social architecture that provides meaning for employees. This leader tries to develop self-esteem and pride among the followers by being less rule-bound, while maintaining a clear vision. The measure of a transformational leader's effectiveness is the success of the followers.[22] Transformational leadership is a values-oriented relationship, which can only occur within a climate of trust and mutuality. In practice, establishing and maintaining both organizational and personal trust with others represents the fundamental strategy of the transformational leader. Only in an environment of trust can people truly be, and act, their best. This form of leadership has been endorsed by many leadership scholars.

A research study by McDaniel and Wolf examined the effects of transformational leadership on work satisfaction and retention on staff nurses.[23] Among the results were "positive work satisfaction and low turnover" among registered nurses where transformational leadership was in place.[24] Despite the limitations of the study, such as a small sample from one institution, transformational leadership produced a positive work environment. Another study conducted by Dunham and Klafehn asked the question: Are nurse executives transformational leaders from their own perception and from immediate staff members' perceptions?[25] The results revealed the sample of executives were very much seen as transformational leaders. In addition, the researchers' data were compared to a study of world leaders, administrators, and managers conducted by Bass.[26] Results revealed the nurse executives' transformational leadership scores were higher than those surveyed in the Bass study.[27] Transformational leadership is a process that encourages the use of capabilities among leaders and subordinates.

Because of the desirability of transformational leadership, recent studies explored its effectiveness, and reported conflicting results. In a study of critical care managers, trends supported that managers with more years of experience were more inclined to use transformational leadership concepts, as well as more involvement in situations where mistakes are likely to occur. Managers who worked in decentralized structures reported significantly greater use of idealized leadership.[28] However, another study examining organizational effectiveness and transformational and transactional leadership found no significant difference in organizational effectiveness upon exposure to both modes of leadership. This is in direct contrast to the variety of studies. The authors conclude that a cultural element may be in play, which reinforces the notion of situational theory.[29]

Connective Leadership

In contrast to transformational leadership, which focuses on cooperation and conflict, another multidimensional leadership model has been proposed that focuses on caring. **Connective leadership**, developed by Jean Lipman-Blumer and based on extensive research with her Achieving Styles Model, creatively connects individuals to their tasks and visions, to one another, to the immediate group, and to the larger network.[30] It empowers others and instills confidence. These strategies produce success, not only in the workplace, but in the interdependent world community. Since health care is moving from fragmentation to a seamless continuum of services, interconnectedness is increasing. Thus, leaders are called upon to exceed their given authority and bridge the gaps and divisions of the organization. It emphasizes the need for a leader to cope with the requirements of multiple constituencies. Health care organizations exist within diverse communities that impact mission and purpose. Connective leadership is seen as an integrative model of leadership that will be appropriate for the 21st century.[31]

Seven Lessons of Leadership

In a book written by David Gergen,[32] he identifies the seven lessons of leadership he observed while serving for four presidents of the United States. Although his experience was political, the lessons he suggests transcend politics and are applicable to any leadership position.

The first lesson states leadership starts from within. This means a leader must gain mastery over self before mastering others. Heraclitus, an ancient philosopher, said "character is destiny." There is an inherent ethical responsibility in leadership as leaders guide others to the common good. The leader's character predicts the integrity of the leader's decisions and actions. Courage may be required of a leader, and only an individual with strength of character will be able to go forward.

A second lesson of leadership is a central compelling purpose or ability to convey a major idea. Nursing leaders will clearly explain the values of nursing, and guide the profession to enact our values. A leader may have high hopes, but if unable to communicate them with succinct and meaningful objectives, the leader will fail.

The third lesson of leadership is that leaders must also have the ability to persuade others. Persuading others is a communication technique similar to "selling." The ability to communicate ideas to others in a personal yet understandable manner is a necessary skill for a leader. It amounts to taking very complex ideas and explaining them in an appropriate way to people who will be affected by those decisions.

The fourth fundamental lesson of leadership states a leader must work within the system. A leader cannot succeed without the ability to work with others in the workplace. In effect, the leader should be in the center of competing forces. The leader must determine the institutional centers of power which can promote or block the leader's plans. It will be necessary for the leader to develop working relationships with the various units through persuasion, communication skills, networking, or cooperation. For example, it will be incumbent on nurse leaders to deal with various elements of the society to generate change in working conditions. These units are the press, the general public, legislators, health care administrators, and members of the nursing profession.

Another lesson of leadership is a sure quick start when assuming a position. In some cases stature builds over time, but it is incumbant on the leader to give the impression of a plan of action early on. If the leader stumbles and doesn't appear to have a sense of organization, the followers will lack confidence and faith in the leader's ability to lead.

The next lesson of leadership is strong prudent advisors. Any individual who wishes to be successful in a leadership role must have trusted and knowledgeable advice. The best course of action will be determined after serious discussions with experts.

Finally, the last lesson of leadership offered is that a leader should be able to inspire others to carry on the mission. The ability to motivate and sustain action is integral to successful leadership. Standing on the shoulders of past leaders allows new people to propel plans at a more rapid rate.[33]

From this overview of leadership theories, many possible explanations for leadership have been postulated that identify its complex nature. A modern perspective suggests the leader is in a position to use appropriate methods to empower the group. Personal characteristics a leader must cultivate to be successful include patience, as moving a group toward an objective takes time and diligence. It is easy to become frustrated when things do not go as you desire. Creativity is a desirable trait in a leader as it fosters and encourages the formation of ideas. It challenges and empowers the group to use personal resources. Self-confidence and self-esteem are qualities that grow over time, but are necessary for a leader to make thoughtful and courageous decisions. Being able to handle setbacks requires the self-confidence to pursue an action, as well as being able to step back and evaluate alternative plans. A leader should also have an ability to see the whole organization but understand the component parts and how it is necessary for them to work together. Lastly, a leader should have a sense of timing, which means identifying a good time to introduce an idea. Timing is believed to be a readiness or openness to commit to a plan of action.[34]

PROCESS MODEL OF LEADERSHIP

For the beginning student, a **process model of leadership** is offered, which summarizes essential factors and activities that comprise a leadership decision or behavior. This model identifies those elements a leader should consider to produce an appropriate, group-oriented, and measurable leadership action. The concepts introduced in the model will be explained more fully throughout the text. See Table 2-3 for a depiction of the process model of leadership. The model is composed of three stages. Stage 1 involves the analysis of the problem, stage 2 includes the determination of an action plan, and stage 3 involves the evaluation of the selected action.

Stage 1—Analysis and Problem Identification

The analysis stage categorizes elements of the problem or event. This categorization provides a framework to select the critical aspects from the broad organizational influences, as well as the actual (problem/conflict) event. The analysis stage is composed of the following variables: (1) the event (problem), (2) the participants and their perceptions, (3) the organization factors (organizational structure and climate), (4) interpersonal processes (locus of power), and (5) controlling forces or limiting factors. The following discussion explains these terms.

TABLE 2-3. Process Model of Leadership

Stage One	Stage Two	Stage Three
Analysis of Events	*Determination of Action*	*Evaluation of Action Plan*
1. Describe the nursing event and state the desired outcome. 2. Identify the participants and how they see the problem and solution. 3. Describe the organizational factors—structure and climate. 4. Describe the quality of interaction between the participants—locus of power. 5. Describe the controlling factors that influence the situation.	6. a. Generate ideas for action to accomplish desired outcome. b. Weigh each alternative. c. Select the best alternative. 7. Identify barriers associated with selected action and plan for managing the conflicts.	8. Monitor. 9. Correct errors. 10. Provide feedback.

The Event

The event can range from an obvious problem to a feeling of dissatisfaction with the status quo. The problem begins the analytic process. A simple question (e.g., Is this an isolated event or does it occur frequently?) will suggest a simple or complex decision-making process. Isolated problems should be treated differently than problems that occur regularly. Eliminating the cause of problems often includes assistance from more than one department. For example, what is the effect on patients when no effort is made to solve the problem of dietary trays always being late? Certainly the effect on diabetic patients goes beyond inconvenience.

The Participants

Next, the participants of the event should be identified. All persons from each department who have a direct impact on a particular activity should be involved in the solution. People perceive their own behavior from their very unique perceptions. It is essential that those involved in the event express their point of view and objectively state "what happened" so that the elements of the event can be commonly understood and an acceptable solution can be reached.

Organizational Factors

Events that occur in organizational settings vary in the scope of how broadly they affect others. Organizations form structures composed of division of labor, authority, and responsibility, which require coordination through the processes of leadership and management. The manner in which the organizational structure connects work, people, and managers impacts how a problem may be solved. The event occurs as people try to work together in an organization that by its very nature separates people so that communication, and ultimately understanding, are more difficult. Thus, the impact of a problem should be considered on the work area as well as on the total organization. For example, does the problem have a time pattern? Do problems occur only during peak vacation months? If so, what is the policy regulating vacations, and can it be modified as part of the solution? In a complex organization, can a policy modification affect only one or two groups, or must the modification include personnel in all departments? What kinds of morale problems might result from such changes? Organization theory offers a variety of theoretical rationales that will be discussed elsewhere in the text for the purpose of explaining the complexities modern organizations hold for incumbents.

The other factor to consider is the climate of the total organization and its influences on the work area. Climate, by definition, is a characterization of the socioemotional effect produced by the emphasis placed on human relationships and work. Problem-solving activities have to consider the existing structure, with its programmed demands, and the climate to produce a solution that is consistent with organizational goals and psychologically satisfying.

Interpersonal Processes between Participants

The interaction between the leader and the subordinates affects the means by which decisions are made. The combination of these processes defines the degree of compatibility seen in the work group. The length of time and effort to arrive at a decision is partially determined by this compatibility, as well as the respect shared by the leader and group. When a group member emerges as a strong, opposing leader with little regard for the formal leader, effort and time are diverted from the main problem and instead focus on the group's internal relationships. Incompatible working relationships develop when people do not recognize the leader's broader organizational responsibilities. The ability to manage conflict situations is an important skill for the nurse leader/manager. (The skills of communication, conflict resolution, and decision making will be addressed in Chapters 3 and 4 of the text.) The concept of power, both as an individual characteristic and force, impacts decision making. A position of power refers to the variety of transactional and legitimate forces that produce the ability to influence others. Power may well be the most critical force in determining an outcome.

Controlling Forces

There must be a basic understanding and agreement to certain rules and regulations that allow the organization to run with efficiency. Controlling factors, such as protocols, procedures, and standards of professional and personal behavior, dictate norms that reduce ambiguity in the workplace.

Stage 2—Determination of Action

Action Plan

After considering the myriad of factors that contribute to the situation, a course of action must be determined. The activities of stage 2 necessitate the use of decision making as discussed in detail in a later chapter. The process, in brief, considers the defined problem and categorizes information about it based on specific information of what, who, and how best to solve the problem. To arrive at the best action, many alternative solutions must be considered, and prediction of the outcome should be attached to each alternative solution. The predictive effort should include the consideration of both positive and negative outcomes of each solution proposed. Selecting the solution offering the greatest overall advantages and least disadvantages is part of the ongoing process. Leadership and management theory offer concepts that make this a selective process. The leader then clearly describes relationships between the desired outcome and each possible alternative.

Stage 3—Evaluation of Action

The last stage of the process model is evaluation of action. Evaluation as an activity makes a judgment that determines worth and value. Its major aim is to reduce subjectivity and to increase objectivity through measurable criteria.

Following implementation of the selected action, the results should be evaluated in terms of actual outcome, even if it is an unexpected outcome based on the established criteria. These criteria should judge the immediate effect of the management decision. In addition, criteria should be included that are sensitive to the total system. The long-range effect of any decision has to be considered to reduce the sources of new problems.

The evaluation criteria should be compared to a variety of issues, such as: (1) the acceptability of action for a particular organization or setting, (2) the psychologic-social acceptance of the selected action, (3) the effect, direct and indirect, on the quality of nursing care, (4) the possible growth for the group implementing the plan, and, finally, (5) the solution's ability to maintain order.

Conclusions on the Use of Process

Nurse leaders are expected to meet professional standards and organizational goals. Using a process model of leadership is one mechanism that highlights the necessary forces in a situation, leader, and followers that influence decisions to achieve successful outcomes. A process leadership model in all its stages requires application of theory to determine the best possible leadership action. The knowledge and skill level of the duly-appointed leader directly and indirectly influence the short- and long-range goals of the organization. Interpersonal relationships significantly influence the possible alternatives that might be generated to solve a problem or to make a decision. The creative leader who possesses innate intelligence, resourcefulness, dominance, and self-sufficiency will be able to facilitate a course of action.

CASE STUDY

Laissez-Faire Leadership

You are a new staff nurse in a sizable ambulatory care setting where 150 to 200 patients are seen each day in 25 specialty clinics. Your reason for joining the staff in ambulatory care is your interest in the nursing functions you believe are essential to the setting (e.g., patient teaching, being an advocate to patients/families in maintaining health and in adapting to changes in their lives imposed by illness, and serving as a liaison and coordinator between patients/families and members of the health care team).

Shortly after your orientation period it becomes apparent to you that these are not consistent functions of the nursing staff in the department. You become frustrated when assigned to receptionist functions, such as logging patients in and assigning them to examining rooms, and to task functions, such as taking and recording vital signs and weights on patients. When you attempt to become more involved in total care functions, you sense the alienation of the other nurses. In addition, it becomes apparent that the organizational structure necessary to carry out giving and documenting total care does not exist. It is difficult to identify a person as the leader. An ineffective, free-reign style seems to be in operation. The lack of visible structure in the department leads you to higher-level nursing administration for assistance in dealing with your professional role conflict.

You make an appointment to see the director of outpatient clinics. Although the director listens to you, she admits this is a new area and that she is in the process of forming a workable structure. The director asks you to submit ideas for change in the setting.

- What changes do you think would facilitate the workflow?
- What style of leadership would be most effective in this situation?
- What attributes should the leader display in this situation?

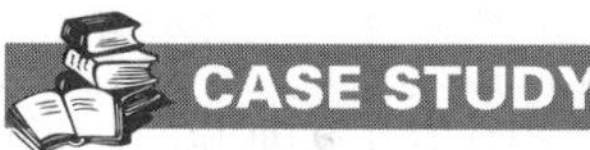

CASE STUDY

Autocratic Leadership

Mrs. Meyers is the nurse manager on 3 South, a very busy general surgery division. Mrs. Meyers is known for "running a tight ship." For instance, Mrs. Meyers makes out all the assignments on the division in a very detailed manner. She prefers to call physicians for new orders and to report problems. Mrs. Meyers consistently provides more structure than the task requires.

Many of the professional nurses have tried to discuss the problem they see with Mrs. Meyers, but the conversation with her goes nowhere. Mrs. Meyers insists that the responsibility of a nurse is great and that without her vigilance, errors would occur. Of late, RNs are asking to transfer from 3 South almost as fast as they are hired. The associate director for surgical divisions suspects that the problem may be Mrs. Meyers' leadership style.

As a result of inquiry and observation, the associate director concludes that Mrs. Meyers is a major factor in the turnover. She offers some alternatives for change to Mrs. Meyers, including a conference about how she sees her role and the role of the staff.

- Is there any hope for an autocratic leader? Is the style of leadership solely a function of personality and thus intractable? Are different behaviorial responses able to be learned in the work situation?
- Is it possible for a person to understand the needs of subordinates and to become more flexible in a leadership style?

NOTE: A leader's behavior is a complex process. It is not just a style but a combination of personality, habits, values, experiences, and motivation.

In order for a leader/manager to be more appropriate in the workplace, she or he must have performance appraisals and positive behaviorial goals emphasized.

Subordinates have the choice of staying, leaving, or coping with the individual.

CASE STUDY

Need for Democratic Leadership

You are a new nurse in an Emergency Department. You observe a very busy area where rooms are filled with patients awaiting attention. The triage nurse is responsible for prioritizing who is seen first. This often necessitates that certain patients are not seen for long periods of time, so that more seriously ill patients may be treated or admitted. You notice that on a regular basis, waiting patients and families become very angry. Often, nurses repeat blood work for patients, and there is general disorganization. You are convinced the head nurse is too laissez-faire. You believe the workplace needs order, and that if the group was called together, solutions could be found that would enhance the work flow.

- What type of leadership style would be effective in this situation?
- What leadership behaviors would be necessary to bring more structure to the flow and treatment of emergency patients?

SUMMARY

This chapter has provided a progressive discussion of leadership from a birthright to a complex process. The various perspectives have provided sequential insights for modern theorists who highlight the need for effective leaders in these unpredictable times. The conceptual basis for leadership is still not fully understood. However, each succeeding theory adds more understanding to the process. Leaders in nursing are suggesting the thoughtful study and implementation of transformational leadership as a congruent method with nursing's values and organization requirements. A process model of leadership was offered to highlight the multiple concepts that need to be understood for a leader to be truly effective.

LEARNER EXERCISES

1. There are two components of leadership. The first is your own personal style and the second is how you choose to lead.

   Use the following checklist to evaluate your leadership style: What Kind of a Leader Am I? (see Appendix A)[34].

   You also may wish to evaluate how you follow others. The way in which we lead is often the way in which we follow others (see Appendix B).

2. To examine how you choose to lead, use the following checklist and see how well you are able to lead others.

The Leadership Behavior Checklist

Directions: Answer honestly how well you deal with people in various situations.

Leadership Behavior	**Yes**	**No**
• Do you have a personal history of helping others to improve their work?	❑	❑
• Do others bring tough problems to you?	❑	❑
• Are you able to work in stressful situations?	❑	❑
• Are you able to get others to cooperate?	❑	❑
• Are you able to get others to accept change?	❑	❑
• Are you able to get others to volunteer easily?	❑	❑
• Do you use encouragement with others ?	❑	❑
• In a conflict situation, are you able to listen to all sides?	❑	❑
• Do you treat everyone fairly and squarely?	❑	❑
• Do you avoid accusing others when something goes wrong?	❑	❑
• Do you keep confidential information confidential?	❑	❑

The extent to which you are able to answer "yes" to the above will demonstrate your ability to incorporate leadership concepts in your professional role.

3. What traits do you admire in leaders and professionals from your own experience? Why?
4. Identify your leadership strengths and weaknesses. How do you plan to address the areas that need improvement?

REFERENCES

1. Hodges, L. (2001). Testimony on Nursing Shortage Before the Senate Subcommittee on Health, Education and Pension, February 13, 2000.
2. Hodges, L. (2001). Testimony on Nursing Shortage Before the Senate Subcommittee on Health, Education and Pension, February 13, 2000.
3. Brown, J.A.C. (1954). *The social psychology of industry*. Baltimore, MD: Penguin Books, pp. 129–130.
4. Peterson, A. (1994, December). The changing management role: Autocratic doer to team facilitator. *Nursing Management,* 2(4), 209–212.
5. Dunham, D., & Fischer, E. (1990). Nurse executive profile of excellent nursing leadership. *Journal of Nursing Administration Quarterly,* vol. 15; 1–8.
6. Murphy, M.M., & DeBack, V. (1991). Today's nursing leaders creating the vision. *Nursing Administration Quarterly, 16,* 78–80.
7. Meigham, M.M. (1990). The most important characteristics of nursing leaders. *Nursing Administration Quarterly, 15,* 63–69.
8. Stevens-Barnum, B. (1994, October). Leadership: Can it be holistic? *Holistic Nursing Practice,* 9–15.
9. Stevens-Barnum, B. (1994, October). Leadership: Can it be holistic? *Holistic Nursing Practice,* 10.
10. Lewin, K., Lippitt, R., & White, R.K. (1953). Studies in group decisions. In D. Cartwright & A. Zander, *Group dynamics,* New York: Harper & Row.
11. Schmitt, W., & Tannenbaum, R. (1964). How to choose a leadership pattern: Skills that build executive success. *Harvard Business Review,* 6(116).
12. Bagott, I., & Bagott, J. (May 2001). Think like a CEO: How to sell your ideas to management. *Metro Edition*, 25–27. Retrieved October, 2001 from the World Wide Web: *http://www.nursingspectrum.com*.
13. Korman, A.K. (1973). Consideration, initiating structure and organization criteria—A review. In P.F. Sorenson, Jr. & B. Hill (Eds.), *Perspectives in organizational behavior.* Champagne, IL: Stripes.
14. Fleishman, E.A. (1951). *Leadership climate and supervisory behavior.* Columbus, OH: Ohio State University Press.
15. Stogdill, R.M. (1948, January). Personal factors associated with leadership in a survey of the literature. *Journal of Psychology, 25,* 35–71.
16. Schmitt, W., & Tannenbaum, R. (1964). How to choose a leadership pattern: Skills that build executive success. *Harvard Business Review,* 6(116), 118–121.
17. Fielder, F.E., Chermers, M.M., & Mahar, L.C. (1976). *Improving leadership effectiveness: The leader match concept.* New York: Wiley.
18. Hersey, P., Blanchard, K., & LaMonica, E.L. (1978, May). A situational approach to supervision: Leadership theory and the supervising nurse. *Supervisor Nurse,* 7(17), 20–22.
19. Hersey, P., & Blanchard, K.H. (1993). *Management of organizational behavior: Utilizing human resources,* 6th ed. Englewood Cliffs, NJ, Prentice Hall.
20. Bennis, W., & Nanus, B. (1985). *Leadership: The strategies for taking charge.* New York: Harper & Row.
21. Burns, J.M. (1978). *Leadership.* New York: Harper & Row.

22. Klakovich, M.D. (1994). Connective leadership for the 21st century: A historical perspective and future directions. *Advanced Nursing Science, 16*(4), 42–54.
23. McDaniel, C., & Wolf, G.A. (1992). Transformational leadership and the nurse executive. *Journal of Nursing Administration*, 22(2), 60–65.
24. McDaniel, C., & Wolf, G.A. (1992). Transformational leadership and the nurse executive. *Journal of Nursing Administration*, 22(2), 63.
25. Dunham, J., & Klafehn, K.A. (1990, April), Transformational leadership and the nurse executive. *Journal of Nursing Administration*, 18–31.
26. Bass, B.M. (1985). *Leadership and performance beyond expectations*. New York: The Free Press.
27. Dunham, J., & Klafehn, K.A. (1990, April). Transformational leadership and the nurse executive. *Journal of Nursing Administration*, 32.
28. Ohman, K.A. (2000, Spring). Critical care manager, change views, change lives. *Nurse Manager*, 28–33.
29. Prenkert, F., & Ehnfors, M. (1997). *A measure of organizational effectiveness in nursing management in relation to transactional and transformational leadership: A study in a Swedish count hospital*. Journal of Nursing Management 5(5): 279–87, Sept. 1997.
30. Lipman-Blumer, J. (1992). Connective leadership: Female leadership styles in the 21st century workplace. *Sociology Perspective, 35*(1), 183–203.
31. Klakovich, M.D. (1994). Connective leadership for the 21st century. A historical perspective and future directions. *Advanced Nursing Science, 16*(4), 52.
32. Gergen, D. (2000). *Eyewitness to power*. New York: Simon & Schuster, pp. 343–352.
33. Gergen, D. (2000). *Eyewitness to power*. New York: Simon & Schuster, p. 343.
34. Appendix.

For more information about the Smart Business Plan, visit *http://www.smartonline.com* or call (800) 791-1000; for Business PlanPro, you can go to *http://www.bplans.com* or call (888) 752-6776, for the American Organization of Nurse Executives, you can go to *http://www.aha. org/aone*, and for Microsoft Project 2000, *http://www.microsoft.com/office/project* or call (425) 882-8080.

Further information about Figure 2–3, Leader Behavior, can be found in:
Hersey, Paul. *The Situational Leader*. Center for Leadership Studies, Inc. Escondido, CA, © 1984, 1997.

Appendix

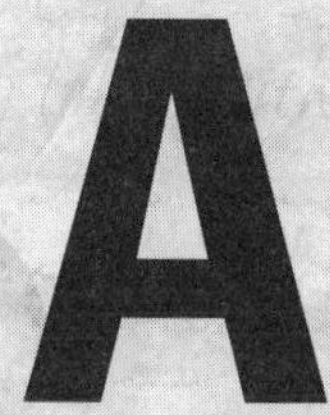

What Kind of Leader Am I?

The quiz below can reveal to you in approximate terms the type of leader you naturally tend to be. You will be able to answer some of the questions without difficulty. A few will require careful thought. Answer all of the questions as accurately and honestly as possible. Where a question has no ready answer from your experience, indicate what you believe you would do in the situation described.

	Yes	No
1. Do you enjoy "running the show"?	❑	❑
2. Generally, do you think it's worth the time and effort to explain the reason for a decision or policy before putting it into effect?	❑	❑
3. Do you prefer the administrative end of your leadership job—planning, paperwork, and so on—to supervising or working directly with a subordinate?	❑	❑
4. A stranger comes into your department and you know he's the new employee hired by one of your assistants. On approaching him, would you first ask his name rather than introduce yourself?	❑	❑
5. Do you keep your people up-to-date on developments affecting the group as a matter of course?	❑	❑
6. Do you find that in giving out assignments, you tend to state the goals, and leave methods to subordinates?	❑	❑
7. Do you think that it's good common sense for a leader to keep aloof from his or her people, because in the long run familiarity breeds lessened respect?	❑	❑
8. It comes time to decide about a group outing. You've heard that the majority prefer to have it on Wednesday, but you're pretty sure Thursday would be better for all concerned. Would you put the question to a vote rather than make the decision yourself?	❑	❑
9. If you had your way, would you make running your group a push-button affair, with personal contacts and communications held to a minimum?	❑	❑
10. Do you find it fairly easy to fire someone?	❑	❑

(*continued*)

	Yes	No
11. Do you feel that the friendlier you are with your people, the better you'll be able to lead them?	❑	❑
12. After considerable time, you work out the answer to a problem. You pass along the solution to an assistant, who pokes holes in it. Would you be annoyed that the problem is still unsolved, rather than become angry with the assistant?	❑	❑
13. Do you agree that one of the best ways to avoid problems of discipline is to provide adequate punishments for violations of rules?	❑	❑
14. Your way of handling a situation is being criticized. Would you try to sell your viewpoint to your group, rather than make it clear that, as boss, decisions are final?	❑	❑
15. Do you generally leave it up to your subordinates to contact you, as far as informal day-to-day communications are concerned?	❑	❑
16. Do you feel that everyone in your group should have a certain amount of personal loyalty to you?	❑	❑
17. Do you favor the practice of appointing committees to settle a problem rather than stepping in to decide on it yourself?	❑	❑
18. Some experts say differences of opinion within a work group are healthy. Others feel that they indicate basic flaws in group unity. Do you agree with the first view?	❑	❑

Taken from: *Techniques of Leadership*, by Auren Uris, McGraw-Hill Book Co., Inc., New York, 1964 (out of print).

Appendix B

What Kind of Follower Am I?

Answer the following questions, keeping in mind what you have done, or feel you actually would do, in the situations described.

	Yes	No
1. When given an assignment, do you like to have all the details spelled out?	❑	❑
2. Do you think that, by and large, most bosses are bossier than they need to be?	❑	❑
3. Would you say that initiative is one of your stronger points?	❑	❑
4. Do you feel a boss lowers himself by buddying around with his or her subordinates?	❑	❑
5. In general, would you prefer working with others to working alone?	❑	❑
6. Would you say you prefer the pleasures of solitude (reading, listening to music) to the social pleasures of being with others (parties, get-togethers, and so on)?	❑	❑
7. Do you tend to become strongly attached to the bosses you work under?	❑	❑
8. Do you tend to offer a helping hand to the newcomers among your collegues and fellow workers?	❑	❑
9. Do you enjoy using your own ideas and ingenuity to solve a work problem?	❑	❑
10. Do you prefer the kind of boss who knows all the answers to one who, not infrequently, comes to you for help?	❑	❑
11. Do you feel it's OK for your boss to be friendlier with some members of the group than with others?	❑	❑
12. Do you like to assume full responsibility for assignments, rather than just do the work and leave the responsibility to your boss?	❑	❑
13. Do you feel that "mixed" groups—men working with women—naturally tend to have more friction than unmixed ones?	❑	❑
14. If you learned your boss was having an affair with his or her secretary, would your respect for him or her remain undiminished?	❑	❑
15. Have you always felt that "he travels fastest who travels alone"?	❑	❑
16. Would you agree that a boss who couldn't win your loyalty shouldn't be a boss?	❑	❑
17. Would you get upset by a fellow worker whose inability or ineptitude obstructs the work of your group?	❑	❑
18. Do you think "boss" is dirty word?	❑	❑

Taken from: *Techniques of Leadership*, by Auren Uris, McGraw-Hill Book Co., Inc., New York, 1964 (out of print).

Appendix C

Scoring for *What Kind of Leader Am I?* and *What Kind of Follower Am I?*

Count the number of "Yes" answers you had for questions in each of the following groups.

Group	Questions
I	1, 4, 7, 10, 13, 16
II	2, 5, 8, 11, 14, 17
III	3, 6, 9, 12, 15, 18

If most "yes" answers are in group I, you prefer an autocratic leadership style.
If most "yes" answers are in group II, you prefer a democratic leadership style.
If most "yes" answers are in group III, you prefer a laissez-faire or free-reign leadership style.

Appendix D

What Scores Mean

High scores—Any category in which you scored from 4 to 6 "yes" answers is one toward which your inclinations are strong:

Autocratic	5
Democratic	3
Free-reign	1

Autocratic tendency strong

Low scores—Score not above 3 "Yes" in any category

Autocratic	1
Democratic	2
Free-reign	3

Most likely an individual without strong impulses toward any of the three types of leadership is probably not self-assertive.

3

Interactive Processes of Leadership

Communication and Group Process

"You can have brilliant ideas but if you can't get them across, your ideas won't get you anywhere."

Lee Iaccoca

INTRODUCTION

Effective nursing leadership is absolutely required to make the necessary changes needed for professional nursing's future. Leadership skills may be developed and learned. It is known that identifying nurses with leadership potential early in their careers and helping them to further their ability has been a successful method. Traditionally, leaders have been developed in the hospital, but in this era of rapid change, opportunities for leadership development need to be incorporated into the new landscape of health care organizations. Leadership development remains of continuing interest to nurses.[1] In a review of the nursing leadership literature, nurse scholars advocate the use of mentorship, networking, and continuing education as valuable methods to develop leadership behavior.[2,3] Fundamentally, leadership skills consist of communication skills and knowledge of group processes. The ability to work in teams is recognized as a necessary skill for all nurses, and this skill emanates directly from group process skills. The objective of this next chapter is to discuss leadership development, focusing on communication and group process skills.

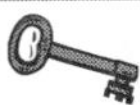

KEY CONCEPTS

Aggressive Communication is a bold, forthright confronting pattern of speaking and dealing with others.

Assertive Communication is a confident pattern of speaking and dealing with others.

Communication is the transfer of understanding from one person to another.

Communication Climate is a general socioemotional feeling (positive or negative) that results from the interplay between a leader and followers.

Communication Process is the means by which ideas are transferred through ideation, encoding, transmission, receiving, decoding, and response.

Group Dynamics are the variety of behaviors and characteristics that are demonstrated in a group and that allow a group to meet a goal.

Lateral Communication refers to a pattern of communication among those of equal rank.

Message represents that which one individual wishes to convey to others.

Nonverbal Behavior is the behavior, expressions, and accompanying gestures that oppose or support the communicated message.

Passive Communication is a seemingly uninvolved, shy, or withdrawn communication pattern of speaking and dealing with others.

Team represents an interdisciplinary group of individuals representing different units of patient care who are able to develop a comprehensive care plan.

Team Building involves a set of activities that strengthen a working team based on the principles of group dynamics.

COMMUNICATION

Leadership is an interactive process in which a leader influences a group. The nature of the leader's influencing process remains an ambiguous topic among leadership scholars. Research efforts have established that leadership consists of personal, functional, and situational variables. Formal educational and training programs have provided a foundation to the belief that leadership skills may be developed.[4] Nonetheless, **communication** is the medium by which leadership is conveyed to the group (see Figure 3-1). Communication, by definition, is the transfer of information and understanding from one person to another. This occurs by means of the communication process, consisting of a sender, message, and receiver, which are influenced by an environment. Each of the components of the communication process is capable of enhancing or inhibiting the understanding of the message.

The Message

The **message** is the idea to be conveyed. A leader should keep in mind that the meaning of words resides not in the message but rather in people who interpret the message. Words do

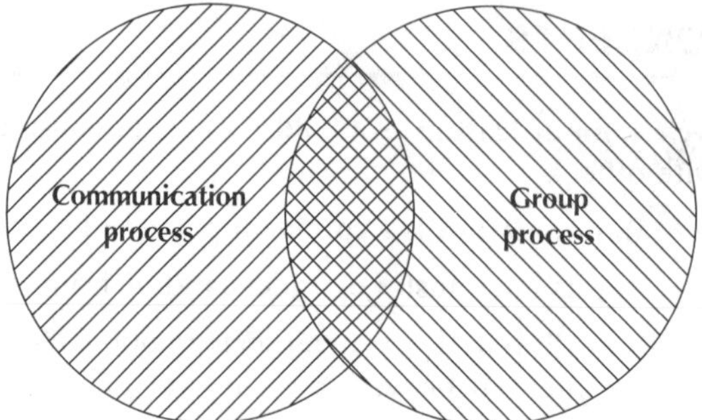

FIGURE 3-1. The main components of leadership: communication and the group process.

FIGURE 3-2. The essential elements of the communication components; the message and the communication climate in which the message is delivered.

THE MESSAGE

1. *Verbal*
   What you talk about
2. *Nonverbal*
   How it is communicated
   Facial expression
   Guarded remarks
   Pauses
   Gestures
   Posture
   Tone of voice
     Accepting
     Rejecting
   Body language

COMMUNICATION CLIMATE

Positive—enhances the message
or
Negative—detracts from understanding the message

mean different things to different people; thus, individuals assign their own meaning, and it may be different from what was intended. The message is composed not only of symbols (words), but also a tone and nonverbal behavior. The tone of the message reflects an emotional level, whereas **nonverbal behavior**, consisting of facial expressions, pauses, gestures, posture, and guarded remarks, reinforce or contradict the primary message. Words become far less important than the tone of the message and the accompanying body language.[5] The message itself is conveyed by means of the **communication process** (see Figure 3-2).

Communication Process

The communication process consists of six steps: ideation, encoding, transmission, receiving, decoding, and response (see Figure 3-3). *Ideation* refers to the message, the idea, or the thought to be communicated to the individual or a group. *Encoding* is the manner

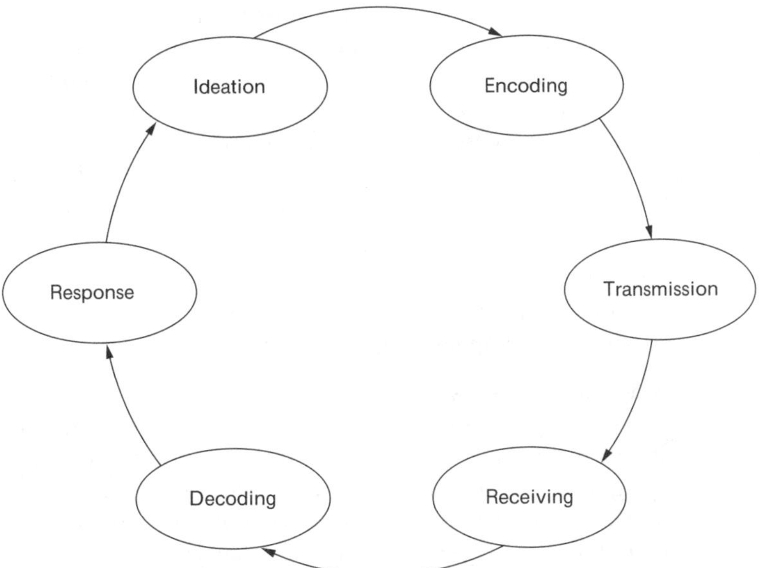

FIGURE 3-3. The conceptual components of the communication process. The circle is used to denote the dynamic and reciprocal properties of the communication process.

in which the message is conveyed. The manner may be something other than verbal, such as a written message or a visual or spoken cue. *Encoding* also takes into account the nonverbal behaviors that accompany the message, such as a gesture or an expression. *Transmission* is the transmittal of the message. For the listener or reader to *receive* the message, intact senses and appropriate ability are required. *Decoding* refers to the mental mechanisms used to receive and, consequently, interpret the message. The *response* or feedback should, in turn, tell the leader if the individual or the group understood the message. The communication process will now reverse for the leader's understanding. Both the leader and followers share responsibility to understand each other.

The nurse leader/manager uses communication skills in all aspects of organizational life. Today, the nursing student is well grounded in therapeutic communication skills. However, different skills are required to communicate effectively with groups of professional workers. The ability to communicate effectively is particularly important today, with the growing emphasis on interdependence in health care. Experts agree: success in the workplace is directly related to human relations skills. Effective communication among professionals is one way to establish and maintain the desired atmosphere of professional competence which ensures quality patient care.

TEN BASICS FOR GOOD COMMUNICATION

Skillful communication is fundamental to successful leadership. The following suggestions are offered to enhance communication in the workplace.

1. **Clarify your ideas before communicating to others.**
   Before speaking to an individual or a group, plan and organize what it is you are going to say. Analyze your thoughts carefully, and keep in mind the objective you wish to meet as well as the unique characteristics of those to whom you are speaking. Provide an opportunity for questions and answers to enhance the clarity of the message. If necessary, return to the objective to increase the likelihood of mutual understanding. The steps to take to assure your message is clear are as follows:
   - Tell them.
   - Have them tell you.
   - Have them write it down.
   - Schedule follow-up meetings or reports.[6]
2. **Consider the physical setting.**
   The physical setting can be either conducive or a serious block to communication. Environmental distractions interfere with the communication process. People may be trying to have a serious conversation when a sudden, distracting noise occurs that directs attention away from the message and toward the environmental stimuli. Consider the following situation: a nurse manager is explaining the medication error policy to a new staff nurse, and the phone rings or there is a knock at the door. This is distracting, and both parties will have to compensate for the interruption before they are ready to continue their conversation. The physical environment should support the opportunity to have a meaningful two-way conversation. This means ensuring a quiet, private, comfortable setting in which all parties will be able to concentrate on communicating.
3. **Consider the psychological environment.**
   The psychological environment is also referred to as the communication, or social, climate. A **communication climate** is defined as the general socioemotional feeling that is produced between the leader and group as a result of the emphasis placed on productivity and human concerns. A psychological and emotional contract results within the work group, producing either a supportive or defensive climate. If you as a leader have created a supportive and open (positive) environment, you will have less difficulty communicating with your staff than you would within a defensive and hostile (negative) environment (see Figure 3-4). A supportive communication climate is characterized by a leader who listens; is empathetic; offers acceptance of individuals; exhibits a shared, problem-solving attitude; is open; and values equality in the workplace. The group members exhibit the same attitudes and behaviors. In a supportive environment, a bond between leader and follower ensures safe, consistent, and meaningful communication. Conversely, a defensive climate is characterized by a leader who may be controlling, punishing, evaluating, advice giving, and who insists on being right. The followers, however, are submissive or hostile, and communication is usually nonproductive.

   The power of a positive communication climate is that it fosters behaviors among the leader and followers that lead to trustful and cooperative working relationships. To a great extent, following the 10 basics of good communication will contribute to

FIGURE 3-4. The characteristics of both a negative and positive communication climate. These behaviors are exhibited by the leader or the followers or both.

Positive climate behavioral characteristics

Listening
Empathy
Acceptance
Shared problem-solving attitude
Openness
Equality

Negative climate behavioral characteristics

Controlling
Punishing
Evaluating
Advice giving
Superiority
Certainty

a positive communication climate. It is much easier to problem solve when working relationships are good.

4. **Consult with others when necessary to be sure your information is accurate.**
   A major mistake for a leader is to communicate incorrect information to the members of the group. If misinformation is given to an individual or to the group, the leader should acknowledge the error and correct the situation as soon as possible. This demonstrates to subordinates and to superiors that the leader deals with mistakes in a direct, honest, and forthright manner.

5. **Be mindful of the tone, as well as the words, of the message.**
   Tone refers to the emotional level of the message. It may be interpreted as angry, friendly, dictatorial, fair, or a number of other emotional reactions. The tone may be opposite from the words that are being spoken. If you say something of a very serious nature and smile and laugh, you are giving mixed messages, making it very difficult for the listeners to know what you are trying to convey. The tone of your voice or written memo should support your message, not detract from it.

6. **Take the opportunity to convey something of help, value, or praise to the receiver.**
   People need to know that their contributions are useful and respected. This is not just limited to subordinates; you also might wish to acknowledge the helpful contributions of superiors. Give credit for the contributions of others when genuinely deserved. It is amazing how powerful praise can be in establishing positive feelings in other people. By giving praise, the leader is actively involved in the development of the followers as well as a good work environment.

7. **Follow-up your communication.**
   Feedback is necessary to make sure that the message was understood as you intended it to be understood. To encourage feedback, watch for nonverbal signs of confusion. Encourage and reward questions from the group. Ask open-ended questions such as,

"What do you think about the plan?" Avoid close-ended questions like, "Is that clear?" Take the initiative by assuming responsibility for any potential misunderstandings by saying, "Sometimes I am not clear. Would you repeat your understanding of what I have just said, so that I can check myself?" Depending on the nature of the communication, you may require serial contacts or meetings. This is all a part of leadership, and you, the beginning leader, are showing your serious and committed effort to help people understand the message.

8. **Nonverbal behavior should support communication.**
   For the most part, nonverbal behavior is unconscious, and since most individuals don't control these reactions, they tend to be extremely revealing. Thus, be sure your actions support your communication in two ways. The first is in the delivery of the message. Facial expressions and body posture should be consistent with the message. Demonstrating self-confidence and erect posture evokes confidence in what you are saying. The second component of nonverbal behavior is with follow-through of the message. If the leader makes a request of the group, the leader should also comply with the request. This promotes trust. If actions and attitude are in conflict, there will be confusion, and people will tend to deny what has been said. For example, if the leader tells the staff that they must be on time for work and then the leader is consistently late, the message will not be taken seriously.

9. **Be an active listener.**
   To improve your listening skills, certain behaviors should be learned and practiced as you interact with people. Active listening begins as you give full attention to the person speaking. This means that you listen carefully with your mind as well as with your gestures and facial expressions. Look directly at the person to whom you are speaking. Direct eye contact conveys your undivided attention to the speaker. It is also a good idea to indicate your desire for understanding by asking for clarification, paraphrasing, summarizing, and requesting information as necessary. The most important aspect of active listening, and also the most difficult, is keeping silent, which shows respect for the other person. Active listening will enhance understanding of messages by facilitating communication through appropriate feedback. Listen to what the person has said, as well as the way it was said. Listening takes discipline, effort, and time to develop. Discipline requires emotional, intellectual, and behavioral control. A leader must develop the self-mastery to be silent when someone else is speaking. This means putting another's ideas before your own. Active listening implies a good faith effort on the part of the leader to understand the message.

   Developing active listening skills includes the following suggestions:

   - *Stop talking.* To be able to listen to another person, stop what you are doing, eliminate distractions, and give full attention to the speaker.
   - *Put the other person at ease.* Try to be relaxed yourself, and open the conversation with a nonthreatening comment such as, "Anything I can help you with?"
   - *Don't interrupt.* This is particularly important if the person is upset. It is important for people to believe that they have been heard.
   - *Empathize.* Indicate by your response that you are concerned. You might ask for help by saying, "I would like to understand your problem. Will you help me?"

- *Paraphrase.* Try to summarize what you have heard and restate it to the satisfaction of the person.
- *Ask open-ended questions.* This form of questioning is indirect and provides for more clarification of points of view. A question such as "What do you suggest we do?" engages the other individual in a meaningful way.
- *Use silence.* Silence in a conversation may produce tension. This tension may be necessary to insist that the other individual respond. Using discriminant periods of silence may enhance the ability to problem solve.
- *Allow reflection.* In many cases, the leader's role may be to act as a sounding board for the group member. This is also called passive listening. The leader will gain a better understanding of the other's views, which enhances the potential for a positive solution.

10. **Be assertive when expressing your view.**
Communication patterns exist on a continuum from passive to aggressive. Assertiveness is the desirable style for the nurse leader and manager. Assertive communication and behavior maintains a balance between aggressive and passive styles. The assertive style considers the rights of all persons involved in the communication process. The Nurse's Bill of Rights, identified by Hermann, and reiterated by Miller and Catalano, states very clearly what these rights are:

- The right to be treated with respect.
- The right to be listened to.
- The right to have and to express thoughts, feelings, and opinions.
- The right to ask questions and to challenge.
- The right to understand job expectations, as well as have them written.
- The right to say no and not feel guilty.
- The right to be treated as an equal member of the health team.
- The right to ask for change in the system.
- The right to have a reasonable workload.
- The right to make a mistake.
- The right to make decisions regarding health and nursing care.
- The right to initiate health teaching.
- The right to be a patient advocate or to help a patient speak for himself or herself.
- The right to change one's mind.[7,8]

The **assertive communication** style is demonstrated by communication that says directly and clearly what is on one's mind. It is also demonstrated by listening to what others say. The leader uses objective words, uses "I" messages, and makes honest statements about the leader's ideas and feelings. Part of an assertive style is the use of direct eye contact, spontaneous verbal expressions, and appropriate gestures and facial expressions while speaking in a well-modulated voice. Assertiveness is also a process that comes with maturing in a role and gaining self-confidence in one's own knowledge and experience. An assertive style is appropriate and is based on self-respect and consideration for other people.

Aggressive communication, however, is concerned only with the rights of one position and is very goal oriented. This style may be characterized as being forceful, and may be inappropriate, or confronting. It may or may not be overtly hostile.[9] This style uses subjective words, makes accusations, and sends "you" messages. It may be confronting, sarcastic, or rude. This individual often belittles others while seeming to take charge of the situation. The rights of all individuals have not been considered.

A **passive communication** style, however, is uninvolved. This style may be withdrawn and shy or purposefully withholding. Women in particular may tend to be silent in group situations, and beginning leaders may have to overcome some hesitation about speaking to groups. Some suggestions that can help include recognizing your value and rights in a professional situation. Try to make one contribution in each group situation. Gradually, you will feel more comfortable speaking in groups. Plan in advance what you wish to say, and if possible speak from a prepared text.

Communication among professionals is an essential hallmark of health care. Keep in mind that the leader and followers have a basic right to give and to receive information in a professional manner. Communication skills grow and develop over time and are the means by which leadership is exercised. It is important to remember that communication does not mean agreement or harmony concerning every issue but rather an understanding of the message between the leader and followers.

BLOCKS TO COMMUNICATION

Blocks to communication refer to obstacles that prevent the message from being delivered or understood. Some of the more common reasons for blocks to communication are poor listening habits, time and work demands, semantics, and different frames of reference.[10] In addition, cultural and gender differences may be responsible for misunderstanding and blocked communication. Blocks to communication are the reasons why people leave meetings with half messages and incomplete or inaccurate information.

Poor listening skills, or the inability to listen attentively to people, result from a variety of sources. Among the reasons are that the leader prejudges the conversation with prior expectations and assumes to know what the speaker is about to say. Some leaders may assume hearing and listening are the same activity. Other reasons for inattention are disinterest in the conversation and allowing the mind to wander. We hear faster than people can speak; thus, active listening will facilitate focusing on the speaker.

Time and work demands also may interfere with the ability to communicate effectively. The stress of the work environment, with all its constraints, minimizes the ability to concentrate. Stress produces an intense reaction and likely will produce a temporary block to communication. The individual stops listening, or may hear part of the message, and the mind is closed to other ideas. Stress is a powerful force that interferes with concentration. Before constructive communication can continue, time has to be set aside and work responsibilities met.

Semantic barriers can also pose problems for communication. Semantics refers to the study of words. In day-to-day conversations, people may use the same words but ascribe different meanings. Since words are symbolic, their meaning is subject to multiple interpretations. The leader should try to be aware of the choice of words or phrases used in conveying a message to avoid misinterpretation or sending the wrong message to the group. In addition, the leader should consider the context of words and their relationship to a particular idea. Using messages in the proper context will enhance communication. For example, suppose a nurse manager wishes to praise the staff because of their outstanding efforts during an extremely hectic period. The nurse manager tells the group, "You are all guilty of doing an unbelievable job!" Unfortunately, it is really not clear what the head nurse is trying to say or for what period of time or particular activity. In this case, there is a great deal of room for misunderstanding the message.

People speak and think from their personal frame of reference and experience. Eliciting feedback allows the leader to judge the listener's understanding. This can be accomplished by asking the right questions, phrasing questions within a frame of reference, and requesting that questions asked of you also be placed in a frame of reference. As always, acknowledge the message and affirm that both you and the speaker have the same understanding. If it is appropriate, thank the other person for being honest and expressing his or her feelings.

Culture and Gender

Currently, the general society is diverse, and the workforce reflects this diversity. The changing demographic includes new immigration groups, maturing of "the baby-boomers", exponential increases of the elderly, and "minorities" are becoming the "majority."[11] The U.S. population is expected to grow by 42 million persons by the year 2010. Of this increase, Latinos and Hispanics will account for 47 percent, Africian-Americans 22 percent, Asians and other people of color, 18 percent, and those of European descent, 13 percent.[12] The challenge to nursing leadership is twofold; the first is to ensure culturally relevant care for patients, and the second is to capitalize on the strength of the diverse workforce.

Since various ethnic and racial groups are employed in health care, patterns of communication may differ among the many cultural groups. Culture impacts communication in several ways since it is a system of customs, beliefs, ideas, values, and behaviors, which in turn affects the creation, sending, storing, and interpretation of information.[13,14] To avoid misunderstandings, knowing more about specific cultural patterns is helpful. In general, cultural differences involving communication patterns (proximity of those communicating, such as different perceptions of personal space and tolerance of touching), body movements, paralanguage (inflections, silences, volume or timbre of voice, and pace of speaking), and density of language are among some of the characteristics that differ among cultures.[15] See the end of this chapter for websites to provide specific information about specific cultural groups.

Gender issues should also be considered to ensure effective communication in the workplace. Within the health care industry, men and women work side by side, and research shows men and women also communicate with different styles.[16] Despite greater cultural and social awareness, men and women are educated by society to speak and act differently based on gender expectations. Wood suggests that men and women are socialized into distinct speech patterns, and learn different rules about the purpose of communication. Women tend to use communication to maintain or establish relationships, share themselves, and learn about others.[17] Men tend to use communication in an instrumental way; that is, to accomplish goals. Research also suggests men tend to be more abstract, theoretical, conceptual, general, and less personal than women.[18]

Women are conditioned to assume a quieter, less forceful, and possibly tentative questioning approach; while men are conditioned to assume a more direct and forceful manner of speaking. The differing use of language may lead to misunderstandings in communication. However, both men and women are capable of speaking forcefully, directly, questioningly, and tentatively.

Suggestions to facilitate communication involve recognizing and accepting these differences. It is possible men and women have different styles of communicating and exhibit unspoken cultural rules.[19] In general, for men to improve communication skills with women, they should listen to women's feelings by attempting to understand their point of view. Men need to avoid interrupting (often acceptable between men) or solving the problem before the woman is finished, and men need to admit if they don't understand the content of the conversation. Women, however, may improve communication with men by being direct, explaining why or how they feel a particular way, and allowing questions and disagreements to be a part of a conversation.[20]

In all instances of culture and gender, no one style or communication characteristic is absolute or inclusive to a particular group; rather, these characteristics have been noted to be dominant in groups being studied. Communication patterns will always vary according to the context or situation. In addition, people have their own idiosyncracies which affect their style and manner. Miscommunication occurs when people expect one thing and experience another. Focusing on the message, rather than the person's communication style, will facilitate the communication process.

For the beginning leader, it is important to be aware of the powerful role communication plays in the organization. Those aspects of the situation and within the leader and followers that contribute to an understanding of the communicated message should help you refine your ability to communicate with the health team. Avoiding blocks to communication will contribute to successful interaction.

COMMUNICATION WITH THE HEALTH TEAM

Good communication builds relationships with the health team that strengthens a leader's position to manage and motivate. The future leader should be prepared to communicate with subordinates, other leaders/managers, and superiors. Given the many demands that are placed on all health care providers, there is a need for effective and professional communication. A relationship between leader/managers and employees or subordinates may be viewed from four stages:

1. Meeting
2. Knowing
3. Enabling
4. Directing[21]

The *meeting* stage is a short phase occurring when people are introduced in order to lay the foundation for the relationship. This phase is essentially an information-sharing exchange. The objectives of this meeting are to learn about the employees' experience, to orient the employee, to create expectations for instruction and feedback processes, and to establish expectations about work attitude and quality of performance. Skills the leader should use are the ability to give information clearly; listen; communicate empathy, respect, and warmth; and role-model expected behaviors.

The *knowing* stage involves gaining insights into the person's attitudes and motivation. The objectives of this phase include learning the employees' ability to perform assigned work, understanding how to help them improve, accepting personal characteristics (pleasant, as well as unpleasant) that are unrelated to the work product, and gaining deeper insights of the employees' person (opinions, attitudes, preferences, goals, and motivation).

The *enabling* stage is the phase when the leader/manager encourages and gives praise, advice, and instruction. The objectives of this phase include increasing productivity and providing opportunities for staff members to grow profesionally through their work.

The *directing* stage is that stage in the process where authority is established with subordinates. When necessary, this phase includes reiterating rules, setting deadlines, giving ultimatums, and taking the necessary disciplinary action. Behaviors used in this phase include forcing, demanding, telling, and, when necessary, coercing. It needs to be understood that use of these behaviorial strategies produces a degree of resistance that will affect the nature of the relationship for the short term or long term duration of the relationship. Leadership skills require a wide repertoire of behaviors, and sometimes it will be necessary to compel others to perform appropriately. When it is necessary to be more direct with subordinates, the role of feedback becomes even more important. Feedback will support clear and open communication (see Figure 3-5).

Communication with other managers is known as **lateral communication.** Communication with those of comparable authority and power also requires effective communication skills. Superiors are those individuals with more legitimate authority, or those people who

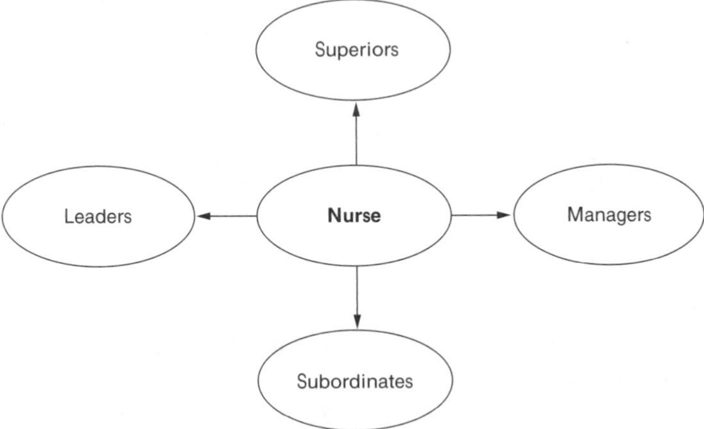

FIGURE 3-5. The members of the health team with whom the nurse communicates on a regular basis.

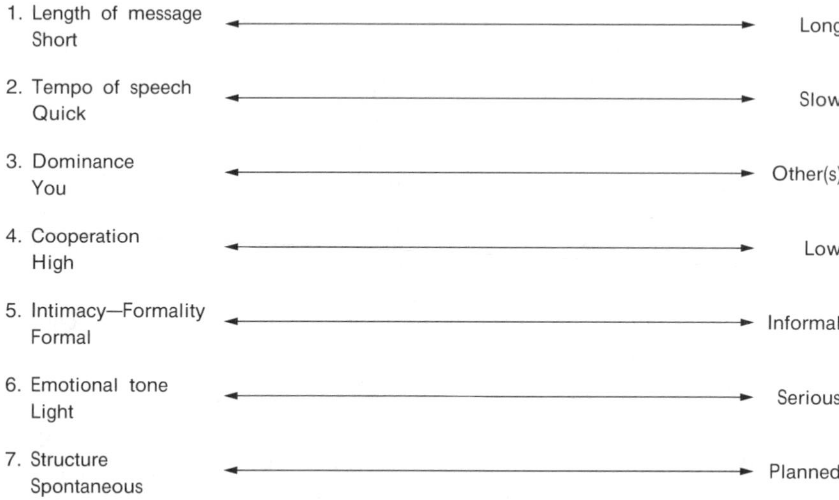

FIGURE 3-6. The factors that need to be considered for the most effective communicated message.

possess more power and status. For the beginning leader or manager, communication with superiors can be threatening and intimidating, because of the social differential between the two. Dealing with those more powerful is a fact of organizational life. For a formal meeting, the new leader will have an opportunity to be prepared for the topic to be discussed. In this case, reviewing the fundamentals of good communication will be helpful in facilitating participation in the meeting. Spontaneous meetings with superiors may be difficult for the beginning leader. However, the same communication rules apply to facilitate the communication process: stay focused on the topic, make sure your message is understood, and listen actively to understand (see Figure 3-6). Despite the different roles played by the various team members and their accompanying levels of status, communication is the critical process that focuses the work of the organization.

Preventing Communication Breakdown

Because of the complexity of the health care system and its various roles, preventing communication breakdown is a major leadership responsibility. Communication problems may result from the personalities of the individuals, or flaws in the system.[22] The areas where communication breakdowns are most likely include failure to clarify physician orders, failure to communicate change of a patient's status, failure to adequately document patient or employee incidents, and failure to understand written job descriptions and organization policies.

Physicians and nurse practitioners who write orders for patients are expected to clarify orders that are unclear or have illegible handwriting. A nurse has a duty to have orders clarified for patient safety. After contacting the appropriate person for clarification of the order, he or she should state clearly and specifically why the order appears improper. For example, "This dose is three times the normal adult dose, is that what you meant to write?" Another approach is, "It is not clear what you have written, and we cannot initiate your medical plan, please clarify your orders." If an improper order is not changed, the nurse has a responsibility to go up the chain of command in the organization to report the problem rather than threatening a patient's health status.

Communication among the health team is especially important when a patient's status has changed. Nurses must not let other demands get in the way of timely care. It is important for the nurse to identify the necessary members of the health team who are responsible for patient care. Preplanning on the part of the nurse to identify the doctor, family members, and others who should be informed of patient changes is a proactive communication method.

Written communication or documentation is necessary to create a history of events that suppport proper managerial or professional decisions. In the case of a manager who is concerned about employee performance, a written record of events will be necessary to support managerial decisions of whether or not to terminate or maintain the employee in question. Without adequate documentation, this becomes a much more difficult, if not litigious, situation.

Communication problems may also develop among nurses and managers when the manager asks or demands that the nurse employee perform activities which the nurse does not wish to do. This may involve being pulled to another area, performing new tasks, or working at unscheduled times. Knowing the job description and policies that regulate performance will reduce workplace misunderstandings on both parts.[23]

Communication with Difficult People

Positive communication is a desirable goal, but problems may arise with certain individuals. In any organization, there may be a few people who deal with others in an unreasonable way. They may be overtly hostile or unwilling to speak at all. Difficult people who consistently interact in an unproductive way cause problems for those who must interact with them.

What are the reasons for impossible behavior? People learn and use behavior that gets results for them. If bullying others gives one power and control, goes unchallenged, and is reinforced, a behavioral pattern develops. While human behavior is a complex phenomenon, responsibility for that behavior belongs to each person. Individuals who continually cause havoc with others' sense of equilibrium may be termed "difficult." Dr. Robert Branson has made a study of personality types that cause the most disruption in the workplace.[24] He has identified them to be hostile aggressives, complainers and negativists, silent and unresponsives, super agreeables, know-it-alls, and indecisives. He has proposed particular coping mechanisms for those who must deal with these individuals. Difficult people make up less than 10 percent of any organization.[25] However, they cause untold problems in morale, turnover, and productivity. The usual ways of dealing with these people include explaining and excusing their behavior or reacting in a defensive and frustrated manner. Dr. Branson offers another response: coping in highly specific ways to the different personalities.

The new leader should consider the underlying coping strategies, which include the following presumptions:

1. **One individual cannot change another's behavior.**
   The behavioral reactions of difficult people are long-standing and well-developed. These reactions are a result of stress, and are used to gain control of the situation even if other people are affected.
2. **Behavior that is not confronted will not change.**
   Individuals who display problem behavior don't use conventional methods of problem solving. Thus, if dealing with these people, leaders must facilitate problem-solving skills.
3. **Coping skills with difficult behavior may be learned.**
   It is more appropriate and less taxing to learn techniques that deal effectively with problem behavior. It empowers the leader to be in charge of potentially emotionally charged situations.

Specific coping strategies that deal with individual personalities follow.

Hostile aggressive people behave as they do when under stress. They typically blame other people for their situation and for triggering their angry, demeaning reaction. The way to cope with this behavior is twofold. The first is to stand up for yourself, and the second is not to engage in an argument. Your statement might include, "I don't agree," or "I see things differently. Let's discuss this further." Do not engage in an argument; it will only make the situation worse. It is very important that you keep an emotional distance from hostile aggressive attackers. This is done by remembering that there is an issue that needs to be addressed, besides the overwhelming behavior. The behavior is the responsibility of the hostile aggressive person. You have a responsibility as a coworker to try to deal with the issue, not the behavior. If at all possible, remove the hostile aggressive person from public view. Suggest that you converse in a private setting or at a later time so that his or her emotions can calm down.

Complainers and negativists are individuals who criticize or are unsatisfied with given situations or decisions. These individuals feel powerless in the face of a problem, as though they have no control over events. Coping strategies include not agreeing with them, and asking for their view on how to: (1) structure the problem, (2) analyze the negative consequences of the final decision, and (3) help them solve or accept the negative aspects of the best solution while reminding them of their role in constructing the solution.

Silent, unresponsive people have learned that, by simply never speaking, they don't have to participate in problem solving. This way, they don't have to take responsibility for decisions. Coping with this behavior includes, after posing your concern, keeping silent until the person speaks. If the individual refuses to speak, repeat your concern and remain silent. If all attempts to engage the person in communication fail, conclude and state that because there is no response, you will make the final decision.

Super agreeable people are those who want to please everyone, even if they can't. They find it highly stressful to explain that they are unable to do something because it might displease the leader. When they fail to do what they said they would do, it becomes a problem. Coping with this behavior requires the leader to assure the persons that it is all right to say if they are currently unable to complete their work. Follow-up and encouragement are also helpful activities for the leader.

Know-it-alls are people who are only impressed with their own views and facts, even if they aren't always correct. To cope with this behavior, the leader must use these persons' own words and facts to dissuade them. The leader should suggest that they review the facts of the situation, and point out discrepancies in those facts. In this way, know-it-alls convince themselves of their error.

Indecisive people have a difficult time making decisions. They feel great stress when choosing a course of action because they see impediments to any given course of action. To cope with this behavior when a decision must be made, the leader should say, "In any plan there are problems. What gets in the way of this one? Please tell us even if you feel it is insignificant." Be assured, what they tell the leader is not insignificant; it is a major block to the decision-making process, and it is up to the leader to offer a compromise.

If leaders can learn to use different communication and behavior patterns that facilitate group members making responsible decisions, working relationships will be highly productive.[26]

Communication Networks

Communication patterns, or networks, form within the organization and among the health team, allowing information to be circulated. These same networks also affect the ways groups solve problems. The actual pattern of the communication network may be as varied as the number of groups in existence. However, common patterns are downward, upward, downward and upward, circular, or multichanneled. Figure 3-7 illustrates the communication networks. In essence, the leader either talks in a downward pattern to the group or there is a sharing, both up and down, with the participants of the group as well as communication that is shared among the participants. The real issue is not whether every participant shares a two-way communication channel with every other member but whether the communication is effective. Open communication patterns are preferable to restricted networks.

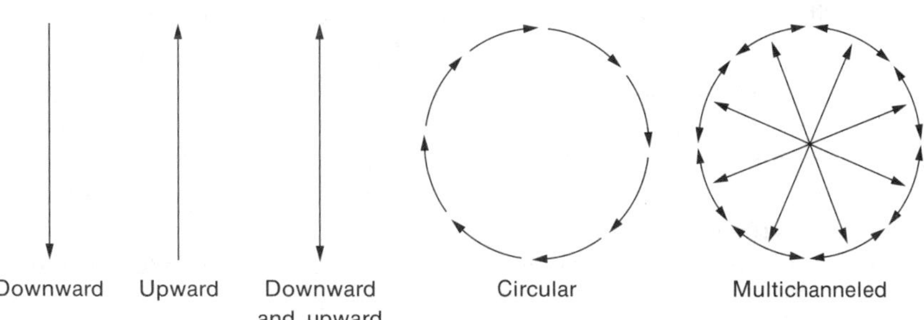

FIGURE 3-7. Some of the ways communication networks can form.

TEAM BUILDING

Professional nurses are educated to make independent decisions. They are taught to behave as autonomously as possible in order to manage patient care. Coincidentally, the new health care environment structures most health care through using **teams.**[27] A requisite skill for the new nurse leader will be the ability to work within teams or interdisciplinary group structures. While communication skills are one aspect of leadership development, equally important is the knowledge of group dynamics. **Group dynamics** include the study of how people form and function within a group structure. The group becomes a unit when it shares a common goal and acts in unison to meet that goal. This is referred to as **team building.** Particular problems in organizations can only be studied through group behavior; for example, a labor and management dispute represents different points of a collective view.

Group Dynamics

A group may be defined as a collection of individuals who interact with each other on a regular basis, are psychologically aware of each other, and who see themselves as a group. Groups are categorized as primary or secondary. Primary groups are composed of individuals who interact on a "face-to-face" basis, and the relationships are personal. In addition, there are no written, formal rules or regulations impacting the group because they are unwarranted. Examples of primary groups are families or groups of friends. In the workplace, primary groups also exist in the form of those who affiliate because of something held in common. Similarity distinguishes this group. For instance, the group members may all be women in the administrative field, all graduates from the same institution, or all of the same ethnic background. Secondary groups are larger and more impersonal. These groups are organized around formal rules, procedures, policies, and other regulations. The workplace is composed of secondary groups that are found in departments and levels forming the work group.[28]

The leader deals with secondary groups in the workplace. Secondary groups may also be categorized as formal and informal groups. Formal groups are the official or legitimate work groups, whereas informal groups form for a variety of reasons. The leader must be able to influence both groups and thus move the work group toward meeting its objectives. Most research on effective leadership behavior focuses on formal leaders in positions of authority. However, there is a growing interest in the role and influence of the informal leader.

An effective work group, composed of formal and informal groups, is characterized by the ability to meet its goals through a high degree of appropriate communication and understanding among its members. This group makes good decisions based on respect for all members' viewpoints. Another characteristic is the ability to arrive at a balance between group productivity and individual need satisfaction. This group is not dominated by the leader; instead, there is a flexibility among the leader and members to use individual talents appropriately. This group is cohesive and can objectively review its work and face problems in a way that balances emotional and rational behavior for a productive group effort. The leader who enhances cohesion and cooperation will be moving the group toward completion of its goals.

Interdisciplinary Teams

An interdisciplinary team is a group of individuals representing different units of patient care and who each contribute to the overall plan for patient care. The configuration of the team will consist of those individuals who are able to assist in the stated goal of the group. Teams are currently viewed as an extremely efficient and effective method for complex decision making. Because teams are specialized groups, information aiding in the understanding of group dynamics also applies to team functioning.

Teams form because of a specific mission or goal. Because the participants are selected, the leader serves to facilitate the flow of information and encourage the active participation of members. The best decision depends on the quality of information and the group's ability to plan the best course of action.

Characteristics of a Group

Group affiliation is a source of need satisfaction. Membership in primary and secondary groups meet social and psychological needs. To a great extent, people choose groups that closely match their values. This can be explained on the basis of group characteristics, consisting of values, norms, and conformity. Groups share a value structure that comes about through the influence members have on one another. For example, some groups value their expertise, friendship, or higher wages. The ability to influence one another may be positive or negative.

Another characteristic of a group is conformity to norms (without some degree of conformity, there is no group or group identity). Norms refer to the expected behaviors within a group. If an individual violates these norms, he or she is at risk of becoming an outcast. Take, for instance, the new staff nurse from fictional University Hospital who has worked with every conceivable medical and nursing advancement. As this individual works with patients in a highly competent way, it is likely the new nurse will be discussed by coworkers who feel threatened. Their discomfort springs from a threat to their knowledge and skill level. The new nurse is a stimulus for a different norm, and the group has several ways of dealing with this challenge. The first may be to minimize the performance of the newcomer and to exclude him or her from the group until the productivity level becomes comparable. Norms of a group are powerful enforcers for human behavior. Compliance to the norm means group membership.

While most group members conform, some individuals do not. The single most important individual characteristic that leads to group conformity is the degree to which the individual finds the group attractive psychologically. For the individual who feels that membership in this group gives status, participation will follow. For those who don't perceive membership as a positive activity, participation will be more doubtful. The leader who understands each member's potential contribution will be able to encourage both conformists' and nonconformists' strengths and orchestrate the diversity. This is accomplished through the different roles and positions available to group members.

Group Processes

Lippitt Summarized how to work more effectively with groups as a result of his extensive work with small groups.[29] He contends that leadership skills can be learned and practiced within a group context, and skill with groups can be developed. Some individuals have a very natural and easy ability to work with other individuals on a one-to-one basis, but the idea of dealing with a group needs special attention. Lippitt contends that to work more effectively with groups, a leader needs to develop the following:

- An awareness of the leader's impact on a group.
- Insight into others' needs, abilities, and reactions.
- A sincere belief in group decision making.
- An understanding of what makes a group tick.
- Ability to diagnose a sick group.
- Flexibility as a leader or member of the group.[30]

Each of the necessary skills to become an effective leader will be discussed below.

LEADER'S IMPACT ON A GROUP

A leader's impact on a group refers to the leader's effect on other people. When dealing with a group, ask yourself: Are you comfortable in group situations, or do you feel a bit insecure? Some individuals enjoy groups while others find working with groups difficult. If you find yourself in the latter categroy, make a conscious effort to objectively evaluate how your behavior, regardless of your feelings, affects the group. Pay attention to: (1) how you act, (2) how much or how little you speak, and (3) what the group's reaction is to you. Does the group listen to you, or do they overlook your silence? Does the group really appreciate your attempts at humor, or do they find such comments irritating and distracting? By developing a sensitivity to the reaction of others, you will become aware of the group members' reactions to you, either in what they say or in what they do (e.g., the subtle expression on someone's face, the tone of a person's voice, or how relaxed or tense the atmosphere of the meeting becomes when you introduce a thought). The consistent reaction of the group to your presentations will be a gauge of your effectiveness. Conversely, you should also consider the reaction that other people and their behaviors have on you. As a leader, it is helpful to focus on communication as opposed to reacting to the individual.

Insight

Insight into the needs and abilities of others is an important leadership group function. It recognizes that people belong to groups for different reasons. Individuals participate in groups to meet their needs. If needs are not being met, the individual will become hostile or apathetic. The wise leader understands that individuals bring different capabilities to group productivity, and the most important activity the leader can engage in is to look for unexpected talent in individuals. The leader allows the member to participate in different ways that broaden the individual and build the participant's ego. This is accomplished by allowing members to participate broadly so that their capabilities may emerge.

Some of the available behaviors that participants in the group may exhibit are broadly grouped as task or maintenance functions. Task functions serve to facilitate and to coordinate group effort in the selection and definition of a common problem and in the solution of that problem. Behaviors that fall in this category are:

- *Initiating*—suggests new ideas or a different way of looking at an old problem; proposes new activities.
- *Information seeking*—asks for relevant facts and feelings about the situation at hand.
- *Information giving*—provides the necessary and relevant information.
- *Clarifying*—probes for meaning and understanding in whatever the group is considering.
- *Elaborating*—builds on previous comments and thoughts and thus enlarges the concept under consideration.
- *Coordinating*—clarifies the relationships among the various ideas and attempts to pull things together.
- *Orienting*—defines the progress of the discussion in terms of goals to keep the discussion in the right direction.
- *Testing*—checks periodically to see if the group is ready to make a decision or to recommend some action.
- *Summarizing*—reviews the content of past discussions.

Maintenance functions are carried out through behavior that maintains or changes the way in which the group is working together. These behaviors seek to allow the group to develop loyalty to one another and to the group as a whole. These behaviors include:

- *Encouraging*—the giving of friendly advice and help. Praising and agreeing with others also define this behavior.
- *Mediating, or harmonizing*—helps others compromise or resolve differences in a positive way.
- *Gatekeeping*—allows the fair and equal participation of all members of the group by such comments as, "We haven't heard from Jane."
- *Standard setting*—the action that determines the yardstick the group will use in choosing its subject matter, procedures, rules of conduct, and, most important, its values.
- *Following*—going along with the group, either passively or actively, during a discussion or in response to the group's decision.
- *Relieving tension*—diverts attention from unpleasant to pleasant matters. Often this behavior smooths the way for constructive communication.[31]

The Group Approach

Fundamental to a successful group is a sincere belief that a group can be effective and productive. Not everyone works well in group situations, and some individuals seek ways to be alone and independent no matter what the circumstances. A group approach enables you to bring a wide variety of experiences, backgrounds, viewpoints, and technical competencies to deal with a problem. Good decisions rely on informed participants, and the leader's attitude has much to do with a successful interaction.

Understanding

An understanding of what makes a group work will enable you to maximize a group's effectiveness. This requires the group to have clear objectives and purposes. Groups exist for specific purposes (e.g., to provide quality patient care, to solve a budgetary problem), and the formal boundaries of the group's jurisdiction should be clear. Group members need to know if their decision is binding or advisory. In addition, the leader should make clear that all members are expected to participate with honesty and candor. Allow the group to do its own best thinking and withhold your own solution to a problem until all members have shared their point of view. The leader should try to elicit as many ideas as possible before beginning the evaluation process; otherwise, alternative solutions will not be considered, and the first few ideas will be the only ideas discussed. To make the group more important than individual members, disassociate ideas from the person who put forward the idea. Keep personalities and personal rivalries out of the discussion. This can be accomplished by giving each idea an impartial title, such as plan A or B.

It is wise to not make decisions until all information is available; try not to guess or to make premature decisions that may have to be changed. As a leader, try to gain consensus rather than take a vote. It is very important that all persons, particularly the more negative members of the group, voice their view.

Diagnose a Sick Group

Sometimes a group just does not work. On the surface, the group may be composed of highly competent people, but for some reason productivity suffers. As the leader, you must try to understand why the group is not operating as it should. The usual reason for a nonproductive group consisting of competent people is that individuals have unexpressed feelings and motivations that cause them to fight among themselves or even to withdraw from a constructive solution. This is often referred to as a hidden agenda, or the real reason that a group member is not participating with the group to solve the immediate problem at hand. There will be no constructive group effort if hidden agendas remain concealed. The leader must try to bring some of these agendas out in the open so that they can be dealt with and not distract from the immediate situation. Without resolve, there is no hope for constructive and effective group action. One very interesting technique to deal with this problem is to enlist the aid of the group to diagnose the difficulty. This can be accomplished through asking for postmeeting evaluations of the process of the meeting, such as an anonymous postmeeting report and suggestions for the next meeting. What you as the leader are trying to do is to make the group conscious of its own procedures and of its own responsibility to criticize and to correct its inadequacies. Without accomplishing this, the group may not succeed and will have to disband. It is a myth to think that every group automatically will succeed; however, much can be done to help it succeed.

Flexibility

Finally, the leader must be flexible. Within a group, members assume a variety of roles. For the most part, people take certain roles and maintain them as they participate in group meetings. It is advisable for the leader to vary roles from time to time. Versatility should energize you and stimulate the group to creativity. In addition, different roles are necessary to elicit alternative actions.

Group processes are the means by which individuals deal with the social interactive component of organizational life. A leader will be in a position to better influence a group if there is some understanding of these dynamics. Today, it is a highly desirable skill to be able to communicate with groups and to influence the outcome of the group effort.[32]

Meetings: A Team Tool

Meetings are a way in which organizational objectives are met through a group's team effort. Typically a meeting brings together a variety of personnel who have the ability to solve problems, meet objectives, and in general advance the work of the organization. Meetings can be very successful in accomplishing work when certain strategies are employed by the leader. These include:

- There should be an established agenda and it should be distributed ahead of the meeting time.
- The items for the meeting should have reasonable goals to allow for the possibility of succesful solutions.
- The number of participants should be limited to those who can advance the discussion or meet the objectives of the meeting.
- The leader should prepare more and meet less. Time is an extremely valuable commodity in today's world, and wasting time at unproductive meetings produces negative feelings among those attending. The most important work done at any meeting is that done in preparation for the meeting. By doing this, the meeting can be focused and brief.
- The leader should control the meeting process. This includes allowing all participants to speak and limiting those who are not facilitating the discussion. (Limit participants to five minutes each, if this is possible.) Choose to discuss only priority items. Non-priority items may be handled in a different way, such as e-mail, telephone calls, or written memos.
- Set a time frame for the meeting and don't go over the time limit. This does not mean important items must be settled in a hurried fashion. It means the time allocated for the meeting is observed and the participants are informed of the time frame necessary for future meetings to complete the project.
- Reports presented at the meeting that exceed three pages should also have an executive summary attached for the members' review.
- Set high expectations for the success of the group's work. It is important for the leader to convey confidence in the ability of the participants to generate valuable solutions or plans.
- Set high standards for admission to the meeting group. It adds status to the process and adds to the self-esteem of the participants.

The leader should consider three questions before the meeting:

1. What is the purpose of this meeting?
2. What do I want to accomplish?
3. What will distinguish success from failure?[33]

Evaluation of Group Effectiveness

An effective group leader is able to evaluate how well the group performed. To facilitate this process, a tool is provided to evaluate group behavior (see Figure 3-8). In addition, problems will be more obvious through the use of an objective measure.

CASE STUDY

Hostile Aggressive Behavior

Dr. Adams is a well-known and experienced surgeon. However, at the very least, he is known to be a difficult individual. He has gained this reputation because he shouts before he thinks, blames before he knows the facts, and generally has a short fuse. Sally Hainer, RN, didn't know Dr. Adams and inadvertently walked onto the unit to transfer a patient. In typical fashion, Dr. Adams couldn't find the laboratory work on the chart and began a temper tantrum aimed at Sally. She looked him in the eye, told him to stop shouting, and, when he could be reasonable, to restate his request. The spectators to this event were speechless.

> The nurses on 7 North, a postoperative surgical division, dread when Dr. Smith is on call for patients who have had major surgery. Dr. Smith does not like to be called for patient problems, especially at night. One evening, a new post-operative patient developed a high fever and shaking chills. Marie Jones called Dr. Smith to inform him of the problem. He screamed in the phone and said how ridiculous it was to bother him. He barked some orders, and said, "Don't bother me anymore."

- What kind of communication techniques are being displayed?
- What should be the nurses' response to these individuals?
- Is there a difference in importance in these two episodes? What is it?
- What can you do when confronted with a powerful colleague who consistently uses hostile aggressive communication patterns?

CASE STUDY

Need for Assertive Communication

Miss Jones, RN, has been invited to represent the nurses' view of case management in an interdisciplinary group composed of physicians, administrators, physical therapists, and the financial officer. Dr. Brown presided over the group's first meeting and called it to order. Miss Jones happened to notice she was the only nurse and female in attendance. Shortly after the meeting was brought to order, Dr. Brown asked Miss Jones if she would take the minutes at the meeting.

- What should she say and do?
- Why was Miss Jones chosen for this task?

Problem (1)	Rating	Productive (3)
ACTIVE PARTICIPATION was lacking, We served our own needs. We watched from outside the group	1 2 3	ACTIVE PARTICIPATION was present. We were sensitive to the needs of our group. Everyone was "on the inside."
LEADERSHIP was dominated by one or more persons.	1 2 3	LEADERSHIP was shared among the members according to their abilities and insights.
COMMUNICATION OF IDEAS was poor; we did not listen. No one cared about ideas.	1 2 3	COMMUNICATION OF IDEAS was good. We listened and understood one another's ideas.
COMMUNICATION OF FEELINGS was poor. No one cared about feelings.	1 2 3	COMMUNICATION OF FEELINGS was good. People cared about other people's feelings.
SINCERITY was missing. We were just acting parts.	1 2 3	SINCERITY was present. We were revealing our honest selves.
REACTION among GROUP MEMBERS was a problem. Persons were rejected, ignored, or criticized.	1 2 3	REACTION among GROUP MEMBERS was active give-and-take
FREEDOM OF PERSONS' IDEAS was stifled. Persons were not free to express individuality. They were manipulated.	1 2 3	FREEDOM OF PERSONS' IDEAS was enhanced and encouraged. The creativity and individuality of persons was respected.
CLIMATE OF RELATIONSHIP was one of hostility, suspicion, anxiety, or superficiality.	1 2 3	CLIMATE OF RELATIONSHIP was one of mutual trust. The atmosphere was friendly and relaxed.
GOALS were fuzzy, contradictory, or just plain missing.	1 2 3	GOALS were clear to all. We had a definite sense of direction.
PRODUCTIVITY was low. Our group was irrelevant; there was no apparent agreement.	1 2 3	PRODUCTIVITY was high. We were digging hard and were earnestly at work on a task. We created and achieved something.

1 = problem
2 = neutral
3 = productive

FIGURE 3-8. Summary of those characteristics of group life that allow a group to either be effective or not. As they are listed, they form an evalulation tool of group effectiveness. The student can categorize the various aspects of the group's behavior as a problem, neutral, or productive.

CASE STUDY

Communication Patterns

Mary Mitchen is a new staff nurse on a general medicine pediatric division. She had completed her senior practicum on this particular unit and was also working as a student nurse. Her first week of work was relatively uneventful, and she was feeling confident about her new position. One day, at the end of her shift, she was about to tape her change of shift report when the nurse manager stopped her and asked her some questions about one of her patients. Mary began to answer when the nurse interrupted her, so Mary tried to continue to answer her questions when it happened again. Every time Mary tried to talk, the nurse manager cut her off. Finally, Mary said, "Please let me finish my thoughts. I am new here and want to learn, and would be interested in how to improve."

- What type of communication patterns were being expressed?
- Analyze Mary's reaction to the interaction. Do you agree with her response?
- What should Mary do if this happens again?

SUMMARY

This chapter discussed leadership development from the standpoint of the interactional, or social, components of communication and team building based on knowledge of the group process. These are the fundamental concepts that the leader should understand and then practice. Since leadership has been defined to be a process, time and experience will facilitate leadership development, as well as following the examples of the leaders in your own organization.

LEARNER EXERCISES

1. Use the various communication networks suggested in the chapter and circulate a message. Which network produced the least distortion in the message?
2. Based on your own individual experiences, compare positive and negative communication climates. Discuss the characteristics in each.
3. Observe the group dynamics in one of your classes or groups. What do you see in terms of roles played by the different participants? What is your role?
4. Try to influence the outcome of your next group meeting by using the fundamentals of communication and by being aware of how groups function. Share with the class your experience.
5. What is your communication style?

Answer the questions on the Communication Style Evaluation to evaluate your personal style (see Appendix).

REFERENCES

1. Fonville, A.M., Killian, F.R., & Tranbarger, R.E., (1998, March/April). Developing new nurse leaders. *Nursing Economics, 16*(2), 83–87.
2. Johnson, J., Costa, L., Marshall, S., Moran, M.J., & Henderson, C.S. (1994). Succession management: A model for developing nursing leaders. *Nursing Management*, *25*(6), 50–55.
3. Manning, G. (1991, December). Invest: A plan for developing new managers. *Nursing Management*, 26–28.
4. Bruderle, E.R. (1994, October). The arts and humanities: A creative approach to developing nurse leaders. *Holistic Nursing Practice*, 68–74.
5. Bass, B.M. (1990). *Bass and Stodgill's handbook of leadership*, 3rd ed. New York: Free Press.
6. Osborne, W.L., & Covits, N.F. (1991, August). Better communication makes more compassionate hospitals. *Nursing Management*, *22*(8), 31–38.
7. Hermann, S.J. (1978). *Becoming assertive: A guide for nurses*. New York: D. Van Nostrand Co., p. 27.
8. Miller, L.M.P., & Catalano, J. (2000). *Understanding and dealing with difficult people in nursing now: Today's issues, tomorow's trends*. Philadelphia: F.A. Davis, p. 302.
9. Johnson, J.R. (1994). The communication training needs of registered nurses. *The Journal of Continuing Education*, *25*(5), 213–218.
10. Newbauer, S. (1995). The learning network: Leadership development for the next millennium. *Journal of Nursing Administration*, *25*(2), 25–32.
11. Bureau of Labor Statistics, U.S. Department of Labor. (1996). *Occupational outlook handbook, 1996–1997 ed.* Washington, D.C.: U.S. Government Printing Office.
12. Bureau of Labor Statistics, U.S. Department of Labor. (1996). *Occupational outlook handbook, 1996–1997 ed.* Washington, D.C.: U.S. Government Printing Office.
13. Carbaugh, D. (1990). *Cultural communication and intercultural contact*. Hillsdale, NJ: Lawrence Erlbaum Associates.
14. Gudykunst, W. (1997). Cultural variability in communication. *Communication Research*, *24*(4), 327–348.
15. Gudykunst, W. (1997). Cultural variability in communication. *Communication Research*, *24*(4), 328.
16. Wood, J. (1997). *Communication, gender, and culture*, 2nd ed. Cincinnati, OH: Woodworth Publishing Co., pp. 7–90.
17. Wood, J. (1997). *Communication, gender, and culture*, 2nd ed. Cincinnati, OH: Woodworth Publishing Co., pp. 7–90.
18. Wood, J. (1997). *Communication, gender, and culture*, 2nd ed. Cincinnati, OH: Woodworth Publishing Co., pp. 7–90.
19. Wood, J. (1997). *Communication, gender, and culture*, 2nd ed. Cincinnati, OH: Woodworth Publishing Co., pp. 80–90.
20. Wood, J. (1997). *Communication, gender, and culture*, 2nd ed. Cincinnati, OH: Woodworth Publishing Co., pp. 70–80.
21. Power, communication and conflict: Two in a series of nurse management certification program. LTU: Healthcare Continuing Education. Chatsworth CA, 1999.
22. Callaway, S.D. (2001). Preventing communication breakdown. Retrieved from the World Wide Web: *http://www.rnweb.com.*, *64*(1), 71–74.
23. Fiesta, J. (1998). Failure to communicate. *Nursing Management*, *29*(2), 22.
24. Branson, R.M. (1988). *Coping with difficult people*. New York: Dell (Doubleday), p. 22.
25. Branson, R.M. (1988). *Coping with difficult people*. New York: Dell (Doubleday), p. 1.

26. Branson, R.M. (1988). *Coping with difficult people.* New York: Dell (Doubleday), p. 4.
27. Drucker, P. (1998, October 5). Management's new paradigms, *Forbes*, 162.
28. Kreitner, R. (1995). *Management,* 6th ed. Boston: Houghton Mifflin Co., pp. 436–437.
29. Lippit, G., & Seashore, E. (1966). *The professional nurse looks at group's effectiveness.* Washington, D.C.: Leadership Resources, p. 4.
30. Lippit, G., & Seashore, E. (1996). *The professional nurse looks at group's effectiveness.* Washington, D.C.: Leadership Resources, pp. 4–5.
31. Lippit, G., & Seashore, E. (1996). *The professional nurse looks at group's effectiveness.* Washington, D.C.: Leadership Resources, pp. 14–15.
32. Silva, K. (1994). *Meetings that work.* Burr Ridge, IL: Business One Irwin/Mirror Press.
33. Kemp, J. (1994). *Moving meetings.* New York: Mirror Press.

WEB SITES ABOUT CULTURAL DIVERSITY

Cultural Diversity for Health Professionals: *http//www.health.gld.gov.*

Perspectives on Language and Cultures: *http//www.literacynet.org.*

Cultural Diversity–A Guide for Health Professionals: *http//www.nwrel.org.*

Relocation Journal: *http//www.relojournal.com.*

Appendix

Communication Style Evaluation

In a social situation, do I prefer to talk to others or do I prefer to listen?

Do I find it necessary to use many descriptive terms when speaking or do I prefer short, succinct sentences?

Do I prefer cause and effect situations as opposed to creative, ambiguous dilemmas?

Do I prefer to be alone or be with others?

Do I prefer to make decisions alone, or do I prefer to work things out with others?

The extent to which you answer these questions highlights aspects of your personal communication style, but a leader should have some skill at all of these actions.

A leader should be able to listen attentively.

A leader should be able to provide information in a variety of ways, sometimes with a great deal of information, and at other times with very short and to-the-point sentences.

A leader will be in a variety of situations, sometimes very structured and at other times very loosely constructed. A leader needs to develop the skills to be able to communicate within both types of situations.

A leader is engaged with other people; communication skills need to be developed to deal with a variety of personality types (including adapting the leader's personal preference to the needs of the followers).

A leader understands that decisions sometimes need to be made alone and communicated to the group, as well as sometimes sharing decision making with the group.

4

Decision Making and Conflict Management

"One of the tests of leadership is the ability to recognize a problem before it becomes an emergency."

Arnold Glasow

INTRODUCTION

The objective of this chapter is to continue the discussion of leadership development through decision making and management of conflict. The two topics were introduced in Chapter 2 during the discussion of the process model of leadership. They are activities people frequently engage in throughout the course of everyday life and range from unimportant to critical. In the current health care economic environment, nurses will be accountable for efficient and effective decision making and conflict resolution as they relate to professional standards of practice. Developing skill in the use of the two processes is, therefore, an important pursuit. In this chapter, both will be explored in some detail. The two topics are presented in the same chapter because of their interrelatedness—decisions cause or prevent conflicts, and conflicts are solved through the decision-making process.

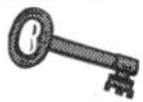

KEY CONCEPTS

Analysis is a critical function essential to sound decision making.

Centering is a form of body relaxation that allows the harnessing of energy to overcome conflict by strengthening one's psycho-physiological state and producing physical and emotional stability when confronted with conflict.

Conflict is an unsettling condition that causes a clash of ideas about what is expected or established. Conflict can be friendly or hostile.

Creativity is a human quality needed to generate ideas in decision making.

Decision is a complex conclusion derived from a set of premises that relate to a situation.

Decision-Making Process is a process of arriving at a conclusion after an analysis of units of related information. It is purposeful and goal directed.

Internal Climate is the dynamic socioemotional milieu that establishes the harmony/conflict ratio among people.

Power is a force within people that shapes the way in which others can function. Two types of power are described in this chapter: (1) **directive power**—a negative force that exploits others by advancing the power wielder's interest, and (2) **synergic power**—a positive force that cherishes others by incorporating their values.

Prediction is an identification of the likely outcomes of a decision given consideration of all known facts about a situation. It is a critical part of selecting a decision.

Premise is a proposition about something that serves as a basis for decisions. A premise can be correct or incorrect and serves as the unit of analysis when evaluating decisions.

Situational Anger results when a legitimate expectation has not been met. It differs from chronic anger and can be energizing and constructive.

DECISION MAKING

In nursing, the quality of decisions is measured in relation to professional standards of practice that emanate from contemporary societal forces. The focus of the decision-making process discussion is on an analysis of situations that require action and on the prediction of outcomes of the several possible choices of action.

Analysis

From the outset, **decisions** must be viewed as highly complex conclusions drawn from multiple **premises.** From such a view, it is understood that the decision itself cannot be analyzed but rather that the units of analysis are the premises from which decisions are formulated. Units are all factors that influence a total situation. The configuration of factors is what differentiates one situation from all others. As an example, Figure 4-1 illustrates a situation in which the quality of change-of-shift reports is being questioned. A variety of possible causes for the problem are shown. The action to be taken to correct the situation depends on which factor, or combination of factors, is identified as contributing to the problem. Each situation will be unique based on consideration of all relevant factors.

According to Simon, two classes of premises make up the basis for decisions in organizations: (1) the criterion of efficiency and (2) identifications.[1] Simon defines *criterion of efficiency* as conserving the scarce resources the organization has at its

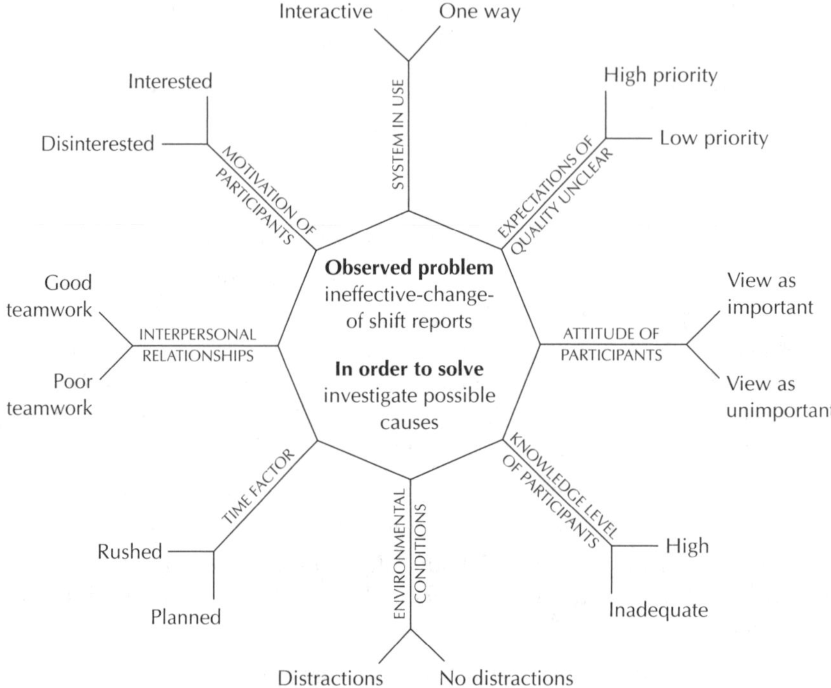

FIGURE 4-1. Illustration of an observed problem with an array of possible causes. In the center of the figure the observed problem is stated, and the reader is directed to investigate possible causes described in the eight spokes that extend out from the center. Each possible cause forks into two possible responses. The choice of responses at the forks provides information unique to a situation that provides direction for decision making about possible solutions to the problem.

disposal for accomplishing its task. He says *identifications* mesh the sub-goals of components of an organization with the goals of the whole organization. Identifications are intangible, psychological loyalties and values that individuals subscribe to that relate to a mission and purpose. Both classes of premises are at play in organizational settings, sometimes as competing forces. Decisions about efficiency issues frequently involve known boundaries. Take, for instance, a budget that has an absolute ceiling. Making rational decisions about spending can be done with relative ease in light of known limits. No institution, however, operates solely on efficiency issues. In the business world, profit is tempered by sensitivity to quality and human values. Companies are satisfied with adequate profits, share of the market, and fair prices in place of a monopoly. Nursing prides itself in being value driven. It is a profession being challenged to maintain its values in an economy of ever-increasing health care costs and limited resources. While the viability of health care agencies depends on the co-operative efforts of all organization departments in conservation efforts, nursing must be proactive in re-establishing itself to its rightful position of importance in the system.

When identifications involve the goals and values of several different departments in an organization, how resources are distributed becomes an issue. It is at this time that nursing must be prepared to identify, in a measurable way, the dollars and services

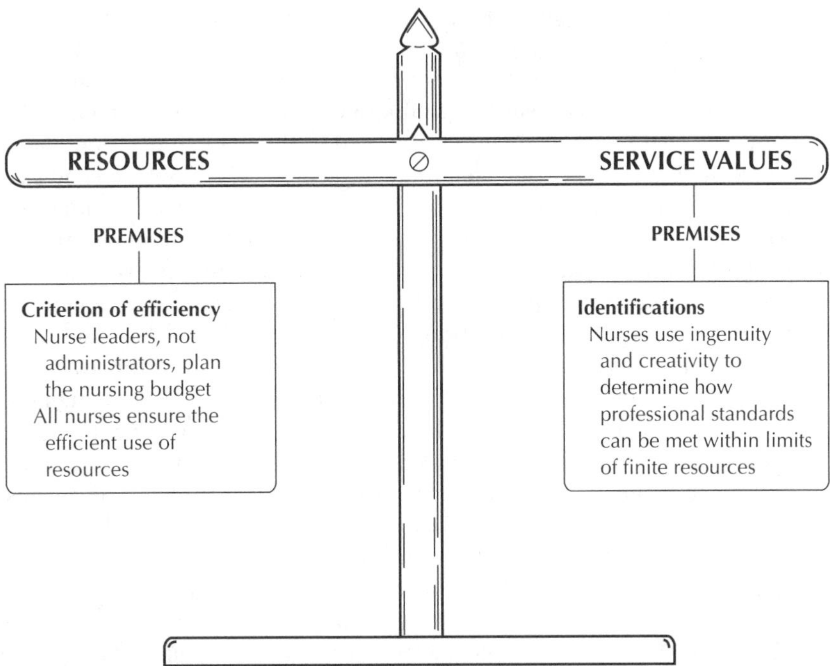

FIGURE 4-2. Illustration of the delicate balance needed to provide quality professional nursing services within the limits of finite resources. Resources should be interpreted to include material supplies, personnel, and time. Nurses' decisions and performance determine balance or imbalance between resources and services.

necessary for the delivery of nursing care. Garre discusses the relationship between decision-making methods and the nature of the problem to be solved.[2] Cost effectiveness is of paramount importance, and it must be accomplished in a way to prevent additional conflicts, such as morale problems, that develop when professional standards are compromised to a point of creating perceived unsafe practice conditions. Decision making about cost must take into account the multiple attributes involved. The need for broader and more active involvement of nurses in organizational operations is relatively new, and it becomes more important as fundamental professional issues come under scrutiny. Efficiency within the overall organization is increasingly a consideration that calls for new ways of decision making. An analysis of nursing decisions must be considered in light of professional standards as well as how they affect the whole organization. Good decisions are the stabilizing force in balancing efficiency and values. Correct premises about both, as they relate to both nursing practice and organizational viability, are essential to arrive at good decisions. Figure 4-2 illustrates how decisions affect the balance of efficiency and service values in nursing.

Prediction of Outcomes

Improving skill in decision making through study and experience is important to the profession of nursing. In organizational settings, nursing decisions affect others, be it staff, patients, the organization, or even society in general. Few, if any, decisions made about nursing issues or events are unimportant. Consider that a decision about the time and place for coffee breaks can have unwanted effects on the morale of the staff, just as do more critical issues, such as staffing needs. In his book *Administrative Behavior*, Simon says that in group situations we need to think about decision making as a way of thinking about issues that concern others, and that there are good and bad decisions relative to any issue a group might encounter.[3] In other words, decisions do not occur in a vacuum, and what is perceived as good by one department might produce adverse outcomes for other departments in an organization. In order to avoid such conflicts, Bragg points out that everyone must understand and abide by the accepted decision-making process in the overall organization.[4]

The best possible decisions result from skills in critical thinking. Critical thinking is a complex fluid activity that takes into account multiple changing factors as they relate to an issue. Understanding that critical thinking is included in the decision-making process is essential to improving outcomes. Well thought-out decisions facilitate the avoidance of the unmanageable, negative consequences of poor decisions. Characteristics of critical thinkers include being inquisitive, open-minded, flexible, fair-minded, honest about biases, willing to reconsider, diligent, and precise. Intellectual traits described by Richard Paul, director of the Center for Critical Thinking in California, include intellectual humility, integrity, courage, and empathy. In the same document, Noreen and Peter Facione state that critical thinkers are truth seeking, open-minded, analytical, systematic, self-confident, inquisitive, and mature.[5]

CHALLENGE TO NURSING

Traditionally, nurses had been involved almost exclusively with meeting the holistic needs of individual patients, leaving budgetary and other business matters to the organization's administrators. Such a position fostered a paternalistic attitude that led to administrative control of the nursing department in much the same way that a head of a household controls spending within the family.

The soul of nursing leadership is to influence decisions affecting the practice of nursing in the organization. Such an influence will facilitate a shift from paternalism to collegiality between nursing and agency administration. Nurses at all levels need to be prepared to knowledgeably engage in decision making in matters that affect all aspects of the profession, while connecting to the overall organizational standards and principles. Improved knowledge of, and skill in, decision making will enable nurses to contribute more effectively to organizational viability. Opportunities exist daily for nurses to study situations that call for decisive action. Analysis of unique factors in situations improves the quality of decisions. Studies indicate that, by increasing the amount of analytic thought in decision making, best practice and outcomes for patients often improve. Practitioners are encouraged to increase their analytical thought while engaged in decision making instead of relying on intuition.[6]

Just as nurses at every level are directly or indirectly affected by decisions that come down from administration (from parking places to available equipment needed in the delivery of nursing care), so too are patients affected by decisions nurses make relative to the delivery of nursing care. As an example, an area in which all nurses can thoughtfully engage in decision making is in determining the pattern of patient care assignment in care settings. It is an area that belongs exclusively to nurses.

There are differences in the patterns of patient care assignments, and analysis of their makeup relative to patient needs and staff competencies leads to critical selection. The pattern selected—case management, team approach, primary nursing care, or functional task approach—is one element in determining low-, adequate-, or high-quality outcomes for patients. Determining the best pattern for any given situation is based on an analysis of multiple considerations, such as:

- The type of organization (primary or tertiary care).
- Credentials of available staff.
- Their level of competency.
- Acuity level of patients.
- Boundaries to be observed.

At times, nursing has operated on the tendency to adopt the newest pattern as the best for all situations. It is clear that such a position can be problematic in terms of quality of patient care and staff morale. The ideal pattern for a critical care unit certainly differs from that for an ambulatory care setting. Analysis of information about a given pattern of patient care delivery in relation to a given set of patient care requirements is needed before a decision can be made to adopt any pattern.

There are stressful situations that arise within nursing that require quick action. An analysis of all information is not possible. Bourbonnais and Baumann describe the effects of stress on decision making.[7] That stress causes an erosion of the general cognitive ability to cope with complexity is a finding of their literature review. As a result, the range of cues used in decision making is altered; initially, peripheral cues are missed, and as stress builds, central cues are not perceived. According to Carnevali and Thomas, a mild level of anxiety produces broad perceptions and increased learning, moderate anxiety produces narrowing perceptions and decreased learning, severe anxiety produces scattered perceptions and an inability to understand, and a panic level of anxiety produces distorted perceptions, making new learning impossible.[8] Decisions made under such adverse circumstances must be revisited when the situation allows for more deliberation.

IMPACT OF DECISIONS

Everyone is affected by the manner in which policies are designed and implemented. Take, for example, the effects on nursing of recent decisions made by top administrators in health care as they sought to create bigger, more cost-effective health systems throughout the country. The loss of focus on the importance of nursing created numerous problems. In an effort to contain costs, administrators inadvertently created conditions that must currently be corrected through costly recruitment and orientation efforts. When rationale for a decision is sound and is presented in such a way as to invite input from all players, potential problems can be prevented, or at least diminished. Many dissatisfactions of nurses come from having had no control over decisions that affect their practice. Now is the time for nurses to exercise active decision making and regain control over their practice, which can lead to higher levels of satisfaction.

The goal of health care organizations to provide the best possible care to clients within a given set of circumstances can be served by well-prepared personnel who are skilled in the decision-making process. Organizations that have knowledgeable individuals at all levels are better able to accomplish their missions. Understanding decision making as a process is basic to this mission and can be studied theoretically through the use of simulation scenarios. Learner exercises included at the end of the chapter are designed to facilitate use of the process in decision making and to eliminate the bias frequently associated with a single-dimensional approach to problems. Students are encouraged to develop their own scenarios from their firsthand experiences. Good decision making hinges on, among other things, good communication skills and knowledge of the group's dynamics. Decision making in nursing is teamwork that calls for both cooperation and coordination. It is not sufficient to agree on a common goal; each participant must also understand the plan. Coordination of group efforts provides stability in the face of differing opinions about an issue. For example, the purpose of signals in football or bidding in bridge is to enable each player to form accurate expectations as to what each teammate is going to do.[9] Group decision making, then, must take place in some structured way with an effective communication flow, agreement on a common goal, and coordination of group activities. A further discussion on this topic appears later on in this chapter under the heading of "Management of Conflict."

SYSTEMS OF DECISION MAKING

How individuals or groups set about making decisions might be similar to how leadership is exercised. Styles range from autocratic or bureaucratic to democratic. An autocratic or bureaucratic approach produces different outcomes than does a democratic approach. Consensus is the ideal as an outcome regardless of approach. The autocratic or bureaucratic system is frequently unattractive to competent groups. Such a system, however, might be best in emergencies such as a ship captain crying out, "Man overboard!" In a crisis event, one individual must be charged with controlling the situation and be assured of the cooperation of others. Crisis situations are not the only instances in which an autocratic system is effective. For example, a symphony orchestra's performance is the result of an autocratic system, and it is by no means a crisis. Both prior examples represent events in which the group freely allows one individual total control. However, control taken by one person without the approval of the group can lead to destructive outcomes. Use of the autocratic system must be carefully reviewed to avoid serious conflicts.

A democratic system of decision making might be highly satisfying to a group that feels it is important for everyone's input to be considered in decisions, especially when all group members have similar professional competencies. It is not, however, necessarily the best system to employ in all situations because every group contains individuals with different strengths. It might be a fact that, because of the nature of an issue, some individuals have nothing to offer in choosing between alternative decisions, whereas they might be experts in other areas. To include them simply out of a commitment to a democratic style is inefficient, time-consuming, and potentially damaging to established group cohesiveness. The nature of teamwork is that, at some point, everyone "sits on the bench." Any style of decision making can be misused, overused, or used appropriately. Each situation determines which style should be selected.

Some decisions are carved in stone and are based on firmly established criteria that are rooted in doctrine, culture, values, and tradition. Many cannot be modified through reason. Others are modifiable but controlled by economic constraints, such as a salary scale. All organizations are influenced, to some extent, by this type of bureaucratic decision making. Nurses seldom have active roles in these types of decisions, but they are affected by them and need to know about them and their sources. These decisions are "givens" in a situation and, as such, do not come under scrutiny in a formal way.

Consensus is a possible outcome of decision making in which all participants satisfy part of their point of view while having to give up some other part. Arriving at consensus is time-consuming, but the final product is mutually satisfying and can be of superior quality. Consensus provides a rich source of new knowledge about an issue and fosters regard for others' points of view.

Skillful decision making is highly useful to groups engaged in a common effort. How a group formulates decisions provides valuable information about their effectiveness in an organization. Through their decision-making activities, untapped creativity is released, potential leaders are identified, and areas needing development are revealed.

THE DECISION-MAKING PROCESS

A group can adopt any of several decision-making models, or can design its own. Symbols used in the construction of a model vary, but essentially they all share the same steps or stages, as follows:

- Identify participants.
- Gather pertinent facts.
- Generate alternative decisions.
- Predict outcomes.
- Plan for managing consequences.
- Select the best alternative.

A brief discussion of each stage follows.

Identify Participants

The configuration of the group charged with formulating a decision should have adequate representation of all who are going to be directly affected by it. Decision makers on a nursing unit should be selected for attributes they possess that can facilitate good decisions. Interest alone, without the other attributes for sound decision making, is insufficient. Interest, however, should be encouraged, and those interested individuals should participate in the capacity of observers until they have sufficient knowledge of the related factors and of the decision-making process to be able to contribute constructively. The experiences they gain can be valuable assets both to themselves and for the group's future use.

Arbitrary assignment of individuals to decision-making teams should be avoided to ensure quality outcomes. Recognition of individual staff members' assets in some organized way, such as anecdotal notes kept by the charge nurse or a periodic collection of data from the staff as to their development and interests, can help improve the utilization of group strengths. Nurse managers must take appropriate steps to design opportunities for staff inexperienced in the use of decision making to improve their skills so that the unit runs efficiently and effectively. Planning staff development exercises for nurses to gain skill through the use of a process model is one way to accomplish this. Expectations of participation and growth in the quality of participation must be clear and understood by everyone, as well as the consequences of non-participation. Nurses beginning their careers should expect to be given opportunities to gain the skills needed to participate effectively in the decision-making process.

Nurses can test their competency for a proposed activity by answering some key questions. Questions included in a decision-making algorithm at Saint John Medical Center in Tulsa, Oklahoma[10] are designed to ensure adherence to standards. Nurses are first asked if they need special education in order to perform an identified function. If not, their participation is warranted, but they are then asked additional questions, such as if the task is within the scope of accepted practice; does he/she have the knowledge and skill for safe performance; can the nurse produce the documented evidence of competency; is there a risk to patients or nurses; and will the nurse assume responsibility for the outcome?

Gather Pertinent Facts

The stage of gathering pertinent facts can be compared to great rivers that draw from many tributaries.[11] Input should be sought from staff at all levels of experience because all contributions, regardless of how small, influence the outcome of this important stage. Ignorance of all factors that relate to a problem leads to poor decisions because premises are then wrong. Poor decisions have to be reversed, which by itself causes a loss of confidence in the decision makers. Communication is a critical skill during the stage of gathering data. The possibility of non-participation as a form of sabotage should be considered, and all individuals held accountable for the roles they play in the process. Sufficient time should be allowed for this step. When the group is satisfied that important facts related to the issue have been thoroughly presented, what follows is the task of prioritizing and arranging the complex bits of information into an effective scheme. Each of these operations calls for analytic and predictive thinking. This step forces balance between the competing forces of efficiency and values. Prioritizing can give rise to serious conflicts as the competing forces collide. In nursing, professional standards must dominate while being tempered by efficiency standards.

Generate Alternatives

The third step in the process is to generate as many alternative decisions as possible. The emphasis is on quantity rather than quality, and judgment about the alternatives is temporarily curtailed. **Creativity** is a valuable trait in idea generation. Free reign should be given to the imagination during this step, and group participants should agree in advance not to criticize any suggestions. Skill in using techniques such as brainstorming, forced association, self-interrogation checklists, think tanks, and the Delphi technique are highly useful. See Table 4-1 for a description of each of these techniques.[12] Time-consuming and sophisticated techniques can be trimmed to suit a situation and still contribute to better quality decisions in the end.

Brainstorming is the oldest and most common of the creative-thinking techniques. Brainstorming involves four principles:

1. Don't judge ideas.
2. Let your mind wander.
3. Aim for quantity.
4. "Hitchhike" on previous ideas (variations on ideas).[13]

Brainstorming is a technique easily used as a group activity or by individuals. Students are encouraged to use two or three techniques from Table 4-1 as learning experiences to generate ideas about solutions to problems they encounter in their daily, clinical nursing experiences.

Predict Outcomes

When group members feel adequately satisfied with the list of alternative decisions, they can move on to **predicting** the outcomes of each. Knowledge of groups and how they are affected by changes is useful during this stage. The realm of a group's possible responses to any decision is an important consideration. During this stage, weighing strengths of the desired and undesired outcomes of each alternative leads to the narrowing of the alternative courses of action. Quality dominates at this stage as the list is condensed and becomes the source from which the final selection will be made.

Select Best Alternative

A process model of decision making appears in Table 4-2. The nature of process is such that stages are interdependent. There is movement back and forth in a cyclical fashion as new information becomes available to be incorporated into the model. Students are encouraged to make use of the model in carrying out activities at the end of the chapter.

Improving the quality of decision making pays high dividends as groups encounter conflicts in the work setting. Dealing with conflicts can be time-consuming. The quality of decisions made relative to a controversial issue can make the difference between managing the conflict and being managed by it.

Plan for Managing Consequences

The group must look at negative consequences with an eye for those that cannot realistically be managed in a way to avoid further, and perhaps more serious, problems. Because each alternative has both desired and undesired consequences, each eliminated

TABLE 4-1. Techniques for Idea Generation

Technique	Description
Brainstorming	Used to generate a large quantity of alternatives to solve problems. Anything goes, and participants are completely free to propose any suggestions. They are encouraged to think without constraint—the wilder the better. Ideas can be toned down later. No judgments, criticisms, or negative statements are allowed during the spontaneous brainstorming session. All suggestions are recorded within a time limit. Analysis and evaluation of the most promising alternatives are done later.
Forced association	This deliberately breaks down habitual associations and seeks new relationships. The item needing action or improvement is stated, and then participants use free association to create a list of 10 words usually associated with it. An entirely different item is then selected and free association is used to create a list of 10 associated words. The two lists of 10 words are written in parallel columns. Participants are asked to make their mind work back and forth between columns, seeing relationships between the original item and the word list of the different item. Ideas are then critically analyzed to choose the useful ones in addressing the item needing action.
Self-interrogation checklist	Questions are used to develop new perspectives on a problem. They stir the imagination, and the writer withholds judgment until all ideas are written down. Questions serve to define and to uncover problems, obtain extra facts, make decisions, and generate ideas for change. Questions might be: (1) Can we do more? (2) Can we streamline and eliminate excess? (3) Can we get information elsewhere? (4) Can we handle the task ourselves? (5) Does it reduce costs? (6) Is it practical? (7) Does it improve efficiency?
Think tanks	Getting a select group of people together to harness imagination and to encourage creativity is one form of think tank. Members must be carefully selected for specific attributes. The group size should range from five to eight members. The right kind of meeting place is essential: often exotic or different places stimulate innovation, and a relaxed atmosphere generates divergent and unusual ideas. A specific problem or goal must be clearly stated for participants to try to solve. Meetings should occur often enough for the germination, pollination, and flowering of ideas. Think tanks are particularly useful for future projections.
Delphi technique	This technique is useful for forecasting, surveying views and attitudes, problem solving, formulating strategies, and airing controversial views. A group of experts in the area being addressed is selected. The experts react to a questionnaire anonymously, expressing their opinions and views. The questionnaires are analyzed, and each expert receives feedback about all the responses anonymously. They are then asked to respond again, taking feedback into consideration. Feedback analysis is again provided. The process is repeated as many times as needed until a consensus is reached about the problem.

alternative represents a loss in terms of the very best, idealized choice; however, the outcome is one that is workable and in the overall interest of everyone.

A final note about decisions based on a consideration of all the elements in the process: Each is uniquely valuable in a specific situation. Skill in the use of the process is therefore very important for quality nursing practice.

TABLE 4-2. Process of Decision Making

1. Participants	2. Gather pertinent facts	3. Generate alternative decisions
Determine qualified decision makers. Select based on: —Nature of issue —Experience —Knowledge —Interest —Personal traits that foster group efforts	Employ fact-finding techniques. Survey others. Remember that each fact is a premise and that decisions are a combination of multiple premises.	Employ techniques that cultivate creativity. Don't judge ideas. Aim for quantity. Entertain what seems ridiculous. Look for variations in ideas.
4. Predict outcomes	**5. Plan for managing consequences**	**6. Select the best alternative**
Recognize desired and undesired outcomes of each alternative. Concentrate on quality. Determine from list alternatives with undesirable outcomes that cannot be managed. Condense list accordingly.	Secure support of the whole group. —Communicate to all who are affected by the decision. —Be honest about pros and cons. —Show how the pros outweigh the cons —Suggest ways to handle undesirable outcomes. —Offer to assist where possible.	Weigh the undesirable outcomes against the value of desirable outcomes of the remaining alternatives. Select the best alternative.

MANAGEMENT OF CONFLICT

Nature of Conflict

Interactive processes of leadership are multifaceted, and the management of conflict might well be the most challenging process of all. Acknowledging the dual nature of conflict as potentially constructive or destructive and recognizing the cues of each is the goal of managing conflict.

Anger is frequently a response to conflict. Lyon[14] differentiates between situational anger and chronic anger. **Situational anger** is energizing and constructive and arises when realistic expectations are not likely to be met. Realistic expectations are those that are likely to be met and involve the following criteria: (1) the expectation has been clearly communicated; (2) persons involved have the capability, knowledge, time, and material resources to meet the expectation, and (3) persons involved are willing to do what is expected. Situational anger is empowering, and Lyon cites Florence Nightingale's anger as an example of how effective it can be in creating opportunities for nurses to practice and improve health care. Nightingale's anger was frequent, situational, data-driven, and about matters that were changeable. She used her anger effectively for action to correct appalling conditions in London's hospitals. Lyon challenges nurses today to empower themselves to change what is changeable through "Nightingale power" (i.e., use of situational anger). It can be used in a variety of situations—in major events or those of less consequence.

When there is concern about an issue, collect data and present it, along with suggestions on how the situation can be turned around, to enhance nursing practice. When nurses follow through with their concerns, they communicate to others what nursing brings to health care that no other discipline can provide.

Keeping conflicts from getting out of control requires communication between participants. Managers need to assure the staff that open sharing can be safe and in their best interest as long as there is respect shown to each other. The open communication should continue until there is consensus.[15]

Not all conflicts are bad. Some conflicts are preventive and reduce hindrances to goal attainment. Effective leaders learn to curtail conflict on one hand and to design or to allow its influence on the other, becoming increasingly astute in determining the need for each. Obsolete practices of entrenched groups can be shaken loose by allowing or imposing conflict events. For example, identifying different expectations that introduce new ideas and ways of doing things can pump new blood into stagnant, but otherwise competent, groups. Members gain new appreciations and readily incorporate changed expectations if the conflict event is managed well. In the case of destructive conflict, early intervention is needed to defuse volatile emotions that threaten an attainment of the group's purpose. Disarming instigators in some way through the use of various techniques is one way of handling destructive conflict. Specific strategies for managing both constructive and destructive conflicts are offered in the following section.

Collaborative conflict resolution is characterized by an approach when people attack problems rather than each other.[16] In order to avoid escalating conflict that can occur when opposing forces hold different perspectives, participants should answer some basic questions before entering into a collaborative effort. An analytic approach includes consideration about: (1) what is essential and what can be given up, (2) what the other person wants, (3) if either side holds false assumptions or incorrect perceptions, (4) what the best strategy is to use, (5) how to handle "hot button" issues should they arise, and (6) what precautions will prevent further conflict? Preparation for collaborative conflict resolution pays valuable dividends in terms of relationships, time, and the prevention of stress. Another technique to enhance collaboration is "**centering.**"[17] It is a method that is valuable in controlling stress during conflict resolution efforts. The goal of centering is to relax the body and open the mind. It strengthens one's psycho-physiological state and produces emotional and physical stability that affects relationships and the environment. It allows individuals to move away from a line of conflict and redirect negative energies.

In settings where conflict has traditionally been viewed as destructive, a new look can broaden perspectives to consider the potential benefits that might result. A simple question (will some change harm or help a situation?) leads to **analysis**, which is the first stage of conflict management. Analysis reveals the nature of the particular conflict, which must be considered within the context of a given situation and point in time to determine its potential outcome.

The degree of conflict in a setting is an important factor to consider when analyzing its effects. Situational factors influence the point at which a conflict is good or bad. Competent groups handle conflicts differently than weak groups. The collective strength of effective groups accommodates weaknesses among its members. Such accommodation is not found in ineffective groups. The style and strength of leadership operating in a specific setting influences individuals' and group's responses to disruptive events. The overall internal climate, therefore, is an important determinant of the outcome of any given conflict. It is important to acknowledge the fluid nature of factors that contribute to **internal climate** so that frequent monitoring of the environment occurs. It cannot be assumed that the cohesiveness of a group is constant.

Conflicts do not fall on a fixed point on a scale from beneficial and growth producing to harmful. Multiple interactive situational factors determine the merit of each. A conflict event might produce the cutting edge needed for growth at one point in time and cause problems at another. For example, in times of organizational prosperity, an announcement of no raises or of cutbacks in salaries will have a very different outcome on the workers than at a time of economic constraint and retrenchment that threatens job security. The same announcement with the same individuals, but with different situational factors, produces different consequences. The assumption that dissatisfaction can be expected from the former situation and cooperation from the latter could be quite accurate depending on the degree of shared information, understanding, and fairness. If cuts only affect the staff, while managers remain completely unaffected, and no explanations are given, a perception of misuse of power is likely, whether or not it is true. Conflicts rooted in misunderstanding, lack of cooperation, misuse of power, and unfairness generally produce detrimental outcomes. At times, skilled negotiators are needed to settle disputes when cooperative efforts within a group fail. Differences in perceptions of events occur from time to time, and it is important that nurses develop an appreciation of conflict as a significant force influencing nursing practice. Failure to understand or handle conflicts appropriately can account for serious internal professional problems.

BASIS OF CONFLICT

Conflict can be of an intra-psychic (i.e., personal), interpersonal, or intradepartmental nature. Nurses encounter varying degrees of each and need to develop understanding and skill in managing them. Individuals can experience serious internal personal conflicts that temporarily force reordering of their priorities. Personal conflicts can put an individual at variance with work goals. In such instances, the collective strength of effective work groups can temporarily compensate for an individual's poor performance, but resolution is ultimately the responsibility of the individual.

Interpersonal influences, such as personality differences and conflicting ideas, produce conflicts that can lead to either positive or negative results. Disagreements between individuals can be good or bad based on the degree of mutual respect shared between them. The outcome of any interpersonal conflict is related to complex, time-related, situational factors surrounding the entire event.

Conflict is frequently associated with felt, unequal distribution of power, status, and resources. It may be real or the result of inaccurate perceptions. In either case, problems arise that must be handled swiftly if complications are to be avoided. The outcome of these conflicts is determined by four critical forces: the issue, power base of participants, cooperation between participants, and communication. Selected courses of action can keep issues to manageable proportion or can escalate them. Power can be used to coerce or to compromise. Individuals can hold onto bias or work to dissipate it. Information can be freely shared or withheld as a means of control, and listening can become an integral part of communication.

Clause and Bailey describe the use of **power** in two ways: directive and synergic.[18] **Directive power** shapes others for the purpose of advancing the interest of the power wielder and is viewed as a negative force. It is an example of unequal distribution of power. **Synergic power,** however, incorporates group values and cherishes other people. Synergic power is an essential element in balancing control in competitive environments. Nursing is in a competitive environment in which bureaucratic goals dominate, putting professional goals and values at risk. Strong cohesive voices from nursing, plus intelligent and articulate nurse representatives, are necessary to keep professional values/bureaucratic efficiency conflicts to manageable proportions in complex organizations. In today's climate of health care delivery, ways must be found to conserve resources and to use wisely what is available. Professional nurses must spend their time providing professional services rather than secretarial and hotel-type activities that frequently consume too many professional nurse hours. An honest look at practices might reveal that some nurses purposely hold on to non-nurse activities because they can provide opportunities for closure of a task, which is satisfying, whereas many professional activities leave nurses with some ambiguity about the outcomes of their efforts. Experience plus maturity allows nurses to handle the ambiguity more effectively.

Recognition of the basis of conflict can be helpful in managing it. Recognizing events that are bound to be problematic can allow for effective interventions to reduce their magnitude or to eliminate them altogether. Decisive action is complex, and analysis of the premises from which action was formed is ongoing and interactive.

Examples of Common Conflicts in Nursing

Nobel and Rancourt present evidence of a lack of cohesiveness in perceptions and values among nurses, which causes major intradepartmental conflicts.[19] They discuss different modes of knowing and knowledge-accessing styles as causes. As a result of the differences, nurses perceive the world of nursing and how they conceptualize legitimate knowledge from opposing viewpoints. Educational preparation was suggested as one factor in accounting for the differences, with university-educated nurses (both staff nurses and nurse managers) being more flexible and broadminded about conflict situations. Nurses with broader educational backgrounds were able to appreciate a variety of perceptions about a situation, whereas non-degree nurses tended to hold on to their own perceptions as being correct. An unwillingness to develop greater flexibility can lead to anger and fear as responses to conflict.

Earlier research by Kramer and Schmalenberg has shown that commonly occurring conflicts in nursing can be categorized according to type.[20] Labels given to the types of conflicts help identify the source and participants of conflict in nursing and provide clues about interventions. Examples of classic conflicts in nursing include professional/bureaucratic, nurse/nurse, nurse/doctor, personal competency gap, competing role, expressive/instrumental, and patient/nurse conflicts. Many nurses will be able to see themselves in each one of these situations at one time or another. How they are managed and what is learned from them is important. A description of each type follows.

Professional/bureaucratic conflicts are the result of an incompatibility of expectations produced by the system and perceived professional standards and responsibilities. An imbalance of power is frequently at the root of such conflicts. As such, they lead to a great deal of frustration for nurses who feel helpless in a situation.

Nurse/nurse conflicts result when differing values toward the philosophy of nursing are held by nurses who work together. The differences interfere with teamwork. There can be ongoing problems between nurses who are consistently task oriented and those who wish to do holistic care. Assignment preferences of task-oriented nurses might be based on procedures to be performed, whereas nurses who prefer holistic care prefer continuity of patient care from admission to discharge. Both approaches cannot exist on the same unit. Recently, nursing has experienced the need for sensitivity training in order to manage staff conflicts that arise out of multicultural issues. Martin, Wimberly, and O'Keefe present a new view of multiculturalism's impact on the health care industry.[21] U.S. standards emphasize the individual, competition, and accomplishment. Nurses strive to assist patients to become more independent in health care matters. Western language is considered to be low context, with many words used to make a point. In contrast, eastern cultures are group oriented, and the individual is subordinated. Harmony is prized, and language is considered to be high context, with only a few words used for necessary communication. Philosophical differences can become sources of misunderstandings that can turn into conflict when planned efforts to improve understanding are neglected.

Nurse/doctor conflicts spring from differing expectations of each other in the delivery of care. The stereotype of physicians dominating patient care has for years submerged nursing. Some nurses continue to feel a need to compete with doctors, and according to Cox and Sofield [22]there remains instances of severe verbal abuse of nurses by doctors. However, some doctors and nurses have worked together and shown mutual respect for each other's expertise and bottom-line care outcomes. A trend toward educating doctors and nurses together for specific areas of learning results in improved collaboration between the two groups. The outcome promotes good practice, fosters respect for each other, and promotes professional satisfaction.[23] There are differences in the "medical model" and the "nursing model." Each emphasizes different aspects of health care that complement each other. Conflict comes about because of an imbalance of power traditionally found in the system. Development of collegial relationships in which there is mutual respect for each other's complementary roles can prevent the time-consuming and senseless problems that take attention away from the shared goals of nurses and doctors. Nurses who take nursing forward through collaboration recognize nurse and doctor contributions to health care as interdependent and equal. They value nurses as full members of health care teams, and identify what is essentially nursing in an overall plan of care. They recognize that incorporating new technologies into health care is essential today and can be done without losing the human element of compassion and ethical caring that meets spiritual and emotional needs.

Personal competency gap conflicts occur when nurses' skill levels interfere with their own expectations of standards of practice for themselves. This type of conflict occurs when nurses are pulled to areas of practice with which they are unfamiliar, especially to intensive care units (ICUs) and trauma centers. The practice of reassigning nurses to different units as a means of taking care of shortages is common and expedient in advancing efficiency. It must be noted, however, that efficiency and effectiveness are different entities. If standards of practice are frequently ignored, some elements of professional/bureaucratic conflict are seen through an imbalance of power.

Competing role conflicts occur when the same person fills the roles of nurse, student, spouse, and parent, all of which exert a pull on that individual's time, energy, and attention. Demands outside of nursing, as well as demands from within nursing, contribute to this type of conflict. Today, to some extent, such conflicts cannot be avoided. Economic conditions can require two incomes to maintain an acceptable lifestyle. Single-parent families require a period of day care for the children, which is not always ideal. The educational level for nurses must be upgraded, however, to meet career demands.

Expressive/instrumental conflicts occur when nurses are torn between technical care demands and the human or expressive needs of patients. Ethical issues, legal issues, patient and family requests and personal values, and the philosophy of the nurse all operate as elements in this type of conflict. Expressive/instrumental conflicts are among the most difficult to manage. They can be a daily source of conflict in ICUs and trauma centers. Nurses in critical care and trauma care settings must work effectively with an expanded professional team and handle sensitive situations with families.

Patient/nurse conflicts result when nurses' goals for care differ from patients' goals for care. When nurses maintain an effective, therapeutic role in caring for patients, this type of conflict can be kept to a minimum. Respecting patients' and families' decisions about their care, especially when their choice is an informed and considered one, is part of holistic care and is an expected standard. It is, however, not easy to accept nontraditional choices, but nurses are sometimes in the position to support them without personal value judgments.

There is another entire category of behavior that comes from increasing violence and crime in our society that can bring about serious patient/nurse conflicts. Daum describes the disruptive antisocial behavior of a patient who is simultaneously a perpetrator and victim of drug trafficking, neighborhood violence, and other criminal activity.[24] They are individuals who have limited ego strength, who act impulsively because of a limited ability to delay gratification of their needs, and who accept violence as a way of life. Recent reports[25] cite violence toward health personnel initiated by patients' family members and intruders who have no legitimate reason for being in the health care setting.

Interpersonal conflicts in nursing are not new, but those that develop into violent behavior are a relatively recent phenomenon. Anderson[26] reports that two-thirds of work-related violence occurs in health care settings. Working in volatile settings, such as psychiatric units and emergency rooms, might increase the chances for violence. Working alone, and working evening and night shifts, also increase the chances of falling victim to violence. They present nurses with challenges formerly not experienced.

Steefel[27] reports that most violence toward nurses is directed toward female nurses, while male nurses are less frequently victims. Where physical violence is a threat, the presence of security guards, or even local police, might be necessary to ensure the safety of patients and staff. Violence is not limited to blatant physical behaviors. The International Council of Nurses (ICN) includes the following behaviors as signs of workplace violence: (1) intimidation, (2) threats, (3) ostracism, (4) sending offensive messages,(5) aggressive posturing, (6) rude gestures, (7) victimizing, and (8) interfering with work equipment. The ICN has created partnerships with the World Health Organization, the International Labor Organization, and Public Services International in an antiviolence campaign. National Nurses' Associations are encouraged to mount zero-tolerance antiviolence campaigns in workplaces, communities, and countries. The ICN Kit 2001 is available to nurses' associations free of charge. It is also available on the ICN website at www.icn.ch for purchase.

Nurses, both beginners and veterans, might have experienced some or all of the types of conflicts described. They appear to be timeless and are a reality in nursing practice. Prevention is the ideal but, when impossible, skill in managing conflicts is aimed at effectively minimizing their effects.

Approaches to Managing Conflict

Valentine[28] compared the use of five conflict management strategies: (1) avoiding, (2) compromising, (3) collaborating, (4) accommodating, and (5) competing as they were used by staff nurses, nurse managers, and deans of schools of nursing in a study of conflict management strategies in nursing. Study results revealed that staff nurses ranked the strategies in order of preference as avoiding, accommodating, compromising, collaborating, and competing. It is speculated that *avoidance* was used most frequently because of the sense of powerlessness associated with the staff nurse role. Half of the nurse managers also selected *avoidance* as the strategy of choice for the same reason, while deans chose *compromising* as their first choice. In the study, *collaboration* was not a popular choice even though it can be the most promising in maintaining positive relationships.

Strategies and techniques for managing conflicts are more easily described than prescribed. At the outset, consider that conceptualizing conflict positively and describing events in positive terms can help produce positive outcomes. Conversely, conceptualizing conflict negatively and describing events in negative terms can cause negative outcomes. Some positive terms are suggested in the Conflict Management Module of Teaching Improvement Projects System (TIPS) developed at the University of Kentucky at Lexington.[29] Positive terms are exciting, creative, helpful, courageous, stimulating, growth-producing, strengthening, and clarifying. In the same reference, Hocks and Wilmot found, however, that more frequently in our society, conflict is depicted in negative terms, such as destructive, confrontational, disagreement, tension, anger, pain, hostility, and anxiety.[30] It would appear, then, that much work is needed in order to foster a positive attitude about the potential that conflict can have. Various strategies can lead to win-win, win-lose, or lose-lose outcomes. Some strategies give rise to legal and ethical problems and must be used cautiously. Situational factors surrounding any conflict are numerous and varied, and planning approaches to solve conflicts is based on situational contingencies. Some techniques for managing conflict described by Booth are confrontation, bargaining, smoothing, avoidance, and unilateral action.[31]

Each technique has its place in conflict management, since situations are uniquely different. A definition of each technique follows.

Confrontation can be difficult and uncomfortable, but its constructive use can be learned. For this approach to be healthy and successful, three prerequisites are necessary:

1. Each party must be motivated to resolve the issue.
2. Each party must have equal power relative to the issue.
3. Each party must have necessary information about the issue.

Successful *confrontation* brings important issues out into the open, facilitates honest and spontaneous sharing of views, and provides information that improves participants' knowledge about the issue. When successful, it leads to a win-win outcome.

Bargaining, as the term implies, involves giving something to gain something in return. A negotiator or arbitrator is useful when bargaining is the technique of choice. The arbitrator must be briefed on the position and preferred solution of each party. The approach is time consuming and expensive, but can yield a satisfying win-win outcome. It is more frequently employed in settling major issues where important matters are at stake.

Smoothing minimizes the importance of differences so that they are not acknowledged and/or respected, and therefore no solution is found. All parties lose, and in time the problem presents itself again. It might be used temporarily as a strategy to gain time while attempting to improve cooperation between rivals.

Avoidance, another no-win technique, sweeps problems under the rug where they are more likely to compound than to go away. It also might be temporarily employed while interaction conditions between parties improve. Avoidance is the technique of choice if the issue itself is too trivial to warrant attention.

Unilateral action implies active involvement by one party while the other is either avoiding action or is helpless in the situation. It might be a power-based conflict and result in a win-lose outcome. This approach creates more problems than it solves and can lead to legal and ethical problems. However, it can also be the technique of choice in certain crisis situations.

Favorable outcomes of conflict situations depend on purposeful selection of the best technique based on the unique circumstances that surround each issue. It is conceivable that any one of the techniques described could be the approach of choice in a given event. Determining the best choice takes place through the use of a structured process. A description of a process follows.

PROCESS MODEL OF CONFLICT MANAGEMENT

The process model of conflict management presented in Figure 4-3 is composed of four stages. Stage 1 has four parts: issue, power, cooperation, and communication. Stage 2 is the use of facilitative techniques. Stage 3 is movement toward resolution. Stage 4 is the implementation of decisions.

In the four parts of stage 1, there are questions to ask about each: Is the issue important? How important? How much time will be needed to arrive at consensus? Is power equal enough for negotiation to take place? Can it be equalized? Is the level of cooperation such that all sides regard others' points of view? Can it be developed? Is

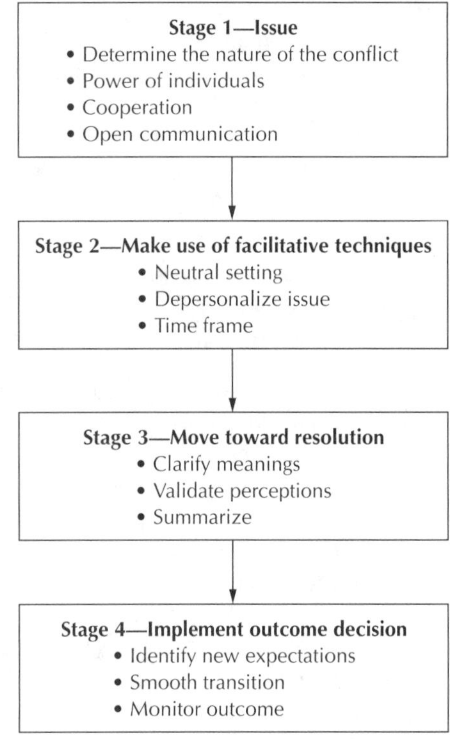

FIGURE 4-3. Process model of conflict management. Stages occur in a one-way sequence. The model is adaptable to a variety of situations involving groups, individuals within groups, or individuals between groups.

communication open, spontaneous, and without hidden agendas? If it is determined that the conflict is legitimately nonnegotiable by virtue of policy, resources, or contractual agreement, group effort is inappropriate and individuals must reassess their own situations and proceed accordingly. However, if the conflict is one for group resolution, proceed to stage two.

Stage 2, facilitative techniques, includes the selection of a mutually agreeable neutral setting so that neither side has an advantage because of space. When possible, and by the choice of those involved, a setting away from the workplace can be helpful. It is important that discussions proceed along depersonalized positions (for example: suggestion A, suggestion B, and so on). Each point is then considered as to its advantages and disadvantages. A realistic time frame should be established in order to ensure forward movement of the process while giving it the importance it deserves.

In stage 3, the group moves toward resolution. Short, frequent exchanges are important and provide a way to clarify and validate terms, restate positions, and validate perceptions. A final definition ends stage 3.

During the fourth and final stage, a plan for implementation is devised. New expectations are described, as well as defining how they will affect others and how a smooth transition can be accomplished. The new practices will be monitored until the new expectations are established. The resolution of some conflicts can be handled quite successfully by staff nurses, such as those that stem from, and are limited to, the operation of a nursing unit. Managing conflicts that have potential legal consequences and those involving several departments in the organization are better left to nurse managers. Managers are recognized as formal leaders, as spokespersons, and as those who have ready access to information not available to others. In any case, it is well to consider Numerof's position that negotiation of conflict is the most difficult aspect of communication.[32] Communication has been covered extensively in Chapter 3. It is of major importance in organizations, and the need for ongoing refinement of communication skills cannot be overemphasized.

CASE STUDY

Nurse/Patient Conflict

Marcus Butler is a 19-year-old patient recently transferred from the surgical ICU to the open surgical unit. He had suffered gunshot wounds to his abdomen and left leg during a gang confrontation in the early hours of the morning four days ago. His condition is stable, but he is expected to be in the hospital for three to four more days. It isn't long before the nurses realize that his behavior presents a real challenge for them. He is demanding, his language is insulting, and his numerous visitors provide him with food items that are not on his restricted diet. Together they play loud music and/or the television late into the night. Nurses have been threatened when they request any form of cooperation from the patient or his visitors. A security guard is stationed on the unit, but his presence seems to make little difference because he is not recognized as a law enforcement agent by the gang members. It is apparent that Marcus does not share or appreciate any of the nurses' values and concern for his health and well-being. Their best efforts have made no difference in his response to them.

- Construct a plan for the care of this patient.
- Define and examine your response to his unconventional behavior.
- Weigh the potential benefits and problems of involving security.

CASE STUDY

Nurse/Nurse Assistant Conflict

On a very busy unit, Mary (RN) asked Bernice (NA) to bathe one of her patients as she had to prepare another patient for a lengthy procedure that would take her until early afternoon to complete. Bernice responded that the patient Mary had asked her to bathe was not her assignment, and she refused Mary's request. Assignments on the unit have always been done in a way to equalize the number of patients each caregiver is assigned.

- Comment on the pattern of patient care assignments.
- Comment on Bernice's reason for refusing to assist Mary.
- How can this problem be prevented in the future?

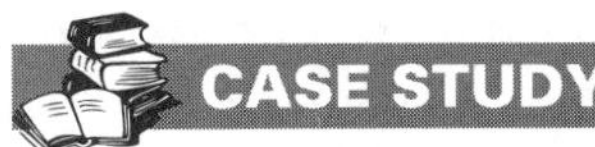

CASE STUDY

Charge Nurse Criticizes Nurse's Decision Making

Ellen, a new graduate assigned to a medical-surgical unit, was assigned to five patients. One patient (Mrs. W.) is very obese and requires three people to assist her with any movement. Mrs. W. was scheduled for wound care by her physician at 9:00 A.M. Ellen made rounds of her other four patients and made sure their immediate needs were met before going into Mrs. W.'s room. Mrs. W. had just had a loose stool and needed to be cleaned. Ellen went in search of assistance when the charge nurse questioned her about her whereabouts since morning report, and why she had not ambulated one of her other patients. Ellen was stunned and explained her activities up to that time. Ellen was told she needed to work on her decision making about priority setting, and to get on with her assignment.

- What is the basis of this problem?
- Comment on Ellen's plan for patient care.
- Comment on the charge nurse's intervention in this situation.

SUMMARY

In this chapter, decision making and management of conflict are discussed. Effective communication improves understanding between parties in complex work settings, and healthy group dynamics facilitate decision making. In turn, quality decision making fosters effective management of conflict. Not all conflict is detrimental, but those that are must be managed and brought under control. Some conflict is growth producing and leads to a revitalization of efforts. Experience in decision making and conflict management leads to heightened precision in communication and improved group relations. Outcomes of both are good or bad, depending on the willingness of participants to work toward success and on improving their skill level. Process models of decision making and conflict resolution are offered.

LEARNER EXERCISES

1. The nursing service department has been asked by administration to select three representatives from the nursing staff to serve on an ad hoc committee that will decide the distribution of widely scattered parking places owned by the hospital. Administration is tired of the bickering about who wants to park where. What criteria would you suggest be used to select the three nurse representatives? Once selected, what method should the representatives use to gain insight into nurses' concerns about parking allocation?
2. The nursing unit is without the services of a ward secretary for a week. The charge nurse wants to be fair to the staff and decides to take her turn at filling in for the vacationing ward secretary. For the full week she serves as the unit's secretary.

Analyze the premises in this decision. Weigh the consequences of the charge nurse's decision relative to patient care issues.

3. Consider the following statements and respond to each with "yes" or "no" according to how you would actually respond, not on how you *think you should* respond.

    1. When I am publicly criticized, I listen calmly and ask to continue the discussion privately later._______
    2. When I am busy and a coworker drops by to chat, I suggest we talk later.________
    3. When I am overwhelmed with work and am asked to do an additional assignment, I ask for help in prioritizing my workload.________
    4. If I have difficulty getting information from a coworker, I remind him or her of the benefits of complying with my request._________
    5. When I am chairing a meeting and an irrelevant topic is introduced, I quickly get the discussion back on track._________
    6. When one of my peers becomes upset, I look for clues to that person's problem._________
    7. When I am having a bad day I try to remember to think before I speak._________
    8. If fellow workers are arguing I do not join in the discussion._________
    9. When someone is acting irrationally, I acknowledge his or her feelings but do not judge the person._________
    10. When I find myself getting defensive, I say that I need time to think through the issue._________

    How many "yes" responses did you make?_________

    How many "no" responses did you make?_________

The "yes" responses indicate that you lean toward being in control of the situation. This exercise can help identify where you are in being objective and rational in potential conflict situations. Reflect on any "no" responses you make for self-improvement purposes.

REFERENCES

1. Simon, H.A. (1976). *Administrative behavior: A study of decision making processes in administrative organizations*, 3rd ed, New York: The Free Press, p. xi.
2. Garre, P.P. (1992, May). Multiattribute utility theory in decision making. *Nursing Management*, 33–35.
3. Simon, H.A. (1976). *Administrative behavior: A study of decision making processes in administrative organizations*, 3rd ed. New York: The Free Press, p. ix.
4. Bragg, T. (2000). Ten ways to deal with turf wars. *Occupational Health and Safety*, 26–30.
5. LeFevre, R.A. (2001, March). Improving your ability to think critically. *Nursing Spectrum*, 2(3), 11.
6. Lamond, D.,& Thompson C. (2000). Intuition and analysis in decision making and choice. *Journal of Nursing Scholarship*, 23(4), 411–414.
7. Bourbonnais, F.F., & Baumann, A. (1985, Spring). Stress and rapid decision making in nursing: An administrative challenge. *Nursing Administration Quarterly*, 85–91.

8. Carnevali, D.L., & Thomas, M.D. (1993). *Diagnostic reasoning and treatment decision making in nursing*, Philadelphia, PA: J.B. Lippincott.
9. Simon, H.A. (1976). *Administrative behavior: A study of decision making processes in administrative organizations,* 3rd ed. New York: The Free Press, p. 71.
10. Hand, E. (2001, June). Tools for the nursing toolbox. *Nursing Spectrum*, 2(4), 22.
11. Simon, H.A. (1976). *Administrative behavior: A study of decision making processes in administrative organizations,* 3rd ed. New York: The Free Press, p. xii.
12. DeBella, S., Martin, L., & Siddall, S. (1986). *Nurse's role in health care planning.* Norwalk, CT: Appleton & Lange, p. 34.
13. Johnson, C., (1988, August). Cultivating your creativity. *Toastmaster*, 8–10.
14. Lyon, B.L. (2000). Situational anger and self-employment. *Reflections on Nursing Leadership*, 3rd quarter, 36–37.
15. Zeidel, N. (Ed.) (2001, April). Management decisions. *RN*, *64*(4), 23.
16. Umiker, W. (1997). Collaborative conflict resolution. *Health Care Supervisor, 15*(3), 70–75.
17. Dawes B, (1999, October). Harnessing energy to overcome conflict. *American Operating Room Nursing Journal, 70*(4), 562–566.
18. Clause, K.E., & Bailey, J.T. (1977). *Power and influence in health care: A new approach to leadership*, St. Louis: Mosby, p. 9.
19. Nobel, K.A., & Rancourt, R. (1991, Summer). Administration and intradisciplinary conflict within nursing. *Nursing Administration Quarterly*, 36–42.
20. Kramer, M, & Schmalenberg C, (1976, October). Conflict: The cutting edge of growth. *American Journal of Nursing*, 19–25.
21. Martin, K., Wimberly, D., & O'Keefe, K. (1994, January). Resolving conflict in a multicultural nursing department. *Nursing Management, 25*(1), 49–51.
22. Stringer, H. (2001, February). Raging bulls. *Nurse Week*, 2(2), 10–11.
23. Ashworth, P (Ed.). (2000). Nurse-doctor relationships: Conflict, competition or collaboration. *Intensive and Critical Care Nursing, 16*, 127–128.
24. Daum, A.L. (1994, August). The disruptive antisocial patient: Management strategies. *Nursing Management*, *25*(8), 46–51.
25. Steefel, L. (2001, May). ICN takes aim at violence. *Nursing Spectrum,* 2(5), 11.
26. Anderson, C., & Stomper, M. (2001, February).Workplace violence. *RN, 64*(2), 71–74.
27. Steefel, L. (2001, May). ICN takes aim at violence. *Nursing Spectrum,* 2(5), 11.
28. Valentine, P.E.B. (2001). A gender perspective on conflict management strategies for nurses. *Journal of Nursing Scholarship, 33*(1), 69–74.
29. Sedlacek, J. (1989). *Conflict management,* University of Kentucky, College of Allied Health Professions: TIPS, 13.
30. Sedlacek, J. (1989). *Conflict management,* University of Kentucky, College of Allied Health Professions: TIPS, 17.
31. Booth, R.Z. (1982, September/October). Conflict resolution. *Nursing Outlook*, 447–453.
32. Numerof, R.E. (1985, April). The manager as conflict negotiator. *Health Care Supervisor*, 1–15.

5

The Ethical Responsibility of the Nurse Leader

> "Nearly all persons can stand adversity, but if you want to test a person's character, give him power."
>
> Abraham Lincoln

INTRODUCTION

In 1980, Flaherty wrote: "Whenever nurses meet, they express concern about the number and complexity of ethical dilemmas that they face and the effect of these on the quality and quantity of their professional practice."[1] More than two decades later, a survey of practicing nurses found that their concerns about ethical issues are still high, particularly around issues of patient advocacy.[2]

Nursing managers are challenged with a health care system that has changed significantly in recent years. Pressures to reduce cost and improve efficiency increase providers' concerns about maintaining the quality of care. A widespread labor shortage and an aging nursing workforce contribute to concerns about the allocation of scarce resources, maintaining quality, and providing a fair and just workplace for employees.

Other issues that will continue to create ethical dilemmas and challenges for all health care providers are the explosion of knowledge in the field of human genetics, issues of confidentiality in the use and sharing of electronic patient health records, and the exposure of high numbers of medical errors in American health care delivery systems. The object of this chapter is to discuss the ethical responsibility of a nurse leader/manager in today's complex health care system.

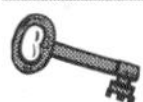

KEY CONCEPTS

Affirmative Action a relatively new ethic written into statutes, provides for employment and promotion opportunities for qualified persons in proportion to the existence of representative ethnic groups in the geographic area.

Autonomy provides for the privilege of self-determination in deciding what happens to one's body in health care.

Beneficence requires that care providers contribute to health and welfare and not merely avoid harm to a patient or client.

Consequentialist Theories define good actions as those of utility.

Deontology Theories presume that one does the good act and avoids evil.

Ethics is that branch of philosophy that examines ideal human behavior.

Ethics Committees are groups designed to educate health care providers in ethical decision making and to provide consultation in resolving ethical dilemmas.

Justice requires that individuals be given what they are entitled to, deserve, or can legitimately claim and that resources are distributed fairly.

Morality is based in values derived from religious precepts, cultural belief systems, or other forms of community expectation or social convention.

Nonmaleficence prohibits deliberate harm and demands weighing risks with the benefits of treatment.

Values are the basis for codes of behavior that affect ethical decisions.

Whistle-Blowing is a cry against wrongdoings; a call for correction of an injustice, abuse, or neglect.

ETHICS

The term **ethics** is used to refer to that branch of philosophy that examines ideal human behavior. **Morality** is a term used to refer to general rules of social and personal conduct and the practices or actions that derive from those rules. While "moral" is sometimes used as a judgment about whether an action is right or wrong, in the field of ethics, "ethical" and "moral" refer not to the rightness or wrongness of actions, but to a category or class of actions that pertain to ethics.[3] Morality is based on strongly held or fundamental **values** derived from religious precepts, cultural belief systems, or other forms of community expectation or social convention. Ethical dilemmas are those situations that present a conflict between two or more fundamental values, are complex and have no apparent solution, and for which all possible solutions have equally undesirable outcomes. While ethical dilemmas confront nurses and nurse managers daily, not all difficult situations encountered by nurses are ethical dilemmas. A situation may have ethical aspects but still be primarily an organizational, communication, or legal problem. For instance, a patient may have a valid living will stating that the patient does not want to be resuscitated in the event of cardiac arrest, but that document is not in the patient's chart. While this situation has ethical implications for the patient's treatment, it is primarily an organizational or legal problem. The Patient Self-Determination Act clearly outlines the hospital's responsibility to assure that advance directive documents be put in the patient's chart.[4]

Ethics is a reflective endeavor in which the individual moves beyond the acceptance and internalization of traditional rules of the social group and moves into the realm of reflecting upon those rules.[5] Ethical decision making for the professional nurse is guided by general rules of social conduct, the nurse's personal values, and the values of the nursing profession. The fundamental values of nursing are expressed in the Code for Nurses.[6] They are the values, such as respect for patient autonomy, acting in the patient's best interest, and maintaining professional competence, that all nurses commit to uphold when they enter the profession:

1. The nurse provides services with respect for human dignity and the uniqueness of the client, unrestricted by considerations of social or economic status, personal attributes, or the nature of health problems.
2. The nurse safeguards the client's right to privacy by judiciously protecting information of a confidential nature.
3. The nurse acts to safeguard the client and the public when health care and safety are affected by the incompetent, unethical, or illegal practice of any person.
4. The nurse assumes responsibility and accountability for individual nursing judgments and actions.
5. The nurse maintains competence in nursing.
6. The nurse exercises informed judgment and uses individual competence and qualifications as criteria in seeking consultation, accepting responsibilities, and delegating nursing activities to others.
7. The nurse participates in activities that contribute to the ongoing development of the profession's body of knowledge.
8. The nurse participates in the profession's efforts to implement and improve standards of nursing.
9. The nurse participates in the profession's efforts to establish and maintain conditions of employment conducive to high-quality nursing care.
10. The nurse participates in the profession's efforts to protect the public from misinformation and misrepresentation and to maintain the integrity of nursing.
11. The nurse collaborates with members of the health professions and other citizens in promoting community and national efforts to meet the health needs of the public.

An important part of professional socialization includes learning to use these fundamental values to guide one's actions in professional situations. Other professional values are more instrumental, in that they are helpful or necessary to achieve the fundamental values expressed in the Code. For instance, nurses value their professional autonomy and the right to control their own practice, because these activities are necessary to assure that patients' best interests are well-served. Nurses value assertiveness because they may find it necessary to confront other professionals or family members if a patient's right to participate in decision making is being threatened.

The first six statements in the Code for Nurses speak to the nurse's relationships with patients and families. New nurses can most easily identify with their individual responsibilities to the patients directly served. As the nurse more fully develops as a professional, there is a greater understanding of, and commitment to, the profession's collective responsibility to society. The last five statements of the Code for Nurses speak to professional activities that help implement and improve standards of high-quality nursing care, provide a sound scientific basis for nursing practice, protect the public from misinformation, and collaborate with others to promote the health of the public. These more socially-oriented goals can only be accomplished when nurses band together in collective activities, such as setting national standards of practice and engaging in political action. The political and economic environment of health care in the 21st century requires nurses to be more aware of the impact of the social context in which they practice. Nurses must not only band together within the profession but also collaborate with other health disciplines and social and political groups to influence social policies related to health care delivery in American society.

Professional values guide nursing actions and motivate one to continue to function within standards and codes. Professional values are developed through education or by observation of role models and mentors. A very important part of the nurse leader's role is to role-model commitment to the individual and collective values of the nursing profession and to mentor other nurses in their growth as professionals.

Ethical Theories

The two categories of ethical theories prevalent in guiding moral decision making are **deontology theories** and **consequentialist theories.** These theories explain reasoned analysis of ethical dilemmas and account for the moral decision of one person as opposed to the moral decision of a second individual. For example, one person may determine that an action, such as telling the truth or keeping a promise, is good in itself and may perform that action regardless of the consequences. A second person may look at the results of the action and determine not to do it. From his or her perspective, it may be hurtful to someone to tell the truth or keep a promise.

Consequentialism is the theory that actions are right or wrong according only to their consequences. The most common form of consequentialism is utilitarianism. In a somewhat oversimplified form, this theory is expressed as "the end justifies the means" or as promoting "the greatest good for the greatest number of people." Thus, the consequences of a specific action assume a very significant role in the decision-making process. Ethical decisions founded on a utilitarian base may be made from the perspective of "act utilitarianism," which judges the consequences or utility of single acts situationally, or "rule utilitarianism," which judges the utility not of single acts but of adhering to certain moral rules. For an act utilitarian, deceiving a patient about a diagnosis may be morally acceptable because, in a particular situation, it satisfies the family's needs and may protect the patient from a possible depression. A rule utilitarian may believe that deceiving the patient is wrong because the greatest good to society comes from adhering to the moral rule, "Do not lie."[7]

Deontological theories are based on the premise that judgments about the rightness or wrongness of actions are based on features other than, or in addition to, the consequences of the action. Deontologic theories presume that one does the good act and avoids evil. Good or right actions honor truth, promises, contracts, and significant relationships, including the nurse–patient and manager–worker relationships. For example, a deontologist may believe that deceiving a patient about a diagnosis is always wrong because deception in and of itself is wrong, regardless of its consequences. Ethical decisions made within a deontological framework are grounded in religious traditions, natural law, or "common moral consciousness."[8]

Ethical Principles

Several ethical principles derived from ethical theories are applicable in health care and nursing situations. The principles most often utilized in resolving dilemmas are autonomy, beneficence, nonmaleficence, and justice.[9]

Autonomy provides for the privilege of self-determination in deciding what happens to one's body in health care. Since the late 1960s, society has affirmed the right of the individual to make decisions about medical care. The President's Commission for the Study of Ethical Problems in Medicine emphasized that the competent adult has the right to decline medical treatments even though it would result in death.[10] Several famous court cases, such as the Nancy Cruzan case, established the patient's legal right to refuse treatment, which was given additional force with the passage of the Patient Self-Determination Act in 1990.[11] The Code for Nurses speaks directly to the autonomy principle in its first and third statements.[12]

Paternalism, in which the physician or health care provider makes decisions about treatment on the basis of what the provider deems best for the patient, is directly opposed to autonomy. The principle of self-determination, or autonomy, requires that patients have adequate information about treatment options to make an intelligent decision and to give informed consent to a specific form of therapy.

Beneficence requires that care providers contribute to the health and welfare of the patient and not merely attempt to avoid harm to the patient or client. Providing for discharge planning early in hospitalization to facilitate rehabilitation or protecting a patient's reputation by maintaining confidentiality of information are examples of following the principle of beneficence.

Nonmaleficence prohibits deliberate harm and demands weighing risks with the benefits of treatment. Not using proper precautions in caring for patients with infectious or communicable diseases, and thus endangering oneself and other patients, would contradict the principle of nonmaleficence. Physically restraining a patient without carefully weighing the benefits against potential risks of restraint could lead to serious problems for the patient, causing more harm than good and thus violating the principle of nonmaleficence. The nurse manager who does not protect the confidentiality of personnel information can do a great deal of harm to a staff member's reputation and professional future.

Justice requires that individuals be given what they are entitled to, deserve, or can legitimately claim. Patients have rights to considerate and respectful care, and nurses are entitled to safe working environments. Generally, physicians deserve to have their orders carried out. Administrators and supervisors can legitimately claim that workers spend their time on the job in productive activities.

The principle of justice has to do with the fair allocation of resources. Decisions about how to allocate become more difficult when resources are limited. As health care reform measures place continued emphasis on containing costs, all health care providers struggle to make allocation decisions that will be as fair as possible for all parties concerned, and still maintain an acceptable level of quality of care. Staff nurses making decisions about how to divide their time among several critically ill patients are allocating the scarce resource of their time, and should examine how they make those decisions.

Barriers to Ethical Decision Making

Several factors relating to individual nurses and the social context in which they practice can present barriers to making sound ethical decisions. Some of these factors are a result of contemporary social conditions from which the nurse leader cannot escape. For instance, over the past few decades, an apathy toward the Judeo-Christian doctrine and moral code has emerged. More individuals reach adulthood having had a limited opportunity to develop strong moral convictions to guide their personal actions. Violence and abuse have become commonplace in American society and seem to reflect a diminished value for human life. As our country becomes more culturally diverse, individuals from other cultures and religious traditions bring different perspectives on ethical issues such as end-of-life decisions and questions of justice and fairness. Ethical decisions regarding care for such persons require an understanding of their cultural belief systems, an understanding that is often lacking.

Many situations have both ethical and legal ramifications. Current social attitudes place emphasis on individual rights rather than responsibilities, contributing to the tendency to turn to the courts to uphold those rights. Within health care, this tendency contributes to the potential for legal actions that may or may not be justified by the facts of a situation. The result is that professionals are cautious in decision making and fearful of litigation. For example, in questions such as whether or not to continue life-sustaining treatments, the ethically good action may be stifled by fears of litigation.

Advances in technology have resulted in such emotionally explosive practices as intrauterine diagnosis or treatment and gene therapy. New technologies have challenged our beliefs about what constitutes life and death. Cost considerations have created concerns about when, and to what extent, society can afford to provide available technology, thus raising the question of whether or not the ethically good action is affordable.

Other potential barriers to moral judgments exist in the nursing practice environment. The nurse leader may not be central to ethical decision making but is subject to physicians and to administrators while being accountable to patients according to codes of ethics. Nurses have overlapping responsibilities with other health care professionals, thus making it unclear exactly where accountability rests and making it difficult to trace and correct errors. There is often inadequate staffing and frequent rotation of nurses, which may place nurses in a position of knowing what is the right thing to do for patients but being unable to fulfill those responsibilities because of a lack of time and situational support.

STRATEGIES FOR ENHANCING ETHICAL DECISIONS IN NURSING PRACTICE

One aspect of ethical decision making over which nurses have control is their own moral development and their perspectives of professional obligations. For example, nurses can determine to what extent they accept traditional male and female roles in health care delivery and understand how these traditional roles affect their ability to advocate for patients. Nurses can make choices that will increase or reduce their risks for experiencing burnout or substance abuse. They can also develop an understanding of how burnout or substance abuse can impede a nurse's ability to carry out professional ethical responsibilities as outlined in the Code for Nurses.

Nurses and nurse leaders may not have received adequate preparation in moral development theory and ethical decision-making models. Despite this, it is their responsibility to participate in ethical decision making. Nurses need to recognize that without adequate education about systematic ethical analysis, their conclusions about the right action in an ethical dilemma are mostly a reflection of what "feels good" to them. What feels good or right for one person may or may not be the best action for someone else. Systematic analysis of situations, applying the tools of ethical theory and ethical principles, helps assure that the values and beliefs of one person are not inappropriately imposed on others. To attain the necessary tools of ethical analysis, nurses can attend courses or continuing education programs in ethics. One study of practicing nurses found that these nurses were very concerned about ethical issues relating to their role as patient advocate. Study participants indicated that in general they had a high-to-moderate need for ethics education in order to practice ethically, and they were particularly interested in education that would help them more effectively advocate on behalf of the patients they served.[13]

Nurse leaders can help provide staff development programs and in-service education to keep staff up-to-date on these and other ethical issues in practice. Professional publications, such as the Code for Nurses with Interpretive Statements or various position statements from the American Nurses Association, can be helpful sources to expand the nurse leader's vision of professional ethical responsibilities.[14] Other activities that facilitate individual development include regularly scheduled nursing ethics rounds or brown-bag discussions. These forums provide opportunities for staff to clarify their legal rights and responsibilities and to begin to deal with the ambiguities and limitations inherent in all ethical dilemmas.

Vigilance against unconditionally accepting the health care decisions of administration and the medical staff will help the nurse leader guard the role of patient advocate in ethical dilemmas. The ability to challenge administrative or medical pronouncements comes with self-confidence in the leadership role based on educational preparation in philosophy, ethics, and moral decision making, as well as management and leadership. Other resources to support ethical decision making include the institution's philosophy and mission statements, patient's bill of rights documents, position statements on ethical issues from professional societies, standards of care, chaplain services or pastoral care departments, and risk-management departments. An ethics hotline can provide anonymity for individual employees with problems that cannot be taken directly to immediate supervisors. Perhaps the most important resource for managing ethical dilemmas is the institutional ethics committee.

The Role of Institutional Ethics Committees

The work of **ethics committees** lies in three areas: education (including education of the committee itself), policy and guideline recommendations, and case review.[15,16] Ethics committees are not established to serve as a second medical opinion, to assume decision making for the patient, or to function as a peer review or grievance committee.

The educational process for the committee members can include a short course in bioethics, reading materials, and attendance at workshops or seminars on ethical issues. Thereafter, education in ethical decision making for the institution, for individuals, and for the community can be provided.[17] Some of these educational experiences will lead naturally to the second objective, which is policy making. The need for more effective communication and clearer definition of roles will dictate specific procedures and policies, reflecting the values of the institution.[18,19] The third function, case review, provides opportunities for persons representing a range of professional and patient perspectives to systematically analyze cases and clarify options for action. Nurses' perspectives on ethical issues should be well-represented on institutional ethics committees. Nurse leaders can encourage and identify well-prepared, articulate staff nurses to serve in this capacity. The nurse leader can help caregivers and families understand how the ethics committee referral process works and encourage them to utilize this system.[20]

THE EMPLOYER–EMPLOYEE RELATIONSHIP

Employer–employee relationships are those that exist between the department of nursing (as represented by the vice president of nursing, or chief nursing executive), nurse managers, and the professional nursing staff. Professional nurses should learn the philosophy and goals of the employing agency. A hospital's philosophy is a statement of beliefs that direct the goals and purposes for which the institution exists. It achieves its aim only when the beliefs are operationalized within each department. Knowledge of the philosophy of the hospital can be compared with personal values and ethics. If the hospital's philosophy and the nurse's values and ethics are congruent, then as ethical issues arise, the nurse can act with the assurance that personal values support institutional values, and vice versa. The individual nurse then has the right and responsibility to "live out" the ethical philosophy and goals of the institution as well as practice somewhat autonomously in relation to position and responsibilities.

Because value judgments and ethics influence institutional policy formulation and implementation, the nurse leader keeps communication lines open with administrators, participates as fully as possible in decision making, and remains committed to identifying with and acting on the values of the organization. This kind of loyal commitment to an institution presumes fairness or justice in employment relationships.

Two very specific fairness issues are job security and equitable treatment of employees. Job security necessitates a contract with four requirements: (1) full knowledge by both parties of the nature of the agreement, (2) no intentional misrepresentation of facts by either party, (3) no enforced entrance into the contract with duress or coercion, and (4) no contract binding the parties to an immoral act. Equitable treatment of employees involves respecting the employees' rights to due process and fair dealings and to achievement of personal growth, fulfillment, human dignity, and emotional health.[21] By understanding issues of fairness and equity, the nurse manager remains sensitive to personnel situations that may involve these principles. The manager's responsibility is to assure that conflicts are resolved fairly, and that employees understand their right to due process and feel comfortable exercising that right.

One way in which organizations express a commitment to the values of justice and fairness is through non-discrimination policies and affirmative action programs. **Affirmative action,** a relatively new ethic currently written into many federal and state statutes, provides for employment and promotion opportunities for qualified persons in proportion to the existence of representative ethnic groups in the geographic area. Considerable controversy surrounds affirmative action laws and programs, particularly in regard to whether or not such programs are fair for all parties involved. Currently, however, with few exceptions, affirmative action guidelines must be followed when hiring and promoting personnel. Similar policies address discrimination on the basis of other characteristics such as age, gender, or sexual orientation. The nurse manager must be aware of such policies and work closely with the human resources or other appropriate institutional departments to assure that non-discrimination policies are closely followed.

Sexual harassment policies are examples of policies designed to uphold the principles of justice and fairness in the workplace. Sexual harassment is morally and legally objectionable; it infringes on human rights and interferes with an individual's privacy and autonomy. Employers have a responsibility to maintain a harassment-free workplace.[22]

Nurse leaders can take the lead in formulating sexual harassment policies and educating everyone in the workplace about sexual harassment.

As an employed professional, the nurse is in a somewhat unique position. All employees hold a certain amount of loyalty to the institution for which they work. This loyalty stems in part from the fact that, when hired, employees make a commitment to accept and support the philosophy and mission of the institution. Employee loyalty also relates to the more practical fact that supporting the goals of the institution helps ensure the employee's paycheck. However, nurses as professionals also have a loyalty to the patients they have promised to serve. Likewise, nurses hold a certain loyalty to other health professionals, such as nursing peers and physicians. While nurses' roles have become increasingly autonomous, assisting the physician is still an important nursing role. Sometimes nurses find themselves in situations in which these loyalties to employer, patients, and other professionals are in conflict. For example, a nurse may be aware of an incident of possible medical negligence. Loyalty to the patient seems to dictate that the nurse take the necessary steps to inform the patient and/or report the situation through appropriate administrative channels. However, loyalty to the institution and to a physician as a colleague may influence the nurse to remain quiet about the incident. These situations are very difficult for nurses to resolve and can create considerable suffering for the nurse. If the nurse acts out of loyalty to the patient and chooses to report the incident, the nurse may be taking on a role of whistle-blower.

Whistle-blowing is defined as a cry against wrongdoing, or a call for correction of an injustice, abuse, or neglect.[23] All possible attempts to solve patient-care deficiencies through open communication and confrontation with the individuals involved should be exhausted before a nurse goes "outside the unit" to call for correction. While blowing the whistle may be the ethically right action, such action places the nurse in a vulnerable position.[24] Whistle-blowers may be fired, demoted, harassed, or shunned.[25] The key to success, in terms of how effective the complaint will be in rectifying the problem, lies in the manner in which the complaint is made. The nurse in a whistle-blowing situation needs to carefully follow the administrative chain of command and thoroughly document all aspects of the situation, keeping personal copies of all documentation.[26] As health care ethicist Emily Friedman advises, "If you need to blow the whistle, and nobody will listen to you inside the organization, then blow it outside. Try not to go to the press unless you absolutely have to because the press might get the story wrong and innocent people can get hurt. The American College of Physicians, the American Association of Family Practitioners, and even the American Medical Association has been far more vocal and visible than has nursing. This is unfortunate. In the individual patient-care situation, it is the nurse who is trusted and knows the patient best."[27]

In some states, whistle-blowers are protected by law. In many instances of abuse, neglect, or incompetence, professional codes or legislation require the reporting of such injustice. Nurse leaders should know the state laws regarding the reporting of abuse.

PEER RELATIONSHIPS

Peer relationships are defined as those that exist between head nurses as colleagues and between staff nurses as colleagues. The informal nurse leader may be either a head nurse or a staff nurse. As a consequence of personal characteristics or knowledge, a staff nurse may be recognized as a leader but not assume a position of authority in the organization.

Mutual respect, collegiality, and cooperative and productive interdependency are essential for effective relationships between nurses and physicians and are equally necessary for healthy and positive relationships with peers.[28] Such working relationships facilitate discussion of the ethical issues that arise from an increasingly complex and technological health care environment. Nurses' daily encounters with critical illness and death, angry and grieving families, and conflicting demands within the workplace can very quickly lead to feelings of burnout. In fact, the burnout phenomenon has been attributed to confronting ethical dilemmas without an arena in which to work through these dilemmas in a reasoned way.[29] Providing opportunities for nurses to ventilate their feelings about difficult patient care situations, or their frustrations about heavy workloads, fears of litigation, or ethical dilemmas may prevent the burnout so prevalent among nurses in today's acute care settings. However, once this ventilation of feelings has taken place, the role of the nurse leader is to help staff members move beyond the focus on emotions and develop productive problem-solving strategies. In the case of ethical dilemmas, one productive strategy is to seek consultation with the institutional ethics committee.

Unfortunately, a common dilemma that nurses face is the unprofessional or unethical conduct of peers. Since the Code for Nurses includes a commitment to safeguarding the client and public from the incompetent, unethical, or illegal practice of any person, awareness of any such activity on the part of peers requires some type of action. Policies are established to guide employee behavior. Blatant disregard for policy requires intervention from the nurse leader.

However, sometimes disregard for policy stems from an ignorance or misunderstanding of the policy. In that case, the role of the nurse leader is to help resolve the misunderstanding or offer opportunities for employees to receive the education they need to overcome ignorance.

An example of how disregard for policy might stem from ignorance or a lack of understanding is the issue of privacy regarding patients' records and information. Safeguarding the privacy of patient information has always been a priority for nurses and is expressed as a key value in the Code for Nurses.[30] However, the Health Insurance Portability and Accountability Act of 1996 (HIPAA) mandates new regulations that govern privacy, security, and electronic transactions standards for health information.[31] These new regulations affect the way in which patient information is shared on the nursing unit and between hospital departments. As these regulations gradually go into effect (beginning in 2002), all health care workers will need significant education to understand these regulations. Having knowledge of the new standards and regulations is a responsibility to be shared by managers and their staff. All nurses, as part of their commitment to the Code for Nurses, should strive to obtain and share only as much patient data as needed to adequately care for the patient and family. However, they also have a legal obligation to adhere to the regulations outlined through HIPAA. The nurse manager is responsible for maintaining standards of privacy and confidentiality on the nursing units. In fairness to employees, the manager must assure that staff members have been adequately educated about new standards or requirements before they are held accountable for putting them into practice.

Psychologists have attributed employees' dishonesty to emotional exhaustion and depression, but such employees are not justified in stealing materials or drugs, damaging property, malingering or wasting time, cheating on time cards, or extending breaks or meal periods.[32] Abusing drugs, falsifying patient records, or acting in ways that compromise patient safety are other examples of unethical or illegal conduct that nurses cannot condone in their peers. A nurse leader as peer could point out these unethical behaviors by approaching the offending party and respectfully confronting him or her with genuineness, honesty, and understanding. Skillful communication of the consequences of such dishonest behavior for the offender, as well as for peers and institutions, is a mark of professionalism. If resolution of the problem does not result from one-to-one confrontation, the nurse leader should carefully follow the chain of command in reporting the offending behavior.

If a nurse suspects that a peer may have a substance abuse problem, the appropriate response involves carefully following institutional policies to assure patient safety and to get the individual into rehabilitation. Most state nurses' associations have a Peer Assistance Program to help and support nurses who depend on alcohol or mood-altering drugs.[33,34] Impairment stemming from alcohol and substance abuse creates huge financial, professional, and personal costs.[35] By knowing the policies and procedures of the employing agency as well as the state laws on the reporting of substance abuse, and utilizing programs such as peer assistance programs or employee assistance programs that offer counseling for impaired individuals, nurse leaders can help reduce those costs.

THE NURSE–PATIENT RELATIONSHIP

The nurse–patient relationship is the foundation for all professional nursing activity. The nurse's obligation to the patient has always been a part of the professional code, but it has assumed increasing emphasis over the years. The first official code for nurses, published in 1950, emphasized a nurse's primary obligation to the physician. In later versions, the emphasis shifted to loyalty to the employing institution. Starting with the 1976 edition of the Code for Nurses, all 11 principles of the Code emphasized the primacy of duties to patients.[36]

In general, nurses' obligations to patients, as outlined in the Code, involve putting the patient's interests before one's own, respecting the patient's right to exercise personal autonomy by taking part in decision making, respecting the dignity and privacy of patients, maintaining professional competence, and engaging in activities that establish and maintain quality patient care. The Code for Nurses serves as a public statement of nursing's commitment to individual patients and to society at large. It serves as a social contract between nurses and their clients. When new nurses enter the profession, they are making a type of public commitment to uphold the obligations outlined in the Code.[37] Nurses also have certain obligations to the institution that sometimes may seem to conflict with their promises or loyalties to patients. For example, in the current environment of cost cutting, the nurse leader may be pressured to reduce nursing staff beyond what the nurse leader believes is adequate for good patient care: Loyalty and appreciation for the needs of the institution conflict with the nurse's professional promise to provide high-quality care to patients. The leader's responsibility is to clearly document and communicate patient care needs and advocate with administration so that care is not compromised.

A situation in which a nurse manager may struggle to balance commitment to the patient with fairness to employees and loyalty to the facility is in the area of medical errors. A report on medical errors published by the Institute of Medicine in October, 2000, put a spotlight on this topic.[38] The report summarized numerous research studies documenting that the rate of errors tolerated in health care is much higher than rates considered acceptable in other industries, such as the airline industry. Numerous publications since the IOM report, including a second Institute of Medicine Report, emphasize that individuals who commit errors are sometimes at high risk to err because of the systems in which they work.[39] In other words, systems and processes within our institutions should be designed to reduce the possibility for human error as much as possible. When this does not happen, individuals are more likely to commit errors, not because they are incompetent or negligent, but because they work in conditions conducive to human error. Experts in medical error reduction recommend that individuals who commit errors not be blamed, but rather that a thorough analysis of the conditions leading up to the error be done and processes be changed to prevent the error from happening again. The nurse manager who is responsible for the safety of patients can face a dilemma when an employee commits an error in caring for those patients. How can the nurse manager hold individual nurses accountable for protecting the safety of patients, while at the same time recognizing the vulnerability of those individual nurses when they work in conditions that increase the risk for error? Examples of such conditions could be a short-staffed unit, nurses pulled to work on units where they are unfamiliar with the medications being given, an illegible order written by a physician who does not answer the nurse's call for clarification, or the nurse trying to administer medications in the midst of numerous disruptions and distractions. In these types of situations, the nurse manager needs to document and regularly re-assess the competence of the nursing staff, to assure that the nurses are accepting their professional responsibility as outlined in the Code for Nurses to maintain professional competence. Once competency is established, a nurse employee who commits an error should not be held totally responsible for that error. The nurse manager should assure that a thorough analysis of all conditions surrounding the error is done. Action plans should be developed and implemented so that processes contributing to the error are changed. In these ways, the nurse manager is fulfilling the obligation to protect patient safety, and keeping individual nurses accountable for maintaining their own professional competence, while at the same time acknowledging the reality of human error and treating employees in a just manner.

Many situations arise in which the nurse leader must advocate to protect patient autonomy. Providing for patient involvement in decision making means taking the time to assure that patients fully understand any consent forms they are signing. It means respecting and facilitating the use of advance directives or helping patients who wish to complete these documents. Respect for autonomy involves respecting the patient's right to refuse treatments, even if nurses, physicians, or families disagree with the competent patient's decision. Nurses in leadership roles often find themselves "caught in the middle" between patients, families, and physicians. While this may seem an uncomfortable position in which to be, nurses are perhaps the best people for such a role. Nurses should feel confident that their strong communication skills, rapport with patients and families, and good working relationships with physicians are just the skills needed to foster the dialogue needed in these situations.

Referring to specific ethical guidelines can help the nurse leader in his or her relationships with patients, families, and other health care professionals. "A Patient's Bill of Rights" and "The Patient's Choice of Treatment Options" are published by the American Hospital Association.[40] Similar Bill of Rights documents are available for nursing home and home care patients. The ANA publishes the "Code for Nurses with Interpretive Statements" and "Ethics in Nursing: Position Statements and Guidelines."[41] The Hastings Center has produced "Guidelines on the Termination of Life-Sustaining Treatment and the Care of the Dying."[42] Addresses for each of these organizations can be found in the end-of-chapter references.

PATIENTS BILL OF RIGHTS
A Patient's Bill of Rights
American Hospital Association
1973

On 6 February 1973 the American Hospital Association's House of Delegates approved a Patient's Bill of Rights. Other historically significant documents in the United States, which predated this Bill of Rights, were a document drafted by the National Welfare Rights Organization (1970) and the preamble to the

Standards of the Joint Commission on Accreditation of Hospitals. The AHA Patient's Bill of Rights, printed in full below, has been influential in the development of similar documents in other parts of the world.

The American Hospital Association presents a Patient's Bill of Rights with the expectation that observance of these rights will contribute to more effective patient care and greater satisfaction for the patient, his physician, and the hospital organization. Further, the Association presents these rights in the expectation that they will be supported by the hospital on behalf of its patients, as an integral part of the healing process. It is recognized that a personal relationship between the physician and the patient is essential for the provision of proper medical care. The traditional physician–patient relationship takes on a new dimension when care is rendered within an organizational structure. Legal precedent has established that the institution itself also has a responsibility to the patient. It is in recognition of these factors that these rights are affirmed.

1. The patient has the right to considerate and respectful care.
2. The patient has the right to obtain from his physician complete current information concerning his diagnosis, treatment, and prognosis in terms the patient can be reasonably expected to understand. When it is not medically advisable to give such information to the patient, the information should be made available to an appropriate person in his behalf. He has the right to know, by name, the physician responsible for coordinating his care.
3. The patient has the right to receive from his physician information necessary to give informed consent prior to the start of any procedure and/or treatment. Except in emergencies, such information for informed consent should include, but not necessarily be limited to, the specific procedure and/or treatment, the medically significant risks involved, and the probable duration of incapacitation. Where medically significant alternatives for care or treatment exist, or when the patient requests information concerning medical alternatives, the patient has the right to such information. The patient also has the right to know the name of the person responsible for the procedures and/or treatment.
4. The patient has the right to refuse treatment to the extent permitted by law, and to be informed of the medical consequences of his action.
5. The patient has the right to every consideration of his privacy concerning his own medical care program. Case discussion, consultation, examination, and treatment are confidential and should be conducted discreetly. Those not directly involved in his care must have the permission of the patient to be present.
6. The patient has the right to expect that all communication and records pertaining to his care should be treated as confidential.
7. The patient has the right to expect that within its capacity a hospital must make reasonable response to the request of a patient for services. The hospital must provide evaluation, service, and/or referral as indicated by the urgency of the case. When medically permissible a patient may be transferred to another facility only after he has received complete information and explanation concerning the needs for and alternatives to such a transfer. The institution to which the patient is to be transferred must first have accepted the patient for transfer.

8. The patient has the right to be advised if the Hospital proposes to engage in or perform human experimentation affecting his care or treatment. The patient has the right to refuse to participate in such research projects.
9. The patient has the right to expect reasonable continuity of care. He has the right to know in advance what appointment times and physicians are available and where. The patient has the right to expect that the hospital will provide a mechanism whereby he is informed by his physician or a delegate of the physician of the patient's continuing health care requirements following discharge.
10. The patient has the right to examine and receive an explanation of his bill regardless of source of payment.
11. The patient has the right to know what hospital rules and regulations apply to his conduct as a patient.

Source: Reprinted with permission of the American Hospital Association, copyright 1992.

No catalogue of rights can guarantee for the patient the kind of treatment he has a right to expect. A hospital has many functions to perform, including the prevention and treatment of disease, the education of both health professionals and patients, and the conduct of clinical research. All these activities must be conducted with an overriding concern for the patient, and, above all, the recognition of his dignity as a human being. Success is achieving this recognition of his dignity as a human being. Success in achieving this recognition assures success in the defense of the rights of the patient.

CASE STUDY

Ethical Decision Making

Mary Kay O'Connor has been working in the intensive care unit (ICU) for over six months. Mary Kay loves her work and finds the staff approachable and competent.

One evening, Mary Kay noted that the narcotic count was off. Mary Kay tried to find out what had happened to the missing narcotic. She reviewed the charts and patient requirements and could not locate the missing morphine. She reviewed the hospital policy for such a problem, called the evening supervisor, and filled out the appropriate forms.

Mary Kay did not give the matter another thought. She assumed it was an oversight, and she was happy to learn how to handle such situations for the future.

A month later, the same thing happened, and Mary Kay was working with the same staff personnel. Mary Kay observed the staff and suspected that one of the new registered nurses might have a drug problem.

- What should she do?
- What are the pros and cons for any action she may take?

SUMMARY

This chapter focuses on the multiple and complex ethical issues that face nurses and nurse leaders/managers. It defines the terms "ethics" and "morality." Values are considered as they affect the nurse personally and professionally.

Two ethical theories, deontology and consequentialism, are contrasted in terms of how they guide thinking and acting in ethical dilemmas. The basic principles derived from these classical theories—autonomy, beneficence, nonmaleficence, and justice—are described and related to the Code for Nurses. Some barriers to the ethical decision-making process are examined and strategies for enhancing good ethical decision making in health care settings are offered.

Specific situations creating ethical dilemmas are explored in the relationship of employer to employee, peer relationships, and the nurse–patient relationship. Examples are included that apply ethics principles as they coincide with the tenets of the Code for Nurses.

To conclude this chapter, student exercises provide opportunities to apply the content to selected ethical dilemmas. A reference list includes up-to-date resources as well as addresses of organizations and associations offering professional and ethical literature.

LEARNER EXERCISES

1. A newly admitted patient continues to ask why she was hospitalized. Her primary nurse wants to tell her that her diagnosis is cancer of the lung. The patient's family insists that the diagnosis be kept from her. Indicate the ethical theories or principles that provide direction for the nurse and for the family. How would you solve this ethical dilemma?
2. A fragile man in his 80s has many sensory and motor deficits from a cerebrovascular accident. When his heart stops, he is resuscitated, and he awakens to find himself hooked up to tubes and machines. He begs to be allowed to die but is repeatedly resuscitated. What ethical principle is being violated in this situation? As his nurse, what steps would you take to be his advocate?
3. One of your coworkers refuses to care for suicide patients in the intensive care, saying, "They wanted to die, so let them." As a peer, how could you appeal to this nurse's moral sense? What principles of ethics are in jeopardy?
4. It is not the practice in your institution to issue contracts to nursing service personnel. How would you, as a nurse leader, initiate a change in this practice? Describe how you would use ethical principles in your arguments in favor of contractual agreements.
5. You discover that one of your colleagues is stealing insulin syringes to take to her diabetic grandmother who cannot afford to buy such disposables. List the steps you would take in confronting her and the ethical principles that would guide you. Role-play this confrontation with one of your classmates.
6. A young couple, who has a newborn with multiple anomalies and deformities, decides against any extraordinary treatment. Using a debate format with another classmate, address these issues: (1) use of differing ethical principles, (2) arguments to support the parents' decision, (3) arguments opposing the parents' decision, (4) allocation of health care resources, and (5) role of the ethics committee.

7. You suspect that one of your staff nurses is stealing patients' drugs for personal use. Her suspicious behavior has also been called to your attention by some of her coworkers. What ethical principles are being violated by the staff nurse stealing drugs? If these drugs are narcotics, what responsibility do you have toward the patient? Toward the nurse?

REFERENCES

1. Flaherty, M.J. (1980). Ethical decision making in an interdisciplinary setting. In K. Sward (Ed.), *Ethics in nursing practice and education*. Kansas City, MO: American Nurses' Association, p. 3.
2. Fry, S.T., & Riley, J.M. (1999). *Ethics and human rights in nursing practice: A multi-state study of registered nurses*. Boston, MA: The Nursing Ethics Network. Retrieved from the World Wide Web: *http://www.bc.edu/nursing/ethics*.
3. Fowler, M., & Levine-Ariff, H. (1987). *Ethics at the bedside: A source book for the critical care nurse*. St. Louis: J.B. Lippincott, pp. 10–15.
4. Barnett, C.W., & Pierson, D.A. (1994). Advance directives: Implementing a program that works. *Nursing Management*, *25*(10), 58–65.
5. Fowler, M., & Levine-Ariff, H. (1987). *Ethics at the bedside: A source book for the critical care nurse*. St. Louis: J.B. Lippincott, pp. 20–25.
6. American Nurses Association (1985). *Code for nurses with interpretive statements*. Kansas City, MO: American Nurses Association.
7. Beauchamp, T., & Childress, J. (1989). *Principles of biomedical ethics*, 2nd ed., New York: Oxford University Press, p. 36.
8. Beauchamp, T., & Childress, J. (1989). *Principles of biomedical ethics*, 2nd ed., New York: Oxford University Press, p. 36.
9. Beauchamp, T., & Childress, J. (1989). *Principles of biomedical ethics*, 2nd ed., New York: Oxford University Press, p. 36.
10. President's Commission for the Study of Ethical Problems in Medicine and Biomedical and Behavioral Research. (1983). *Deciding to forego life sustaining treatment*. New York: Concern for Dying.
11. Office of the Inspector General. (1997, June 15). *Implementation of the patient self-determination act: Executive summary*. Department of Health and Human Services. Retrieved from the World Wide Web: *http://oig.hhs.gov/oei/summaries/b68.pdf*.
12. American Nurses Association. (1985). *Code for nurses with interpretive statements*. Kansas City, MO: American Nurses Association.
13. Fry, S.T., & Riley, J.M. (1999). *Ethics and human rights in nursing practice: A multi-state study of registered nurses*. Boston, MA: The Nursing Ethics Network. Retrieved from the World Wide Web: *http://www.bc.edu/nursing/ethics*.
14. American Nurses Association. (1985). *Code for nurses with interpretive statements*. Kansas City, MO: American Nurses Association.
15. Agich, G.J., & Younger, S.J. (1991). For experts only? Access to hospital ethics committees. *Hastings Center Report*, *21*(5), 17–25.
16. Dalgo, J.T., & Anderson, F. (1995). Notes from the field: Developing a hospital ethics committee. *Nursing Management*, *26*(9), 104–106.
17. Nelson, R.M., & Shapiro, R.S. (1995). The role of an ethics committee in resolving conflict in the neonatal intensive care unit. *Journal of Law, Medicine, and Ethics*, *23*(1), 27–32.

18. Agich, G.J., & Younger, S.J. (1991). For experts only? Access to hospital ethics committees. *Hastings Center Report*, *21*(5), 17–25.
19. Dalgo, J.T., & Anderson, F. (1995). Notes from the field: Developing a hospital ethics committee. *Nursing Management*, *26*(9), 104–106.
20. Nelson, R.M., & Shapiro, R.S. (1995). The role of an ethics committee in resolving conflict in the neonatal intensive care unit. *Journal of Law, Medicine, and Ethics*, *23*(1), 27–32.
21. Drake, B., & Drake, E. (1998). Ethical and legal aspects of managing corporate cultures. *California Management Review*, *30*(2), 107–123.
22. American Nurses Association. (1993). *Sexual harassment: It's against the law*. Washington, D.C.: American Nurses Association.
23. Bandman, E. (1985). Whistle-blowers take risk to halt wrongdoing. In C. Murphy (Ed.), *Ethical dilemmas confronting nurses*. Kansas City, MO: American Nurses Association, p. 18.
24. Sheehan, J. (1996). Advice of counsel: Putting advocacy for patients against job security. *RN*, *59*(1), 55–56.
25. Tammelleo, A.D. (1995). Refusal to "cover up" death: Whistleblower is terminated. *Regan Report on Hospital Law*, *36*(3), 2.
26. Dimotto, J. (1995). Whistle-blowing: Seven tips for reporting unsafe conduct. *Nursing Quality Connection*, *4*(4), 8, 12.
27. Brown, C. (1999). Ethics, policy, and practice: Interview with Emily Friedman. *Image: Journal of Nursing Scholarship*, *31*(3), 259–262.
28. Rotkavitch, R. (1989). The power of the nurse executive. In B. Henry, C. Arndt, M. DiViscenti, & A. Marriner (Eds.), *Dimensions of nursing administration*. Boston: Blackwell Scientific, p. 21.
29. Davis, A. (1980). Ethical decision making: Considerations for future activities. In K. Sward (Ed.), *Ethic in nursing practice and education.*. Kansas City, MO: American Nurses Association, p. 21.
30. American Nurses Association. (1985). *Code for nurses with interpretive statements*. Kansas City, MO: American Nurses Association.
31. OCR. (2001, Winter). OCR to enforce new health care privacy protections, OCR update. Retrieved from the World Wide Web: *http://www.hhs.gov/ocr/newsletter/wi01.html.*
32. Rosenthal, T. (1987). White uniform theft. *Nurse Management*, *18*(4), 89–90.
33. Soalri-Twadall, A. (1990). Peer assistance: One person's experience. *Addictions Nursing Network*, *2*(3), 17–18.
34. New York State Nurses Association (1995). Obligations and rights of nurses whose practice is impaired by addictive diseases: NYSNA's peer assistance for nurses (SPAN) program. *Journal of the New York State Nurses Association*, *26*(2), 14.
35. LaGodna, G.E., & Hendrix, M.J. (1989). Impaired nurses: A cost analysis. *Journal of Nursing Administration*, *19*(9), 13–18.
36. Carroll, M.A., & Humphrey, R.A. (1979). The nurses' professional code of ethics: Its history and improvements. In *Moral problems in nursing: Case studies*. New York: University Press of America.
37. Quinn, C., & Smith, M. (1987). *The professional commitment: Issues and ethics in nursing*. Philadelphia: Saunders, 180.
38. Kohn, L.T., Corrigan, J., & Donaldson, M.J. (2000). To err is human. *Institutes of Medicine Report*. Washington, DC: National Academy Press.
39. Institute of Medicine Round Table Discussion and Report: Crossing the Quality Chasm. (2001). Washington, DC: National Academy Press.
40. American Hospital Association, 840 North Shore Drive, Chicago, IL 60611.

41. American Nurses Association, 600 Maryland Avenue, S.W., Suite 100 West, Washington, D.C. 20024-2571.

42. Hastings Center, 255 Elm Road, Briarcliff Manor, New York, NY 10510.

SUGGESTED READINGS

American Nurses Association Commission on Nursing. (1985). *Human rights guidelines for nurses in clinical and other research*. Kansas City, MO: American Nurses Association.

American Nurses Association Committee on Ethics. (1980). *Ethics in nursing practice and education*. Kansas City, MO: American Nurses Association.

American Nurses Association Committee on Ethics. (1985). *Ethical dilemmas confronting nurses*. Kansas City, MO: American Nurses Association.

American Nurses Association Committee on Ethics. (1988). *Ethics in nursing position statements and guidelines*. Kansas City, MO: American Nurses Association.

Aroskar, M. (1985). Ethics important in allocating health care resources. In C. Murphy (Ed.), *Ethical dilemmas confronting nurses*. Kansas City, MO: American Nurses Association.

Benjamin, M., & Curtis, J. (1992). *Ethics in nursing*, 3rd ed. New York: Oxford University Press.

Canon, B.L., & Brown, J.S. (1988). Nurses' attitudes toward impaired colleagues. *Image*, *20*(2), 96–101.

Cooper, M. (1989). Gilligan's different voice: A perspective for nursing. *Journal of Professional Nursing*, *5*(1), 10–16.

Davidhizer, R. (1988). Confronting employees. *American Operating Room Nursing Journal*, *48*(2), 319–322.

Davino, M. (1995). Advice of counsel: When the nurse with an addiction is your boss. *RN*, *58*(8), 55.

Davis, A.J. (1982). Helping your staff address ethical dilemmas: Formats for ethics rounds. *Journal of Nursing Administration*, *12*, 9–13.

Ethical decisions via rounds and consults. (1986). *Hospital Ethics*, *2*(5), 14–15.

Fowler, M. (1988). Acquired immunodeficiency syndrome and refusal to provide care. *Heart and Lung*, *17*(2), 213–215.

Gilligan, C. (1982). *In a different voice*. Cambridge, MA: Harvard University Press.

Krekeler, K. (1987). Critical care nursing and moral development. *Critical Care Nursing Q*, *10*(2), 1–10.

Mitchell, L. (1995). Resources for ethical decision making. *Journal of Cardiovascular Nursing*, *9*(3), 78–87.

Oddi, L.F., & Cassidy, V.R.(1990). Participation and perception of nurse members in the hospital ethics committee. *Western Journal of Nursing Research*, *12*(3), 307–317.

Raines, C. (1988). Personal value systems: How they affect teamwork. *American Operating Room Nursing Journal*, *48*(2), 324–330.

Silva, M.C. (1992). The ethics of whistle blowing by nurses. *Nursing Connections*, *5*(3), 17–21.

Weeks, L., & Gleason, V., & Reiser, S. (1989). How can a hospital ethics committee help? *American Journal of Nursing*, *89*(5), 651–654.

Windle, P.E., & Wintersgill, C.L. (1994). The chemically impaired nurse's reentry to practice: The nurse manager's role. *American Operating Room Nursing Journal*, *59*(6), 1268–1269.

UNIT 2

An Overview of Organizations and Management

6

Organization and Management Theory

> "Failing organizations are usually over-managed and under-led."
>
> Warren G. Bennis

INTRODUCTION

In this fast-paced environment of new health care organizations, past understanding of organizational behavior is outdated. Today, health care organizations are forming different structures, serving new functions, and require relevant policies. The hospital is no longer dominant in the delivery of health care. Instead, the focal point of the new system is primary care. Despite the reorganization of health care institutions, nurse leaders/managers are expected to coordinate levels of employees and facilitate services for patients. How a complicated web of people function together to meet an organization's goal is explained through sets of concepts known as organization theory. The objective of this chapter is to discuss organization and management theories and their relevance to modern health care organizations.

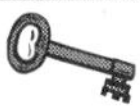

KEY CONCEPTS

Chaos Theory is a way of finding order among random events by identifying trends through mathematical analysis.

Contingency Design is the process of determining the degree of environmental uncertainty and adapting the organization and its subunits to the situation.

Cost Centers are locales of service to which a fixed or preset fee is allocated.

Division of Work is the specialization of effort to produce more, and integrated, work output.

Organization is a social system composed of individuals playing interdependent parts to meet a common goal.

Organizational Chart is a graphic depiction of an organizational structure.

Organizational Learning is a view of the organization as a living and thinking open system capable of changing based on interpretation of environmental stimuli.

Organizing is the establishment of a formal structure of authority through which work subdivisions are arranged, defined, and coordinated for the achievement of defined objectives.

Power is the possession of control, authority, or influence over others.

Social System represents groups of interdependent individuals in social relationships possessing standards and behaviors necessary for the group to meet a common goal.

Span of Control refers to how many, and what levels, of personnel are needed to achieve objectives; the number of subordinates managers manage.

Structure is the internal differentiation and patterning of relationships; the bony skeleton of an organization.

Unity of Command refers to whatever actions or orders come from one command superior only.

Unity of Direction refers to one head, one plan; focus in same direction.

OVERVIEW: ORGANIZATIONAL DYNAMICS

Organizations are a part of everyday life. The social units of family, church, and government are forms of organizations, as well as businesses and health care institutions. An **organization** is defined as a **social system** deliberately established to carry out some definite purpose according to some agreed-upon rules. The purpose, or mission, is carried out efficiently and effectively using both human and nonhuman resources.[1] Since organization theory is the foundation for the management process, management authorities build on the above definition of an organization while emphasizing the pattern of structured relationships, including interpersonal and interdepartmental relationships. People routinely function within organizational structures, and while their behavior is orchestrated, it is often counterproductive to organizational goals. Management then becomes a necessary activity to ensure that organizational goals are met. The task of management is to direct the workforce and available resources within the existing structure. The task of leadership is to provide insights and inspiration to accomplish the work with enthusiasm. Leadership of and by itself is a part of management; however, it is not total management. A good leader can be a weak manager because, although the strong leader gets others to follow, there is no indication that the groups are being led in the proper direction. A manager is required to plan a course of action to reach a goal, wherein the leader's primary responsibility is to challenge the group to follow. Organizational dynamics are those activities that comprise this coordinated social behavior to meet formal goals. It is in this sense that organizational dynamics interact with management and leadership processes. For example, a nurse manager is confronted with the task of reorganizing a department as it merges with another nursing unit. The leader understands that the staff must be led during a period of change and disorganization while managing the day-to-day operations. Knowledge from organization and management theory will help the nurse manager be as effective as possible under trying circumstances.

CLASSICAL THEORY

Organization theory provides a **structure** to understand coordinated and purposeful human behavior and as a foundation for the development of management policies. When people group together and perform different but interdependent work to meet a common objective, this is organized human behavior. The elements of this process are differentiation of labor, a hierarchical structure, and coordination of effort. Early theorists, in the beginning of the 20th century at the time of the Industrial Revolution, developed assumptions about society, people, and management. Classical organization theory, a set of traditions, beliefs, principles, and techniques, studied organized behavior in industry starting in the early 1900s. Classical theory is conveniently divided into three categories: scientific management, administrative management, and the bureaucratic model. Contributors to early theory identified the organization's essential elements, including a common purpose for the organization and its subdivisions; division of labor, or the use of interdependent skills and responsibilities; and a hierarchy that determines privileges, power, and authority. This discussion will limit the study of organization theory to its relationship with the management process.

Scientific Management

The founder of the scientific management movement was Frederick W. Taylor (1856–1915), an engineer and management expert. Taylor proposed a set of techniques that greatly enhanced the efficiency of the manufacturing organization. He developed techniques for systematic job study, time studies, and wage incentives, as well as standardizing methods for different types of industrial work. Scientific management focused on the organization from the manager's perspective and contributed to a more efficient organization.[2]

Administrative Management

Administrative management, another aspect of classical theory, also looked at the organization from the perspective of the administration and management, or from the top down. The primary leaders in this movement were Henri Fayol, a French industrialist;[3] Luther Gullick, an academician and public administration specialist; Lyndall Urwick, a British consultant; and James D. Mooney and Alan C. Reiley, General Motors executives. Fayol's set of universal principles of organization and management are the most commonly reported in the literature; however, all contributed to administrative management's body of knowledge. Between scientific management and administrative management, a group of principles was offered. Each theorist expressed his set of principles differently, but the following represent a synthesis of the main propositions and principles of an organization.

Organizational Principles

The following is a synthesis of organization principles:

- Communication
- Unity of command
- Span of control
- Delegation of authority
- Similar assignments
- Unity of purpose
- General rules

1. **Communication**
   Since a manager has to communicate with so many different persons, communication is a large part of his or her responsibility. In fact, communication consumes about half of each supervisor's work day. Therefore, the need for effective communication is paramount. To ensure effective communication, follow these guidelines:
   - The nature of each position, its duties, authority, responsibilities, and relationships with other positions should be clearly defined in writing and available to all concerned.
   - A clear line of authority should exist from the supreme authority to every individual in the group.
   - Channels of command should not be violated by staff units. A subordinate should never be criticized in the presence of executives or employees of equal or lower rank.
   - The interest of those under you should be promoted when reporting to those over you.
   - Adequate reports must be made, and adequate records must be kept.
2. **Unity of Command**
   When managerial duties overlap, there exists dual command, which confuses workers. The opposite is **unity of command**, wherein workers are responsible for a single area of responsibility and for reporting to one supervisor immediately above the employee (**unity of direction**). To achieve unity of command, observe the following general rules:
   - In any organization, provision is made for centralization of authority and responsibility to the chief executive.
   - No person occupying a single position in an organization should be subject to definite orders from more than one source.
   - You should know to whom you report and who reports to you.

3. **Span of Control**

   Many factors that need to be taken into consideration when determining the number of employees that one supervisor can effectively and efficiently manage. Some of these are the level of managerial experience of the manager, the skill level of the employees, the stability of the work unit or department, the volume of work within the unit or department, the level of morale among the employees, and, lastly, the type of work managed. To determine **span of control**, keep the following guidelines in mind:

   - There is a limit to the number of subordinates that a supervisor can effectively inspire, animate, direct, and coordinate.
   - The supervisor should be responsible for the actions of subordinates.
   - Too few immediate subordinates will result in oversupervision: too many will result in undersupervision.

4. **Delegation of Authority**

   Delegation refers to the designated work within each position. Some amount of participation is an essential part of management. Therefore, responsibility and authority should correspond in every position, as follows:

   - Accomplishment of responsibilities should be limited to only a few delegations after it reaches the operating level.
   - All personnel and activities must be systematically arranged so that authority and responsibility for specific, well-defined duties can be delegated.
   - Orders should never be given to subordinates over the head of a responsible superior.
   - No change should be made in the scope of responsibility of a position without a definite understanding of the effects on all persons concerned.
   - There must be no overlapping of authority (two or more supervisors having control of the same function).

5. **Similar Assignments**

   The responsibilities assigned to a particular unit of an organization are specifically clear-cut and understood, as follows below:

   - A function should not be assigned to more than one independent unit of the organization. Overlapping responsibility will cause confusion and delay.
   - Definite and clear-cut responsibilities should be assigned to each member of the organization.
   - An organization should never be permitted to grow so elaborate as to hinder work assignment.
   - Every necessary function of an organization must be assigned specifically to an individual.

6. **Unity of Purpose**

   Definite plans must be formulated that are based upon the objectives, policies, standards, and work procedures previously accepted by the organization.

   - Every component should work toward unity of effort.

- Authority and responsibility for action are decentralized to the units and individuals responsible for the actual performance of operations.

7. **General Rules**
   - An adequate number of qualified personnel (staffing) is necessary to carry out the plans and to achieve the aims of the organization. Maximum results must be obtained with a minimum of time, effort, supplies, and equipment.
   - Consistent methods of organizational structure should be applied at each level of the organization.

The modern organization continues to implement many of the aforementioned principles because they allow work to be done efficiently. We will see, however, that because people and goals are very complex, some of these rules have been modified for today's health care agencies.

Barnard, an influential thinker, contributed to administrative management through a discussion of authority and its exercise in the organization.[4] Barnard proposed authority to be the right of the superior and maintained that authority is only effective when it is accepted and communicated within the subordinate's "zone of indifference," or willingness to comply. Barnard's work paved the way for the consideration of interactional phenomena, which is the hallmark of the modern behavioral school.

The Bureaucratic Model

The last component of classical theory is known as the bureaucratic model, which describes a particular type of structure. The prominent contributor to this theory, as well as the individual who coined the name, was a German sociologist by the name of Weber, who described the characteristics of a bureaucracy that he felt was the most efficient form of structure for complex organizations.[5] This type of organizational structure is known for the use of extensive rules and procedures to govern the work of the employees. Positions of the employees are arranged in a hierarchy with a given amount of authority and responsibility for each incumbent; positions are defined through job descriptions. To be promoted to a higher level, the employee must demonstrate a level of performance prescribed by an objective criteria. According to Weber, a bureaucracy is a rational structure in which to organize people and tasks, and it demands adherence to principles.

The bureaucratic structure exerts a constant pressure upon its members to be methodological and disciplined to attain a high degree of reliability of behavior and conformity to patterns of action. If the bureaucracy is to function appropriately, discipline is necessary. Herein lies the basic criticism toward this structure: The emphasis is on the task as opposed to the individual. Other structures for the modern organization have evolved to deal with the deficiencies of the bureaucratic structure while trying to retain its stability and unified focus on objectives.

Contribution of Classical Theory

Classical theory offered a highly structured way to create policies for management. However, these same principles have been criticized as being intellectual inventions and not the result of empirical work. More recently Peter Drucker, a renowned management scientist, expressed rigid adherence to these principles will lead modern management astray. In particular, the following assumptions about an organization are out-of-date:

- There is only one right way to organize a business. Structures of an organization must be relevant to meeting the mission of the organization. It is conceivable within any one organization that departments will and should be organized differently.
- There is a single right way to manage people. In the past, emphasis had been on a top-down perspective. Later, decentralization became the norm of management, and currently the team approach is considered appropriate.
- There is no overlap among organizations. This refers to the misconception that each industry exists in a vacuum with its own mission, services, and end-points. Today there is a high degree of interaction among people and a connectedness among different industries. For example, health care is highly connected to insurance companies and legislators (regulators of health care policy).
- Management's job is to run the business or be internally focused. In this current climate, it is also necessary to be externally oriented or aware of the forces that surround the organization.

To suggest the organization is not affected by international concerns is misguided. This assumption is no longer relevant as U.S. health care technology and knowledge are interactive and shared internationally. Drucker explains the new reality of today's world demands abandoning rigid ways of applying organizational principles.[6]

MODERN THEORY

Modern organizational theory represented a new way of viewing people in organizations. The emphasis was on the individuals rather than concentrating on the work or the organizational structure. Modern theory is so designated because of its contribution to organizational theory rather than its chronology. In fact, modern theory originated in the late 1920s and continues through today. It is also referred to as behavioral, or humanistic, theory. To understand the rise of this thought, a review of the sociopolitical background is necessary. The late 1800s to 1920, saw a rapid growth of American industry. This growth, however, was accompanied by poor working conditions, low wages, cheap immigrant labor, high profits for the owners, and the Great Depression.[7] Public sentiment moved from pro-management to pro-labor, and Congress passed the Wagner Act of 1935, which allowed for the formation of labor unions.[8] Thus, the threat of unionization, the Hawthorne Studies, and a philosophy of industrial management were the forces that focused interest on the worker.

Behavioral Science

The contributors to the behavioral school were psychologists and sociologists who studied the workings of private industry. From 1927 to 1932, Mayo and his colleagues at the Hawthorne Works of the Western Electric Company in Chicago ushered in the beginning of the behavioral school. The Hawthorne Studies were the result of Mayo's work. These studies indicated that a group can exert a powerful influence on an individual's productivity. In fact, the ability of the group to influence individuals has come to be known as the Hawthorne effect. In addition, these studies investigated group pressure, social relationships, and supervisory attitudes.[9]

Other leaders in the field who are closely associated with management theory and who made worthy contributions include Douglas McGregor, Renis Likert, Frederick Herzberg, Warren Bennis, and Chris Argyris. More recently, Thomas J. Peters, Robert H. Waterman, Jr., and Stephen Covy have provided insights into personal and organizational success. Each of their specific contributions are discussed under appropriate sections of management topics. This group, with different and interesting insights for modern organizations and management theory, shared a common, optimistic view of the worker in the workplace. They believed that the individual had the potential to be self-directed and capable of enhancing productivity. The emphasis on people was a positive step for organizational theory, but as in classic theory one size does not fit all. There should be a blend of structured principles and a climate to allow individuals to perform. Hierarchy and authority must exist in an organized way to ensure the right of final decision making. The organization is a tool for making people work productively by working together. While this was an important and positive perspective, it stimulated the next step of the modern view, which integrates the worker and the work through systems theory.

General Systems/Social Systems Theory

The social nature of organizations allows the individual to have patterned relationships and to play a specific part in the overall mission of the organization. Social systems theory is a convenient and insightful way to understand the modern organization and how people accomplish the organization's goals. The difference in systems theory and the aforementioned perspectives is that systems theory discusses the organization and worker as a whole rather than as separate entities. A system is defined as an organized combination of united parts or events forming a complex or unitary whole that is coordinated to accomplish a set of goals.[10] This general view of a system provides the necessary overview from which a narrower definition of a social system may be derived. A social system consists of the patterned activities of people that are complementary or interdependent with respect to some common output or outcome, are repeated, are relatively enduring, and are bounded in space and time. A social system is concerned with an individual's participation in society.[11]

When groups of people are thought about in terms of systems, the concept of a social system emerges. This participation may be viewed as groups of individuals joined together in a network of cooperative and conflicting social relationships to achieve common goals developed around a value system, using an organized set of practices and methods to regulate the behavioral standards of the groups.[12] A group has specific patterns of associations and activity in which most persons share their abilities and talents on a day-to-day basis. This is also descriptive of modern organizational behavior. An organization is a social system that permits a structuring of events (or happenings) that have no structuring apart from their functioning. When this social system ceases tofunction (i.e., people stop working),

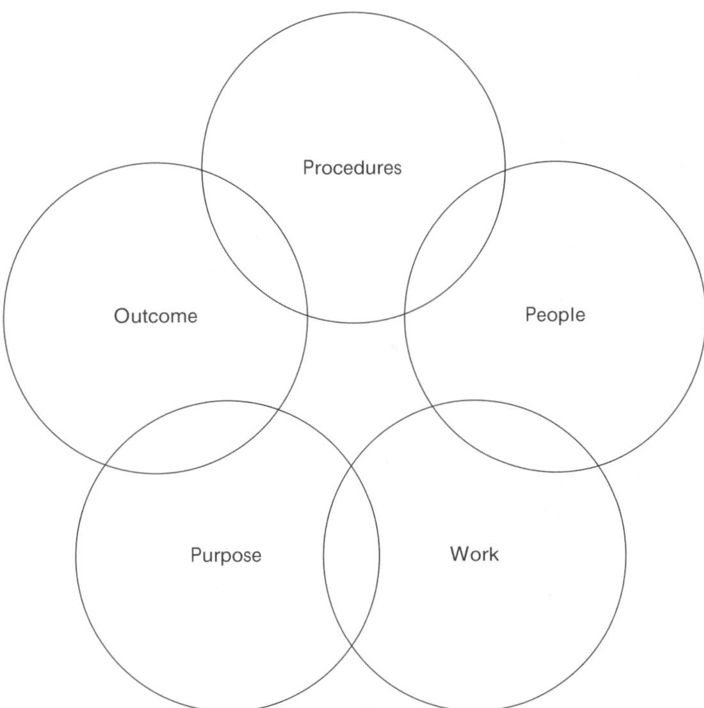

FIGURE 6-1. A graphic representation of the various components of a social system that are also interrelated.

there is no identifiable structure. It is a tendency to think of organizations as buildings or products; yet, the essence of modern systems thinking recognizes that people are the functioning unit of an organization. Without the patterned behavior of the group, there is no social system and, thus, no organization (see Figure 6-1).

Many people have contributed to our current understanding of social systems as an underlying explanatory theory to understand the modern organization. This discussion will focus on a few. Theorists such as Katz and Kahn, and Tosi and Carroll, break down the modern organization into subparts that comprise a whole.[13,14] These subsystems exemplify both the real and behavioral components of the organization. This perspective combines human social behavior and the formal organization structure (see Figure 6-2).

The first conceptual subsystem is known as *Production*, or *Technologic*, and it refers to those activities that are responsible for the end product of the organization, whether that be teaching in a school system, providing patient care in a hospital, or assembling an automobile in a factory. It identifies the major activity of any organization. This particular subsystem is commonly the most responsible for classifying an organization and directs the coordinated activity of the people involved to produce or to meet the goal of the organization.

The next subsystem is called *Supportive* by Katz and Kahn, and *Boundary spanning* by Tosi and Carroll.[15] It involves environmental transactions, such as procuring input for production or disposing of the output. The departments that represent this subsystem are

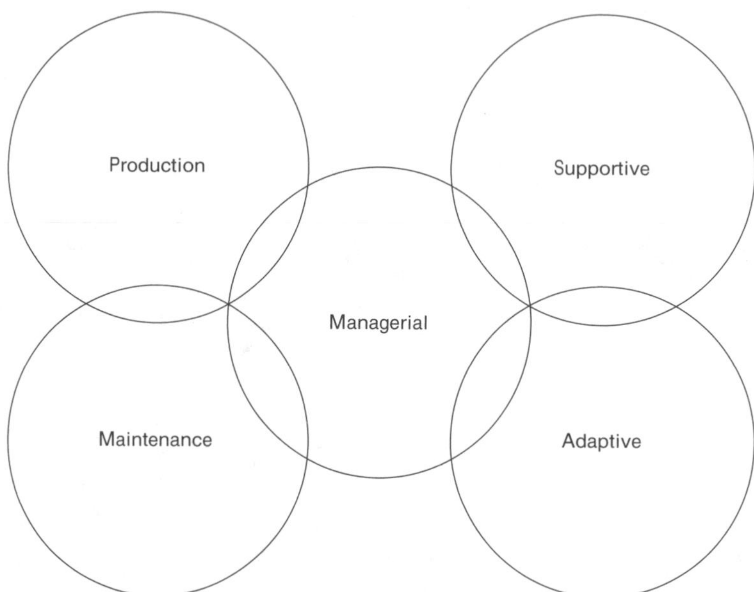

FIGURE 6-2. The various subsystems of an organization that are also interrelated.

purchasing, marketing, or the committee that deals with dangerous waste disposal. These activities involve interaction with the greater social system and acknowledge that the system or organization is open to the forces of change in the world outside.

Maintenance subsystems refer to the upkeep of the equipment or education of the personnel to make sure the work of the organization is properly executed. This might be continuing education or a staff development department. This subsystem keeps the organization functioning and up-to-date.

The next subsystem is the *Managerial*, which refers to the major activities of controlling, coordinating, and directing people, as well as the other subsystems of the organization. Every organization needs the activities of management for the completion of the work.

The last conceptual subsystem is known as the *Adaptive* subsystem, which refers to those activities that ensure organizational survival in a changing environment. Nowhere is this more true right now than in health care. An example is an administration's attempt at strategic or long-range planning.

Modern Systems Theory Models

Because of the influence of the systems approach, a variety of models based on systems theory have been proposed. **Organizational learning,** one such model, views the organization as a living and thinking open system.[16] Since open organizations depend on environmental input and feedback, organizations are said to learn from the interpretation of this input. Thus, organizations engage in complex processes such as anticipating, perceiving, envisioning, and problem solving. This parallels systems theory from the perspective that learning is beyond an individual and includes all persons working together to process this new information for meaningful change. The other, **chaos theory**, also depends on environmental feedback.[17]

Chaos theory, another systems perspective, attempts to find order among seemingly random events. The assumption is that behind every complex system is a set of rules, with its own orderliness and boundaries. The interaction and interconnectedness of the subsystems are the basis of prediction. While seemingly unrelated, all parts of the system are behaving appropriately to ensure the survival of the total system. Two mathematicians, Edward Lorenz and James York, have suggested that this order may be translated into mathematical principles, and the rules of probability.[18]

The Modern Team Concept

Today's organization is relying on, and using, teams to address the complex problems and work of the organization. This concept also evolved from open systems theory which takes into account internal and external forces and a dynamic interplay among units of the organization. Teams take into account the individual expertise of the membership. Nursing is well suited to function within teams, as team nursing (see chapter 7) was a major nursing care delivery system for many years, and nursing has always functioned well within interdisciplinary teams. Teams, as exemplified by the previous examples, may be very diverse in purpose, organization, membership, and rules which govern its implementation.

A *team*, by definition, is a motivated group of people who work together to share resources, are committed to a common objective through coordinated efforts, and produce a product or service far superior than that of an individual alone.[19] The team concept of organizations represents a fundamental change from the way work is structured and organized. It is assumed teams require a different management paradigm and that they are destined to revolutionize the workforce. The benefits of a team within the organization include:

Increased productivity.
Improved quality of service or product.
Enhanced work environment.
Reduced costs to the organization (shared resources, emphasis on efficiency).
Reduced turnover and absenteeism of employees.
Reduced conflict among departments and individuals.
Increased motivation of employees.
Increased adaptability and flexibility among managers and employees.[20]

The essence of team functioning includes an emphasis on processes rather than on individual tasks. Teams require an ability to see outcomes as a group effort rather than an individual's accomplishments. The decision making in teams involves all the participants, and solutions to problems seek to find the root causes rather than an immediate and quick one. Because the nature of the team depends on its mission, there are a variety of team structures. Even this is viewed as a strength, identifying the inherent flexibility of the team model. Teams are interesting ways to achieve organizational goals, but there are potential problems. The most noticeable is the possibility of multiple managers. A staff member may be involved in several teams in the organization, confusing the line of authority in case of a conflict.[21]

Social systems theory, and its variations adapted to the study of organizations, is a way to explain how organizations function through a dissection of the units of purposeful and necessary behavior.

All the preceding theoretical perspectives of organization and management theories share a goal to facilitate the work of the organization. Yet to understand the practical nature of an organization, classical, humanistic, and modern theory contribute to the ability to form organizations that function. It is conceivable to have within one industrial complex a department that is highly structured and another that functions using teams. Despite theoretical differences, there are some organization concepts that are also common to organizational functioning.

Interactional Phenomena

Organizations are so named because of the activity of organizing. **Organizing** is the establishment of a formal structure of authority through which work subdivisions are arranged, defined, and coordinated for the achievement of defined goals. This occurs through interactional phenomena, which emanate directly because of the hierarchical arrangement of interdependent people doing diverse activities. These special phenomenon include power, authority, and status, as well as the process of delegation. Classical theory identified interactional phenomena but modern scholars have studied them. The following section will define the interactional concepts and consider modern contributions.

Power

Power is a force to meet goals and get things done. Powerful people are dominant, and as their power increases, they move upward in the group; conversely, as their power lessens, they move downward. Power is commonly discussed through the five power bases identified by French and Raven: coercive power, reward power, legitimate power, expert power, and referent power.[22] Later, Raven and Kruglanski added a sixth power base, referred to as information power.[23] Hersey and Blanchard identified a seventh base known as connection power.[24] Since power is a transactional process to influence and requires the voluntary support of the group, it is not unlike leadership and is equally elusive. The different types of power emanate from a variety of sources and thus influence people in various ways. Definitions of the power bases follow:

Coercive power is exercised when fear is used to ensure compliance from subordinates. A nursing administrator may state that if the group does not comply with the new staffing policy, then group members will be subject to transfer to a different area of the institution.

Reward power is exercised when the leader or manager uses a position to provide something of value to the employee. A head nurse may be in a position to offer a financial reward, such as a raise, or a personal reward, such as a change in working hours, to the employees. Rewards are a very positive aspect of organizational life.

Legitimate power is comparable to authority. It is the officially sanctioned right of the superior to exact rights and obligations from subordinates. This exercise of power can be used because of the position held by the leader. When power is used in this way it is because the followers are aware of the leader's position and will respond accordingly.

Expert power is the use of superior knowledge and experience to have others do as the leader suggests. The best use of expert power is demonstrated by clinical specialists who do not have line or legitimate authority in their particular institution. Rather, their clinical knowledge allows them to be influential.

Referent power is largely based on a leader's capacity to inspire others to be similar to the leader. It is a type of power that is associated with a leader's personality and the special traits the leader possesses (charisma). A head nurse who is an exceptionally skilled practitioner may be an inspiration to the staff to emulate excellence in nursing practice.

Information power is based on the leader's knowledge of, or access to, information. Followers want or need the information the leader holds. It has been said that knowledge is power, and in this case it is.

Connection power comes from association with a powerful figure. For example, the president's wife has power by virtue of her association with her spouse. In the health care institution, an employee who is a very close friend, or a family member, of the chief operating officer may have the ability to influence a group's decision because of the leader's association.

Management experts are interested in power because it is an interactional process that can be very effective in accomplishing necessary goals. Power can be gained in a variety of ways. To help the leader or manager in the acquisition of power, suggestions have been offered in the form of a chart (see Table 6-1) that summarizes this information.

TABLE 6-1. Skills and Ways to Acquire these Skills for the Purpose of Gaining Power in the Organization

Credibility	Is gained through hard work, gaining skill and becoming competitive in your work, and being very honest in your relationships with other people. Be well-informed and current through professional journals, meetings, and educational conferences. Be well-prepared for presentations using all at your disposal. Audiovisual aids, charts, and graphs provide the basis for a well-researched and documented presentation.
Interpersonal Relations	Good working relationships have to be developed with all coworkers. The suggestions offered for leadership development will help you gain good working relationships because they are built on respect and sensitivity to yourself and others.
Persuasion	To be able to convince others of the appropriateness of your point of view, your argument must be logical and show that your way of thinking is a positive solution. In addition, deal with the issues that are most appropriate for the group you wish to influence by using words that are most familiar to the group you wish to convince.
Membership	Be in a position to speak with, and thus influence, the group. Volunteer to be on committees and to work within the known organization's hierarchy.
Communication Network	Formally and informally talk with people on all levels of the organization. Information comes from many different sources from within the organization. Develop trusting relationships with people, be capable of discretion, and hold confidential information sacred.

Authority

The legitimate right to seek compliance is authority, whereas responsibility dictates the legitimate boundaries of work. There is a direct relationship between the two; thus, they should exist in equal measure. It would be a difficult situation to have responsibility for a task and not have the authority to complete it. Authority by definition is the legitimate right of the superior to exact rights and obligations from subordinates. Authority is an integral part of the fabric of the organization and will be dispersed throughout the organizational structures by virtue of the process of delegation.

There are two ways of delegating authority within the organization: centralized and decentralized. *Centralized* refers to the authority of decision making remaining at the administrative level or central office. *Decentralized* refers to the assignment of decision making away from the central office and close to the operational level.[25] In nursing, this means close to the actual unit level or patient care division. Decentralized authority eliminates the need for levels of management because the nurse manager assumes responsibility for managerial decisions that influence both the patients and staff.

Within the organization are two types of authority. Both forms of authority, when exercised, are able to influence members of the organization. One type is called *line authority*; the other is referred to as *staff authority*. Line authority is the formal, legitimate right of superiors to exact performance from subordinates. It is represented by straight lines on the organizational chart. Staff authority is a consultative or advisory process and is represented as broken lines on the organization chart. Classical theory tended to view line authority as a commodity distributed to positions in measured amounts and did not prescribe a particularly important role to staff authority. The modern organization, however, uses line and staff authority effectively. The use and reliance on consultants demands the integration of experts to deal with modern complexities.

Responsibility

Responsibility, also integral to organizational dynamics, is the obligation to perform according to position requirements. It is an inward obligation to perform so that the entire organization benefits. It is the corollary of authority, as well as its natural consequence.

Status

Another interesting aspect of organizational dynamics includes the awarding of status. Status is the recognition by others that an individual possesses a superior talent or resource. The uniqueness of the organization's hierarchy rewards individuals with varying degrees of importance. Status is a unique concept that serves as a reward, a motivator, and a goal.

Process of Delegation

The process of delegation is the means by which responsibility and authority are entrusted and assigned to the various individuals throughout the organization. These concepts are discussed in greater detail in Chapter 8.

The above-named, briefly presented concepts are the interactional phenomena that occur because people work together in an organized structure. They provide the basic explanation of how individuals take an active part in the operations of the organization. These same concepts also influence the establishment of the formal and informal structure the organization assumes. A structure provides the internal differentiation and patterning of relationships among people, and especially manager and staff.

ORGANIZATIONAL CONCEPTS

Organizational Chart

An **organizational chart** represents the formal organization and all its diverse relationships. It is a visual representation of the chain of authority, **division of work**, levels of management, and functional communication pattern from chief executive to each member of the organization. This view of the organization demonstrates the scaler chain of authority that is represented by the vertical lines clearly showing how line and staff authority has been distributed. See Figures 6-3 and 6-4 for examples of organizational charts.

Organization Structure

The organizational chart is a useful tool that shows us how the modern organization is structured. An organizational structure is the internal differentiation and patterning of relationships. It is the bony skeleton of the organization. The categorizing of an organizational structure is based on the characteristics of the organizing process. Structures of organizations may be categorized as tall, flat, matrix, or contingency. Organizational structures provide the means whereby the organizing process can be accomplished for the organization to meet its goals (see Figure 6-5).

Tall or *vertical* represents an organizational structure that forms when the span of control is small and may also be referred to as a pyramid, or a bureaucracy. This means that managers have fewer subordinates who report to them and likewise report to one superior. This arrangement will produce a hierarchical arrangement, regular assigned activities, written directives, and policy guidance for behavior. This particular structure was and is commonplace in health care because of the scope of responsibility and the diversity of work. In addition, this structure provides for the control of activities of employees. Communication, however, may be distorted because the message, even if written, is sent through the various layers of the organization in a long line.

This structure has characteristically less rigid controls, and more freedom is available to the employees. The manager is able to communicate with less distortion through fewer levels but is not as available to the employees for consultation or supervision because of the wide span of control. Currently, health care institutions are adopting this structure in the department of nursing. This is referred to as flattening the organization by removing levels of management. This activity results in administrative staff with wide spans of control and nurse managers with increased authority. For this structure to be useful, authority must be decentralized to the necessary personnel.

Matrix organizations are similar to team organizational structures. The formal organizational structure may be a bureaucracy, or tall structure, as well as a flat structure. This structure creates groups (or teams) within the organization that belong to different departments but that share common goals that affect the organization as a whole. It basically creates permanent or semipermanent departments within a structure because the needs or goals of the organization require specialized and diverse work. Organizations today are very complex, and the problems faced by such institutions are not always able to be solved within traditional structures. This is because the functional relationships and communication patterns prohibit meaningful problem solving. A matrix structure

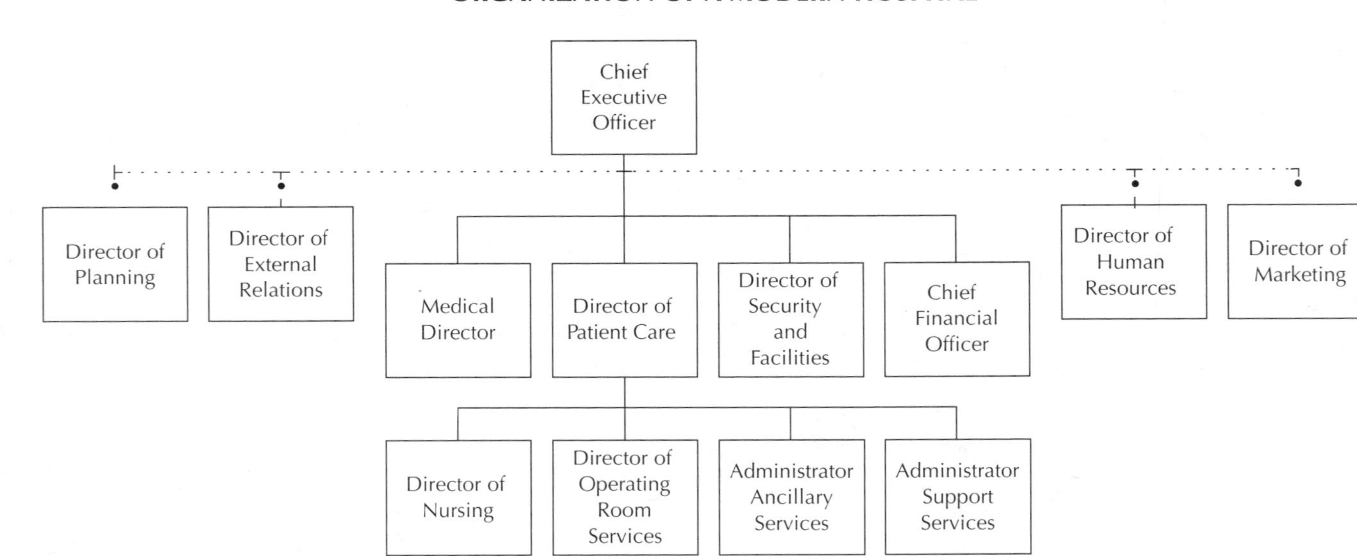

FIGURE 6-3. An example of the organizational chart for an entire hospital.

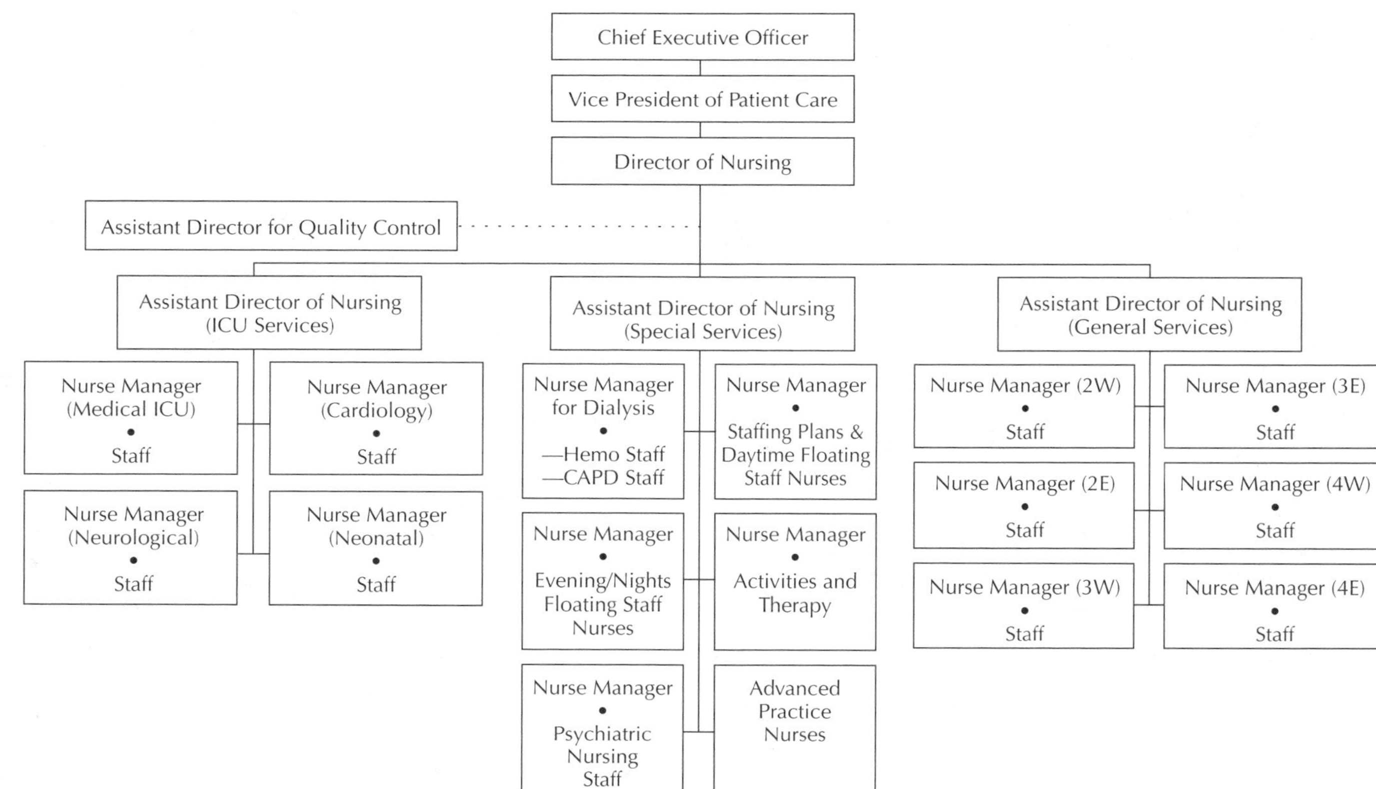

FIGURE 6-4. An example of a department of nursing.

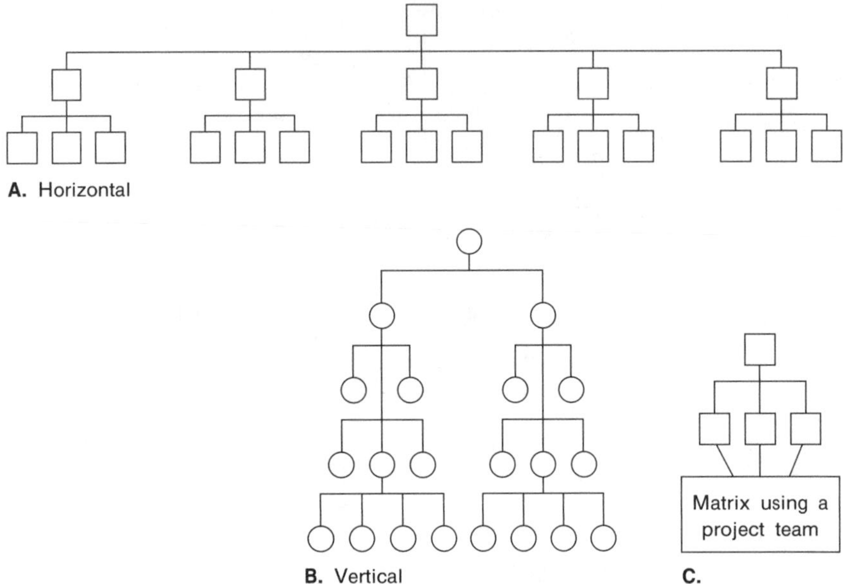

FIGURE 6-5. A variety of organizational structures: (A) horizontal or flat structure, (B) a vertical or tall structure, and (C) a matrix structure.

provides for the creation of a group that would be instrumental in doing the highly complicated problem solving that is necessary. The formation of the new department brings together a group that ordinarily would not be in a position to relate or to communicate because they represent different factions of the organization. This structure is often operationalized through the establishment of project teams with a project manager. The employees are now responsible to the project manager just as they are to the manager of their division. This structure enables organizations to develop solutions to complex problems with the right group of individuals.

Contingency Structure

The contingency structure evolves in response to demands from the situation. The major factors that determine the contingent structure are forces in the environment (or market) and forces within the organization (or technological core consisting of dominant activities). These forces are either stable or volatile (highly changeable). The resulting **contingency design** is the process of determining the degree of environmental uncertainty and adapting the organization and its subunits to the situation.[26] The types of organization structures that evolve are as follows:

- A stable environment and technological core lead to a stable structure such as a flat or tall bureaucratic organizational design. This design, if you remember, works well where conformity to rules and regulations are expected.

- A volatile environment and stable core lead to a market-dominated structure in which much of the energy and resources of the organization are aimed at the marketplace. Examples of these activities would include public relations to determine public views about the service or product.
- A stable environment and volatile technological core lead to a technologically dominated structure in which the organization would have to continuously conform to changing technology. Major resource allocation would be aimed toward keeping the core technology current.
- Volatile environment and technological core lead to a flexible dynamic organization in which change dominates and the structure which forms is able to adapt to information coming from either within or outside the organization. For example, at one time the market concerns would be paramount, and at another time, the technological component would be. The organizational structure would be one that could readily adapt to changing priorities.

INTEGRATED HEALTH CARE SYSTEM

The changing economic, social, and political climate (a volatile environment) has led to transformation of the health care organizations. The issues that are driving the reorganization are quality care (improving patient outcomes), reduction of health care cost, and ensuring patient satisfaction (technological issues). Traditional health care organizations, such as the hospital, are now a unit within a large integrated network (resulting structure). An integrated health care system is a complex network of services to meet the consumers' health care needs. The objective is to keep people healthy and to treat them in the lowest cost setting, of which primary care will be pivotal. The restructuring of health care institutions and reengineering of the work require inventing and managing new systems to meet the needs of the future. Some of the reengineering processes include the elimination of extraneous jobs, determining work to be directed at specific outcomes of the organization, and retraining individuals to have multiple skills rather than hiring highly specialized practitioners with limited skills.[27] Another technique is to reduce the number of managers and levels of management. It is desirable that decisions about work be made by the professional accountable for that decision. This is usually at the level of the operative employee. In addition, increasing the quality and utilization of data will enhance the decision-making process. Thus, decisions will be made on information rather than on circumstances.[28]Currently, the health care system is consolidating its services in preparation for managed competition. The characteristics of this process are the formation of HMOs and PPOs, which provide cost-effective care. Primary care is emerging as the dominant delivery strategy, with health care clinics hiring primary care physicians and nurse practitioners. Patients or clients are being offered incentives to participate in formal groups where capitation is prominent and risk-based reimbursement is provided. Hospitals are joining together by linking acute care services, clinics, and ambulatory care services. To survive this massive reorganization, hospitals

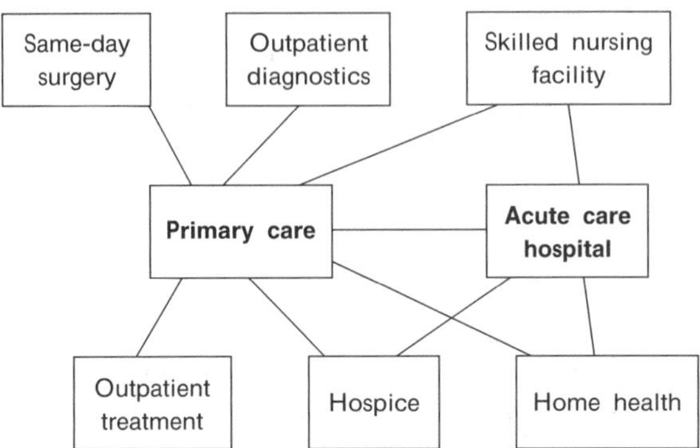

FIGURE 6-6. A graphic depiction of the units of an integrated health care system.

have had to become part of integrated health care networks, share in the financial risk of care, downsize or rightsize, and reduce personnel (see Figure 6-6).

Once consolidation efforts are complete and managed competition is the dominant health care strategy, integrated health care systems will compete for covered lies. All units of this delivery system will be **cost centers**, and the value of care will be systematically evaluated by standardized measures of quality, cost, and patient satisfaction. Organization theory explains these dynamic changes by systematically evaluating the conceptual components of an organization and relating them to the forces that are driving the changes. Organizational models assist in this process.

Organizational Model

Organizational models provide a representation of the conceptual areas of an organization. These components are the subsystems that together explain how and why an organization functions. Similar to a road map, organizational models assist the manager to consider the effects of an action on the organization as a whole (see Figure 6-7). Throughout this text, emphasis has been placed on the importance of: (1) practicing leadership and management based on a comprehensive analysis of factors found in the greater social system or the present situation and (2) forces within the participants which influence the situations. A model is offered that preserves this view by identifying those aspects of organizational dynamics that enhance or inhibit the achievement of goals. The following discussion defines the components of the model and relates them to the turbulence in the health care system.

The greater social system provides direction and definition to the organizational goals as well as the standards to judge the effectiveness of the work. The goal of the particular health care agency is determined by which aspect of health care is being addressed. For instance, the hospital will provide acute care to the patients. To a great extent, the current reorganization of health care has occurred because of the action and attitudes of the greater society. The need for cost containment, emphasis on health (not sickness), and growing partnerships between the health care community, providers, and consumers have revised the health care delivery in which prevention dominates and primary care is the central delivery mechanism.

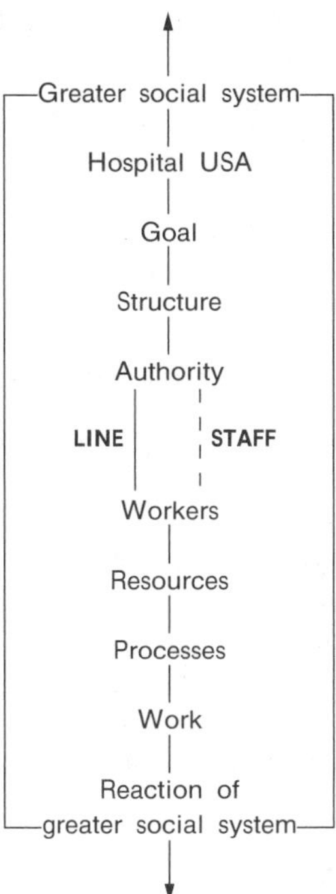

FIGURE 6-7. An organizational model with its components. The arrows represent the reciprocal relationship that exists between the organization and the social environment it serves.

The structure of the organization is directly related to the complexity, level, and diversity of necessary services and individuals needed to meet the particular goal or mission of the organization. The structure can take the form of a traditional bureaucratic organization, matrix, or contingency. The organizational structures within the new health care delivery system represent interdependent and integrated units of care whose aim is to provide a seamless health care delivery system. The structure provides the means whereby the mission of each aspect of the system, as well as the system itself, is operationalized.

Authority represents the fundamental process that brings logic and order to the work of the organization and is integral to organizational dynamics. This authority will either be line or staff, which represents different modes of influence and different sources of power. Line authority is represented in the scaler chain. Authority, known as staff, refers to a form of influence used by specialized individuals who hold unique roles in the organization and who, while not directly responsible for employees, are involved with the outcome of the employees' work. These individuals serve as consultants or advisors to the staff and in some situations may have legitimate authority over the personnel. An example is the clinical nurse specialist who has a staff position in relationship to employees. The authority in the new health care climate is shared with the patient and decentralized to the operative employee who participates with the patient for shared decision making.

The worker or individual who performs in a particular way prescribed in part by the organization and in part by self-direction plays a unique role in organizational dynamics. The orchestration of all members or workers in the total organization, in combination with available resources and the variety of processes, produce the work of the organization. The outcome of the coordinated effort that uses the variety of people in a range of roles to complete the work of the organization is subject to further evaluation by the greater social system, representing the recipient of the service.

Organization and Management Link

This attempt to organize and to classify human behavior within the organizational context gives direction to the study of management. Organizational theory, in a broad and conceptual sense, tells us what is involved when people come together for a similar purpose. Management theory gives us the practical knowledge and tools to meet the demands set by the goals of the organization. Specifically, management maintains the internal structure of the organization that effectively gets the job done. In addition, the manager deals with the human side of the organization: the people and their concerns. The manager also must be the leader ready to adapt to change from within and outside the organization and all for the purpose of meeting specific goals.

Properties of an Organization

Organization theory and management theory, while different, are related. There are properties of an organization that relate directly to management. These properties, as summarized by Caplow and reiterated by Peter Drucker, are as follows:[29, 30]

- All organizations closely resemble each other so that much of what is learned by managing one can be applied to others. These characteristics include a history, a collective identity or image, specialized activities and procedures, a set of formal rules undermined by informal rules, a special vocabulary, and division of labor which affords status.
- Every organization, except the very smallest, is a cluster of suborganizations of varying size. Systems theory explains the interpersonal and social character of the workplace. The need for the various aspects of the organization to function interdependently produce the work output.
- Problems of managing a large organization are similar to those of managing smaller organizations. The role of the manager is to maintain a balance between cooperation and conflict. For a social system to thrive, conflict must be managed, meaningful communication must be encouraged, motivation opportunities must be offered, and evaluations must be provided.
- During any given interval in an organization's history, it will be growing, stable, or declining. Critical to the survival of any organization is regular and systematic evaluation. The cycle of an organization is to grow, stabilize, and decline. Without a concerted effort to keep an organization sensitive to its mission and constituency, it will fail. Periodic evaluations of how effective the organization is performing is necessary to objectively consider change. Despite efforts to keep the organization flourishing, most organizations develop crises from time to time. The manner in which these episodes are managed either ensures survival or hastens decline.

- Most organizations find it easier to satisfy some of their goals more than others for reasons beyond their control. The complexity of people and their motivation often complicates the predictability of the work outcome. However, unexpected results sometimes are extremely helpful and good for the organization.

CASE STUDY

Head Nurse Power

Mrs. Jackson is the nurse manager on a coronary care step-down unit. She has a habit of dictating solutions to her staff whenever a problem arises. She also publicly degrades and demeans her staff, using a rather superior attitude. Unfortunately, she also shows favoritism to some members of her staff. Those who she likes get the best hours and vacation time. The rest of the staff are intimidated by her, and those who dare to confront her to discuss their problems are assigned the worst hours or shifts, and their requests for change are ignored. The stress and tension on the division is great. For instance, Mary Jones, a nursing assistant, asked Pat Polk, an RN, for assistance with her patient. Pat responded, "No, that's not my patient." Conditions on the division have deteriorated, and Mrs. Jackson's response has been to be even more dictatorial.

- What type of power is being utilized in this situation?
- What are the consequences of a strong negative leader?
- What could the staff do with a situation just described?

CASE STUDY

Authority and Responsibility

A small neurosurgical unit, which up until recently displayed good interpersonal relationships among the nurses and nurse aides, has suddenly developed problems. Because other hospitals in the vicinity have closed their neurosurgery units, the census of this unit has continued to increase and is usually maximally occupied. In the past, the nursing staff worked cooperatively, but recently the staff stopped working as a team. The nurse aides are expected to take eight patients, and the nurses are assigned five patients. The nurse aides have stopped completing their job responsibilities, such as bathing patients and changing beds. The nurses subsequently have had to complete the nurse aides' work. This has led to poor working relationships between the two groups. The nurse manager spoke to the nurse aides at the request of the nurses a number of times. Each time, the nurse aides improved their performance for a day or two, and then fell back into the same pattern of not completing their work. The tension between the nurses and nurse aides continues to rise and the situation remains unresolved.

- Who is most responsible to correct this situation?
- What forms of power are being used in this situation?
- Would creating a work team composed of specific nurses and nurse aides be helpful?
- What situational forces led to this situation? Can they be addressed?

CASE STUDY

Organizational Policy

A new policy was posted on the nurse's station of the nursery. The sign read: "To protect patient privacy and confidentiality, no families or patients are allowed beyond this point." The evening nurse read the policy and proceeded to care for the babies. It was an especially busy evening, and one of the infants, whose family had a difficult time coming to the hospital, needed attention and a feeding. The nurse, who was behind in charting, decided to take the infant to the nurse's station and chart while holding and feeding the baby. She was approached by the charge nurse, who informed her of the policy and to kindly comply. The nurse took the baby back to its room for care, and stayed overtime to finish charting and work.

- What do you think of the policy?
- Do conditions change the interpretation of a policy?
- What else could have been done in this situation?

NOTE: Some policies, while well intentioned and appropriate, have to take into consideration the existing work climate and culture. Modifications may need to be in order, such as the time of enforcement or providing barriers to allow the work to be done properly while maintaining the confidentiality of individuals.

SUMMARY

This chapter discussed organization and management theory, looking first at classical theory's contribution and then at modern theory, with special emphasis on social systems theory. The modern organization is a source of complex relationships and functions. An organization model was presented to bring together the key concepts that define the organization and represent the source of analysis for studying organizational behavior and its consequences. To illustrate the model's usefulness, the forces that influence health care reform were used to illustrate the components of the model. Organization and management theories are presented as fundamental to the development of a manager. The relationship between organization and management theory was presented as a way to link abstract concepts to the process of management.

LEARNER EXERCISES

1. Draw the formal organization chart at the agency you are currently working at as a student nurse.
2. Examine the chain of authority in your clinical agency. Draw a representation of who influences whom. Does this match the formal chart of your agency?
3. Distinguish between the different types of power. From your clinical experience, identify individuals who use each type of power. What position does each hold and what behavior does each exhibit? Are the behaviors different?

4. From the following checklist, identify if working teams (from your experience or observation) are effective or ineffective:

Aspect		
Working Conditions	❑ Informal, relaxed	❑ Bored, tense, indifferent
Discussion	❑ Focused, shared, mutual	❑ Unfocused, dominated by a few
Objectives	❑ Understood and accepted	❑ Unclear, undercurrents
Listening	❑ Respectful	❑ Judgmental, and interrupting
Conflict	❑ Comfortable and open	❑ Uncomfortable, aggressive, or hostile
Decision Making	❑ Consensus and shared	❑ Premature, majority vote
Criticism	❑ Constructive, frank, direct	❑ Embarrassing and personal
Leadership	❑ Shared	❑ Autocratic
Assignments	❑ Clear and accepted	❑ Unclear and resentful
Feelings	❑ Freely expressed	❑ Hidden, explosive, and inappropriate
Self-Regulation	❑ Frequent, productive, continuous	❑ Infrequent or outside of meetings

Adapted from McGregor, 1960.

REFERENCES

1. Kast, F., & Rosenzweig, J.E. *Organization and management: A system approach.* 4th ed, St. Louis: McGraw-Hill, p. 108.
2. Taylor, F.W. (1911). *Shop Management.* New York: Harper & Row.
3. Fayol, H., & Storrs, C. (trans.). (1949). *General and industrial management.* London: Pitman and Sons.
4. Barnard, C. (1938). *The functions of the executive.* Boston: Harvard University Press.
5. Weiss, R.M. (1983). Weber on bureaucracy: Management consultant or political theorist? *Academy Manage Revue, 8,* 242–248.
6. Drucker, P. (1998, October 5). Management's New Paradigms. *Forbes,* 177–182.
7. Kreitner, R. (1995). *Management,* 6th ed. Boston, Toronto: Houghton Mifflin Co., p. 51.
8. Kreitner, R. (1995). *Management,* 6th ed. Boston, Toronto: Houghton Mifflin Co., p. 51.
9. Stephen, R., & Jones, R.G. (1990, April). Worker interdependence and output: The Hawthorne studies revisited. *American Sociologic Review, 55,* 176–190.
10. Von Bertalaniy, L. (1968). *General systems theory foundations, development, application.* New York: Braziller.
11. Kast, F., & Rosenweig, J.E. (1985). *Organization and management: A system approach,* 4th ed. St. Louis: McGraw-Hill, p. 108.

12. Kast, F., & Rosenweig, J.E. (1985). *Organization and management: A system approach*, 4th ed. St. Louis: McGraw-Hill, p. 109.
13. Katz, D., & Kahn, R. (1978). *The social psychology of organizations*, 2nd ed. New York: Wiley.
14. Tosi, H., & Carroll, S. (1975). *Management: Contingencies, structure, and process.* Chicago: St. Claire Press, p. 156.
15. Tosi, H., & Carroll, S. (1975). *Management: Contingencies, structure, and process.* Chicago: St. Claire Press, p. 158.
16. Kreitner, R. (1995). *Management*, 6th ed. Boston, Toronto: Houghton Mifflin Co., p. 52.
17. Kreitner, R. (1995). *Management*, 6th ed. Boston, Toronto: Houghton Mifflin Co., pp. 52–53.
18. Wheatley, M. (1992, December). Searching for order in an orderly world: A poetic for post-machine age managers. *Journal of Management Inquiry*, 340.
19. Fisher, K. (1993). *Leading self-directed work teams: A guide to developing new team leadership skills.* New York, McGraw-Hill.
20. Fisher, K. (1993). *Leading self-directed work teams: A guide to developing new team leadership skills.* New York: McGraw-Hill, p. 50.
21. Fisher, K. (1993). *Leading self-directed work teams: A guide to developing new team leadership skills.* New York: McGraw-Hill, p. 54.
22. French, J.R.P., & Raven, B. (1968). The bases of social power. In D. Cartwright & A. Zander (Eds.), *Group dynamics research theory* (pp. 259–269). New York: Harper & Row.
23. Raven, B.H., & Kruglanski, W. (1975). Conflict and power. In P.C. Swingle (Ed.), *The structure of conflict* (pp. 177–219). New York: Academic Press.
24. Hersey, P., & Blanchard, K. (1988). *Management of organizational behavior.* 5th ed. Englewood Cliffs, NJ: Prentice Hall, p. 214.
25. Kreitner, R. (1995). *Management*, 6th ed. Boston, Toronto: Houghton Mifflin Co., p. 54.
26. Porter-O'Grady, T. (1994, December). A systems approach to managing transformation. *Seminars for Nurse Managers*, 2(4), 191–195.
27. Porter-O'Grady, T. (1994, December). A systems approach to managing transformation. *Seminars for Nurse Managers*, 2(4), 191–194.
28. Porter-O'Grady, T. (1994, December). A systems approach to managing transformation. *Seminars for Nurse Managers*, 2(4), 191–194.
29. Caplow T. (1976). *How to run any organization.* Orlando, FL: Harcourt, Brace and World.
30. Drucker, P. (1998, October 5). Management's new paradigms. *Forbes*, 160–170.

7

Overview of Nursing Management

"A manager is like a sailor who can't control the wind, but may adjust the sails."

Author Unknown

INTRODUCTION

Today, there is a need for a new and fresh approach to management. Nurse managers are challenged to define the expected outcomes and organize the resources of the organization to attain those results which will also be evaluated outside of the organization. Nurses are practicing in new settings and organizations that require different and expanded roles. Entry-level nurses need management skills to perform their responsibilities with patients and personnel. Clinical management of patients and clients involves the maintenance of quality patient care, judicious use of scarce resources, and provision of cost-effective nursing services. Simultaneously, nurses will be required to supervise unlicensed and certified caregivers within their scope of authority. The time, energy, and resources spent on developing management skills are worthwhile investments in the future of health care. The dividends are great in terms of successful patient care outcomes, as well as motivated and competent employees

Today's health care system and tomorrow's challenges provide opportunities for nursing management. To become a manager, a new process must be learned, new skills must be acquired, and new attitudes must be adopted. Much of what is known about professional management has been derived from work in other disciplines. However, the nursing profession is developing its own unique and innovative management strategies as nurse researchers and administrators study the management process. This chapter will provide an overview of the management process and what it entails.

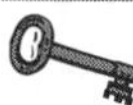

KEY CONCEPTS

Controlling is the management function that regulates activities with plans according to standards.

Coordinating is the management activity that assembles and synchronizes people and activities so that they function harmoniously in the attainment of organizational objectives.

Directing is the management activity that gets work done through others by: (1) giving directions, (2) supervising, (3) leading, (4) motivating, and (5) communicating.

Management is a process with both interpersonal and technical aspects through which the objectives of an organization (or part of it) are accomplished by efficiently and effectively using resources.

Organizing is the management function that provides the relationship between people and activities in such a way as to fulfill the organization's objectives.

Planning is the primary management function that decides in advance what needs to be done and charts the course for future action.

Staffing is the management activity that ensures the proper ratio of workers to work.

Systems of Nursing Care are the organizational and professional structures that provide delivery of nursing care. They are: (1) the case method, (2) functional nursing, (3) team nursing, (4) job redesign (primary nursing), and (5) system's redesign (case management)

MANAGEMENT PROCESS

Management is considered a discipline and a process. Management, as a process, uses both interpersonal and technical aspects through which the objectives of an organization (or part of it) are accomplished efficiently and effectively by using human, physical, financial, and technological resources.[1] The management role is dedicated to facilitating the work in the organization through one's own efforts and the efforts of others. Transition to a management role means assuming a position of authority, with its inherent complexity. The new manager is cast into a role whose tasks are conceptual.[2] The problems that are experienced are often long term, and satisfaction also becomes delayed and abstract. Just as was stated in the previous chapter, there is no one way to structure an organization; therefore, management skills will, of necessity, be varied to accomplish the goals of the organization. This is accomplished through the management process, which consists of:

- Establishing the organization's objectives.
- Developing plans to meet the stated objectives.
- Assembling the necessary resources.
- Supervising the execution of the plans.
- Evaluating the progress or outcome of the stated plan.

Renes Likert's Four Systems of Management

System One	System Two	System Three	System Four
Exploitive-Authoritative	Benevolent-Authoritative	Consultative	Participative

Leadership
Motivation
Communication
Decisions
Goals
Control

FIGURE 7-1. Likert identified four systems of management. The differences among the systems were based on the way managers dealt with the above factors.

Management is an essential activity for organizations. Systematic study of what managers do and how the manager uses this process provides the necessary information to increase the overall efficiency of the organization.

LEVELS OF MANAGEMENT

Managers are expected to make decisions about how others will use their time and be responsible for the supervision of others. Professional nurses and other members of the health team (operative employees) who are not managers are expected to perform those activities that constitute the work (or part of it) for the organization. It is in this capacity that the professional nurse will either manage employees or care for patients. Since the organization is a hierarchy, the work of management is divided into levels of responsibility. Managers at all levels (top, middle, and front line) do the work of management. Top management, or the administrative level, is composed of the board of directors, the president, and the vice presidents. The vice president of nursing is among this group whose responsibilities include managing managers. Middle management includes division heads and directors of nursing (and evening and night supervisors). This group manages front-line managers. Front-line, or lower-level, managers (sometimes called unit managers) are nurse managers (head nurses, charge nurses); they manage staff employees. The various levels of managers use the management process in accord with their scope of responsibility. These levels are pictured in Figure 7-1.

MANAGEMENT SCIENCE

Management has been studied by scholars from business, sociology, psychology, and the military. Different theorists offered frameworks to study the process of management and administration, resulting in a general body of management concepts. For instance, McGregor and his Theory X and Theory Y approach to the supervision of people suggests that there are two classes of supervisors.[3] Theory X assumes that people hate work and as a result have to be coerced, controlled, and directed by their supervisors. Theory Y, however, assumes that people take to work like play and as a result are self-directed, responsible, and capable of solving problems. Other theorists elaborated on this work by placing emphasis on positive relationships between the superior and subordinate.

Herzberg provided assumptions about the motivations of people, namely that most people are motivated by intrinsic factors rather than extrinsic factors.[4] Intrinsic factors are associated with self-actualization on the job and include achievement, recognition, responsibility, growth, and advancement. Extrinsic, or maintenance, factors are those that had been traditionally perceived by management to be motivators, and include company policy, supervision, working conditions, salary, and job security. Both McGregor and Herzberg are discussed in Chapter 10.

Argyris looked at the effects of organizational life and motivation to facilitate a consistency between the organization's and the individual's goals.[5] In his book *Integrating the Individual and the Organization*, Argyris stated his concern with the employee's psychological growth. The concern centered around the employee's ability to self-actualize within a system that, by and large, was in conflict with this need. Argyris argued that the challenge to modern organizations was to allow the maturing person to grow in an environment that was basically immature.

Likert set out four detailed systems of management that ranged from the highly autocratic to the highly participative.[6] The four systems include:

- *System 1*: Exploitative–authoritative
- *System 2*: Benevolent–authoritative
- *System 3*: Consultative
- *System 4*: Participative

The system of participative management has been suggested to be one of the most successful, and those companies that have employed it report positive results (see Figure 7-2). Nursing researchers have attempted to provide empirical data to evaluate the effectiveness of management styles, using Likert's systems and staff reaction. Results overwhelmingly support the participative style of management as the most desirable style that produces staff satisfaction and retention.[7]

Top	Vice presidents	Board of Directors President	Vice presidents
Middle	Supervisory staff Department heads		Directors of nursing service Supervisors
Front line			Head nurses Staff

FIGURE 7-2. The various levels of management: top, middle, and front line.

Peters and Waterman, two well-known management scientists, conducted a study of the 62 best-run companies in America, and concluded eight principles of excellence.[8] This has become known as the excellence approach. While not all eight attributes were present in every successful company, a preponderance of them were reported. The proposed attributes of excellence are as follows:

1. "A bias for action" refers to involved managers. Managers are visible and close to the work unit. These managers are ready and willing to become involved.
2. "Close to the customer" refers to a need to seek customer satisfaction above all else. Active input is sought on a regular basis from those who are served.
3. "Autonomy and entrepreneurship" refers to the encouragement of risk taking, and the tolerance for failure among employees.
4. "Productivity through people" concerns the emphasis of respect for individuals in the workplace. Enthusiasm, trust, and a family feeling are fostered.
5. "Hands-on value-driven" refers to a clear company philosophy that is disseminated and followed. The organization's belief system is reinforced. Leaders are positive role models, not rigid authoritative managers.
6. "Stick to the knitting" means managers manage and employees do what they do best. Emphasis is on the internal growth of the company.
7. "Simple form, lean staff" refers to decentralizing authority as much as possible. Management staffs are kept to a minimum, and talented employees are at the work site.
8. "Simultaneous loose-tight properties" refers to stringent strategic and financial control counterbalanced by decentralized authority, autonomy, and opportunities for creativity.[9]

The various insights represented by the different management theorists have been both praised and critiqued in the management literature. Nevertheless, they share some common assumptions, and may be summarized by the following:

- Managers must trust the employees to be responsible for the performance of their jobs.
- Organizational structures must be flexible enough to allow the employees to function well.
- Managers must have some input and control over the employees' work for the work to be effective.[10]

These beliefs have guided the development of managers in all fields, including nursing. Based on the assumptions of professional management, nursing has expanded the role of manager to include patient welfare.

MANAGEMENT IN NURSING

A philosophy of service is what differentiates nursing management from professional management in other fields. Because of nursing's social responsibility toward the health and illness of individuals, families, and communities, a unique approach is required. The quality of care to be delivered is as important a consideration as the staff and resources used. Thus, success depends on the quality of service as well as the ability to deliver care within a given set of resources. This dual goal of management demands thoughtful and specific professional strategies.

In a recent study conducted by the Nursing Administration Research Project (NARP), a set of priorities was proposed. The top ten of these important research concerns address the uniqueness of nursing management:

1. Effects of the managed care environment on patient outcomes.
2. Impact of organizational change(s) on patient outcomes.
3. Development of tools to measure nurse-sensitive patient outcomes.
4. Impact of administrative practices on patient outcomes.
5. Effect of nursing interventions on patient outcomes.
6. Role of informatics in measurement of outcomes.
7. Effect of changing skill mix on patient outcomes.
8. Identify nursing's contribution to the bottom line.
9. Development of outcomes that can be used across the care continuum.
10. Quality care and its key outcomes.[11]

Evolution of Nursing's Management Role

In the new health care environment, the role of management and manager is changing. The middle management level has been dramatically downsized, and the administrative level is often responsible for a multiple of units within a network. Downsizing and flattening the organization have stimulated reconceptualization of the manager's role. In the past, nurse managers supervised one or two levels of employees, and often relied on an authoritative style. This style emanated from legitimate organizational authority and positional power. The majority of these managers learned their skills by watching their immediate supervisor. They believed there was a need for control and felt an overwhelming sense of responsibility for everything that happened. This control method was a readily accepted practice during these earlier times, and keeping people in line became the norm of a manager's work life.[12] It was an illusion of control and power over employees.

In the mid-1980s, a new concept known as shared governance introduced the idea of shared decision making. This concept suggested that decisions be reached by consensus, not by vote. Staff members were invited to share their views and give input into problem solutions. Despite some hesitation and problems, this methodology was viewed as a transition to a positive and inspiring managerial style. Contrary to past belief, the more staff knew, the better (and more informed) were the decisions. The activities that cultivated shared decision making created a profound impact on the managerial role. Managers needed to learn methodologies that would facilitate staff participation and staff development.[13] Instead of controlling the staff behavior, managers were expected to help staff be responsible for their own behavior. Thus, managers needed education to cultivate a style that would empower the staff. In the current system the manager is expected to be a team facilitator.[14] This means managers have the responsibility to help the staff become successful in their endeavors, which is the work of the organization. This approach to management conforms with the leadership theories that empower the employee.

OBJECTIVES OF NURSING MANAGEMENT

Nursing, a service field, is highly labor-intensive, making nursing management particularly challenging because of the wide variety of experience and educational backgrounds of the employees in the health care setting. The types of work, as well as the workers, challenge the nurse manager to create the kind of environment that facilitates quality nursing practice. The nurse manager has specific responsibilities to the organization and to the staff. The staff, in turn, have responsibilities to the organization and to the manager. The beginning nurse will contribute to the success of the unit's efficiency by being aware of the manager's role. In general, the manager has certain responsibilities. They include:

- Accomplishing the goals of the organization or nursing division.
- Maintaining the quality of patient care within the financial limitations of the organization.
- Encouraging the motivation of the employees and the patients in the area.
- Increasing the ability of subordinates and peers to accept change
- Developing a team spirit and increased morale.
- Furthering the professional development of the personnel.[15]

These objectives are met in varying degrees of efficiency and effectiveness, depending upon the same framework espoused throughout this text. The successful manager is one who is keenly aware of those forces that are relevant to the managerial situation.

The manager should accurately understand the goals, the relationship between the manager and employee, the special abilities of the employee, and those relevant organizational and social factors that impact the situation. Analyzing the managerial situation and using the appropriate management tool will assist in accomplishing the organization's goals. A managerial assessment tool is offered at the end of this chapter to highlight essential factors so that positive action can be taken. The managerial role involves making good decisions based on the management process and the use of management functions.

MANAGEMENT FUNCTIONS

Success of management depends on an individual's talent, motivation, and opportunity to manage. The first step in developing talent is to become familiar with the traditional management functions (see Figure 7-3). These functions, which are expected of managers, include planning, organizing, staffing, directing, coordinating, and controlling. Managers develop skills in the implementation of these functions as they gain experience in the role of manager. Nurse managers also use the same functions as they fulfill their responsibilities.

Planning

The most basic and essential activity of management is **planning.** Planning is the primary management function that decides in advance what needs to be done for the day,

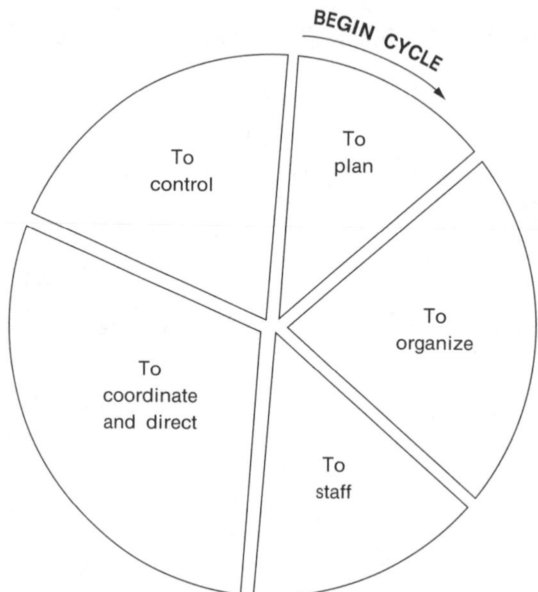

FIGURE 7-3. A graphic depiction of the management functions.

month, or years ahead. It charts the course for future action. Planning is also an activity of the practitioner. To manage care for a patient or a group of patients, planning will facilitate the use of time, activities, and resources. If there is a deviation from the overall plan of care (similar to a critical path), understanding the problem and what to do will be greatly assisted. Just as a patient's condition alters activities for the practitioner, so too will unusual events change the plan for the manager.

Planning will provide the overall structure to accomplish necessary work and, properly, should include possible problems. Specifically the reasons for planning are:

- To focus attention on objectives.
- To offset uncertainty and chance.
- To gain economic operation.
- To facilitate control.

Planning requires a thoughtful reflection of what it is you want to accomplish and how to accomplish it within a given set of resources. Careful analysis of the managerial situation will provide the basis for a well-developed plan for action and will reveal problems that require solutions. Analysis is the related activity that provides the leader or manager with essential elements of the plan. The greater the analysis, the better the plan. Experience and knowledge facilitate the acquisition of this skill.

Types of Planning

Various types of planning strategies are available to the manager, namely standing, strategic, and long range. The most basic is a standing plan, or a stable plan, which lists daily or standard activities. The practitioner uses standing plans similar to a nursing care plan. The manager will use standing plans as a way of organizing time and activities. This may include monthly meetings, weekly staff sessions, and daily review of the patient/client services. This type of plan will provide the manager with a general framework for the purpose of allocating time.

Strategic planning is market- and future-oriented, intended to provide a plan for the life of the entire organization or network. Such planning is part and parcel of an organization's attempt to remain competitive. This kind of planning occurs at an administrative level or at top management and includes an in-depth analysis of those factors within and outside of the organization. Today, strategic planning is involved with methods to increase revenue, consolidate services, reduce loss of profit, and provide income-producing services.[16] Administration alone has the authority to initiate and to commission such comprehensive plans. However, since the mid-1980s, middle- and front-line managers are more frequently being involved in strategic planning efforts.

Long-range planning is also a form of future-oriented planning but is more general and provides a direction for organizational growth. A plan of this nature elaborates 1-, 5-, and 10-year goals. The goals are subject to change as relevant circumstances change. The administration of organizations routinely have long-range planning meetings to continually develop goals for the future. All managers (front line, middle, and top level) will use planning as an important tool but will keep in mind that different types of planning will be determined by the responsibilities of the manager. The vice president of nursing who has a broad scope of responsibility uses planning differently than the new front-line manager or head nurse.

Organizing

Organizing is the management function that relates people and activities in such a way as to fulfill organizational objectives. An organization provides a mechanism through which this can be accomplished, known as vertical and horizontal differentiation.

Vertical differentiation refers to the establishment of a hierarchy, or number of levels, needed to do the work of the organization. Management must decide on a tall or flat structure. *Horizontal differentiation* results from the need to separate activities for more efficient and effective performance. This occurs by forming departments within an organization, enabling work to be accomplished through differentiation of labor or the provision of different services. Take, for instance, the number of units necessary to provide care for surgical patients. The laboratory, radiology, preoperative, and postoperative nursing divisions are but a few. Then consider outpatient as opposed to in-house surgical services. Through the process of integration, both levels of differentiation succeed in meeting the needs of the surgical patients and organizational goals.

At the unit level, the manager maintains the structure that facilitates nursing care. The manager does this by using the system of nursing care adopted by the organization as a whole. Team nursing, primary nursing, modular nursing, and case management are some of the possible models for nursing care delivery. The manager is responsible for the integrity of the model that had been chosen and also for the evaluation of its general effectiveness. Case management as a nursing care delivery system has the capability of being a very efficient method for organizing health care services. Traditional boundaries are crossed when the hospital-based services are arranged to respond to the hierarchy of patient needs. The organization and monitoring of services provided by case management ensures both the vertical and horizontal integration of the necessary departments. The above-named models are discussed under the heading of "Systems of Nursing Care Delivery."

Staffing

Staffing is the management activity that provides for appropriate and adequate personnel to fulfill the organization's objectives. The nurse manager decides how many and what type of personnel are required to provide care for the patients. Usually the overall plan for staffing is determined by nursing administration from among several models. The nurse manager is in a position to monitor how successful the staffing pattern is as well as to provide input into needed change. Staffing is a complex activity that involves ensuring that the ratio of nurse to patient provides positive patient outcomes.[17] An ideal staffing plan would provide the appropriate configuration of caregivers for patients based on data that predict the census. In addition, this same pattern would eliminate or minimize the problems of overstaffing or understaffing while providing flexibility for the individual needs of the staff members. Staffing is discussed in greater detail in Chapter 14.

Directing

Directing is a function of the manager that gets work done through others. Directing includes five specific concepts: giving directions, supervising, leading, motivating, and communicating, as described below:

1. *Giving directions* is the first activity and suggests that directions should be clear, concise, and consistent, and should conform to the requirements of the situation. The manager should be aware of the tone of the directive. Different types of situations require different emphasis. For example, an emergency situation calls for different inflections of voice than does a routine request. Whenever possible or appropriate, the reason for the directive should be given.
2. *Supervising* is concerned with the training and discipline of the work force. It also includes follow-up to ensure the prompt execution of orders. Fourteen qualities necessary for a highly successful supervisor were identified by Dr. Eugene Jennings of Michigan State University in his now-classic work. A successful supervisor consistently demonstrates the following:
   a. Gives clear work orders; communicates well.
   b. Praises others when deserved.
   c. Is willing to take the time to listen.
   d. Remains cool and calm most of the time.
   e. Has confidence and self-assurance.
   f. Has appropriate technical knowledge of the work being supervised.
   g. Understands the group's problems.
   h. Gains the group's respect through personal honesty.
   i. Is fair to everyone.
   j. Demands good work from everyone.

   k. Gains the group's trust by representing their view to higher management.
   l. Goes "to bat" for the group.
   m. Is approachable, friendly, and yet retains some distance.
   n. Is easy to talk to about concerns.[18]

3. *Leading* has been discussed in Chapters 2 and 3 as the ability to inspire and to influence others to the attainment of objectives.
4. *Motivating* is the set of skills the manager uses to help the employee to identify his or her needs and finds ways within the organization to help satisfy them. Motivation will be discussed in Chapter 10.
5. *Communicating* is the last activity and involves the what, how, who, and why of directives or effectively using the communication process. Communication was discussed in Chapter 3.

Coordinating

Coordinating is by definition the act of assembling and synchronizing people and activities so that they function harmoniously in the attainment of organizational objectives. In essence, coordination is a preventive managerial function concerned with heading off conflict and misunderstanding.

Think about the situations in your own life when you have had to coordinate the multiple activities for an important event. A school or community event involves the process of coordinating just as completely as formal managerial situations. The manager is aware of who is doing what and what the outcome should be and has the responsibility to make sure the specific and interrelated tasks are accomplished. This is not the easiest activity to accomplish, but accompanied by a thorough knowledge of the staff's responsibilities, the manager is in a good position to meet the appropriate goals.

Controlling

Controlling is the regulation of activities in accordance with plans. Controlling is a function of all managers at all levels. Its basic objective is to ensure that the task to be accomplished is appropriately executed. The three basic elements of control include standards that represent desired performance, a comparison of actual results against the standard, and, if necessary, corrective action.

STANDARDS

Sets of standards are available for the nursing profession to establish a standard for excellence. Standards for organized nursing services were developed by the American Nurses Association (ANA) Task Force on Standards for Organized Nursing services to provide a framework for nurse managers and administrators.[19] These standards, exhibited in Table 7-1, guide and direct nursing practice by the establishment of a professional and positive environment. In addition, the ANA developed standards for the different practice domains. For instance, the standards for cardiovascular nursing regulate, in a general way, what is expected of nurses caring for patients with cardiovascular problems. These standards serve as

TABLE 7-1. Scope and Standards for Nurse Administrators: The ANA, 1995

Standards of Care
Standard I. Assessment The nurse administrator develops, maintains, and evaluates patient/client and staff data collection systems and processes to support the practice of nursing and delivery of patient care.
Standard II. Diagnosis The nurse administrator develops, maintains, and evaluates an environment that supports the professional nurse in analysis of assessment data and in decisions to determine irrelevant diagnoses.
Standard III. Identification of Outcomes The nurse administrator develops, maintains, and evaluates information processes that promote desired, client-centered outcomes.
Standard IV. Planning The nurse administrator develops, maintains, and evaluates organizational planning systems to facilitate the delivery of nursing care.
Standard V. Implementation The nurse administrator develops, maintains, and evaluates organizational systems that support implementation of the plan.
Standard VI. Evaluation The nurse administrator evaluates the plan and its progress in relation to the attainment of outcomes.
Standards of Professional Performance
Standard I. Quality of Care and Administrative Practice The nurse administrator systematically evaluates the quality and effectiveness of nursing practice and nursing services administration.
Standard II. Performance Appraisal The nurse administrator evaluates his/her own performance based on professional practice standards, relevant statutes and regulations, and organizational criteria.
Standard III. Education The nurse administrator acquires and maintains current knowledge in administrative practice.
Standard IV. Collegiality The nurse administrator fosters a professional environment.
Standard V. Ethics The nurse administrator's decisions and actions are based on ethical principles.
Standard VI. Collaboration The nurse administrator collaborates with nursing staff at all levels, interdisciplinary teams, executive officers, and other stakeholders.
Standard VII. Research The nurse administrator supports research and integrates it into the delivery of nursing care and nursing administration.
Standard VIII. Resource Utilization The nurse administrator evaluates and administers the resources of organized nursing services.

a general guide to focus attention on the important responsibilities entrusted to the nurse. The various sets of professional standards serve to facilitate control of nursing practice. In addition, individual organizations or institutions modify or elaborate on the expectations of a nurse's performance through institutional standards of nursing care. This is intended to make clear the expectations held for the professional nurse. This in turn facilitates the manager's function of control by knowing what is expected of the staff nurse's performance.

POLICIES

Standards that specifically deal with conduct are sometimes referred to as policies. Within the organization, these policies are rules and regulations that regulate both broad and narrow aspects of an employee's position. The broad category includes the interpretation of legislation, or Labor Law, that impacts all employees, including nurses. Usually this kind of policy interpretation is handled through the legal/personnel department. Nursing as a profession is also subject to a nurse practice act that differs in wording from state to state but represents the legal boundaries for professional practice. Interpretation of this act by nursing administration committees with legal advice provides for general policies for nursing practice within institutions. Thus, the professional nurse who is employed in an organization is subject to general labor laws and to the state's professional nurse practice act.

The narrow aspects of what the professional nurse is expected to do are stated through the establishment of policies regarding nursing practice. These policies are derived from the profession's standards and the nurse practice act. Laws, standards, and policies are the basis for job descriptions and performance appraisal systems. Deviation from a stated, expected behavior alerts the manager to a problem. Since regulation of behavior is a part of management, control is exercised when the manager corrects the problem.

The functions of management are the skills the nurse manager uses to facilitate the mission, goals, and work of the organization. Management is a process, and as such knowledge and skills are developed over time. Throughout this text, information is provided that elaborates on these functions. However, nurse managers and vice presidents of nursing make management come to life.

SYSTEMS OF NURSING CARE DELIVERY

Effective management makes the organization function, and the nursing manager of today has a heritage of nursing care delivery systems that demonstrate ways of organizing nursing's work. Within these systems are advantages and disadvantages for quality of care, use of resources, and staff growth. In reviewing the history of nursing, **systems of nursing care delivery** evolved from the existing social and professional environment of the time. Each nursing system was organized as a means of managing the delivery of care, and because these systems existed in an organizational setting with its various characteristics, management was an essential ingredient. These systems of nursing care are presented in chronological order and, though different, the systems share the unique perspective of nursing management that combines the concern for quality of care with the best use of available resources.

Case Method

The case method, traced back to Florence Nightingale, began in the early days of the nursing profession. Individuals were assigned to give total care to each patient, including administering medications and providing treatments. The nurses reported to the head nurse, who was their immediate superior. The disadvantages of this system were that all personnel may not have been qualified to deliver all aspects of care, and depending on the structure, too many people were reporting to the head nurse (overextended span of control).

Functional Method

The functional method evolved as a way to deal with multiple levels of caregivers. Assignment of tasks rather than patients was the way in which care was provided. Each caregiver performed one certain task or function in keeping with the employee's education and experience. Nurse aides gave baths, fed patients, and took vital signs. Professional nurses were responsible for medications, treatments, and procedures. The head nurse was responsible for overall direction, supervision, and education of the nursing staff. The obvious problem with this system was the fragmentation of care. This complicated the process of coordination leading to reduction in the quality of care and a high level of dissatisfaction among the staff.

Team Nursing

A dramatic change occurred after World War II following 1945. The level and number of auxiliary personnel began increasing, and the professional nurse was assuming more and more of the management functions. Because of the changing configuration of the work group and the dramatic social upheaval, a study was commissioned to devise a better way to provide nursing care. Dr. Eleanor Lambertson of Columbia University in New York and Francis Perkins of Massachusetts General Hospital were the authors of the system known as team nursing. Team nursing was developed to deal with the influx of postwar workers and the head nurse's overextended span of control. This was accomplished by arranging the workers in teams. The teams consisted of the senior professional nurse becoming the team leader; the members of the team were other registered nurses (RNs), licensed practical nurses (LPNs) or vocational nurses, and nurse aides and orderlies. Each was given a patient assignment in keeping with the employee's education and experience. The team leader made the assignments, delegated the work through the morning report, made rounds throughout the shift to make sure patients were being cared for properly, and conducted a team conference at the end of the shift to evaluate the patient care and plan and update nursing care plans. By 1950, team nursing was becoming a popular way to structure nursing care.

Team nursing was a pattern of patient care that involved changing the structural and organizational framework of the nursing unit. This method introduced the team concept for the stated aim of using all levels of personnel to their fullest capacity in giving the best possible nursing care to patients. The structural and organizational changes necessary for this method included the introduction of the nursing team, with the team leader assuming responsibility for the management of patient care. The head nurse decentralized authority to the team leader to direct the activities of the team members. The head nurse was no longer the center of all communication on the division because the members communicated directly with the team leader. The team leader had the responsibility for synchronizing the abilities of his or her team members so that they were able to function effectively in a team relationship. Emphasis was placed on the ability of all participants of patient care to plan, administer, and evaluate patient care.

The team approach to patient care represented more than a reorganization or restructuring of nursing service. Instead, it was a philosophy of nursing and a method of organizing patient care. This particular model was widely used and, like all models, was adapted for individual organizations. The difficulty with this method was the nurse's absence at the bedside; the nurse was directing the care of others and thus not using nursing's specialized knowledge as the best provider of patient care. Today there is a renewed interest in the team concept rather than team nursing. The value of committed people working together for a shared goal is viewed as a very effective health care delivery system.

RESTRUCTURING NURSING CARE DELIVERY MODELS

Nursing service has always been challenged to redesign the work of nursing to deal with the demands of the health care system. Based on organization theory, two categories of restructuring nursing care delivery models have been offered: (1) job design and (2) systems redesign.[20]

Job Design

Job design is based on classical theory that shapes a particular job(s) within an organization to optimize worker productivity.[21] Essentially, job design restructures the division of labor within the nursing unit based on job enrichment strategies to develop organizational commitment among nurses, allow for differences in positions because of work requirements, greater support for nursing autonomy, and includes nursing in policy-making, strategic planning, and monitoring of quality patient care.[22] Early examples of job design are primary nursing and the total patient care model.

Primary Nursing

In the 1970s, primary nursing care moved the care of the patient from the team to the individual caregiver. Primary nursing as a system of care provided for quality comprehensive patient care and a framework for the development of professional practice among the nursing staff. Primary nursing was a logical next step in nursing's historic evolution. By definition, primary nursing is a philosophy and structure that places responsibility and accountability for the planning, giving, communicating, and evaluating of care for a group of patients in the hands of the primary nurse. Primary nursing was intended to return the nurse to the bedside, thus improving the quality of care and increasing the job satisfaction of the nursing staff.

Definitions related to primary nursing are:

- *Primary nursing*—the hospital unit organization and philosophy that places on the RN responsibility and accountability for the planning, giving, communicating, and evaluating of care for a caseload of patients.

- *Primary care*—the community contact by a patient seeking entrance to the health care system. He or she may see a physician, nurse practitioner, dentist, and so on and have his or her care given in the office or clinic or be referred into a hospital.
- *Primary nurse*—an RN, usually full time, who is assigned specific patients to whom he or she will provide primary nursing care during their stay in the unit.
- *Associate or secondary nurse*—any nurse caring for patients whose primary nurse is off duty; he or she provides total, 8-hour care.
- *Total care*—the provision of all professional nursing care needed by the patient during an 8-hour shift. This includes medications, treatments, hygienic and comfort measures, teaching, support, charting, reporting, and changing the care plan if necessary.

The basic concepts of primary nursing include fixed, visible accountability of the nurse for the care of assigned cases and inclusion of the patient in his or her own care. The primary nurse is expected to give total care, to establish therapeutic relationships, to plan for 24-hour continuity in nursing care through a written nursing care plan, to communicate directly with other members of the health team, and to plan for discharge. The patient's participation is expected in the planning, implementing, and evaluating of his or her own care. Perhaps the best aspect of primary nursing is the improved communication provided by the one-to-one relationship between nurse and patient. Associate nurses are involved with this method by caring for the patients in the absence of the primary nurse. Their responsibilities include continuing the care initiated by the primary nurse and making necessary modifications. Conceivably the primary nurse for a group of patients may be an associate nurse for other patients. The role played by the professional nurse is determined by the assignment of patients, which is made by the front-line manager or head nurse.

Primary nursing was adapted in organizations to fit the staffing patterns and general nursing philosophy. Because of the need for a high percentage of professional nurses, other modifications of the system were developed, such as modular nursing. See Table 7-2 for the responsibilities of the primary and associate nurses.[22]

Total Patient Care

The model of total patient care was similar to primary nursing care. The difference was total patient care was offered but limited to the duration of the shift as opposed to primary nursing care, which extended responsibility for care throughout the patient's hospitilization period.[23]

Differentiated Practice

Differentiated practice, another model of job design, from the work of Primm and Rotkovich,[24,25] identified different levels of clinical expertise. This perspective suggested two levels of nursing practice: (1) the professional nurse level, a BSN-prepared nurse (with all the responsibilities of the primary care nurse and consideration of the cost of care), and (2) the associate nurse level, an associate-degree nurse who assists the professional nurse. The cost management component of this model includes awareness of supply costs, fiscal implications of therapeutic interventions, and flexible staffing to deal with manpower and caseload needs. This has been an ongoing issue in nursing as both BSN and AD nurses are professional nurses with similar responsibilities. With a

TABLE 7-2. Responsibilities of the primary and associate nurses in the primary nursing model

Primary	Associate
1. Patient and family teaching • Carries out necessary aspects of patient care. • Delegates and ensures continuity through care plan. • Documents, evaluates, and changes plan. 2. Nursing care plan • Assesses patient initially and continually to write care plan. • Updates, evaluates effects of care. • Confers with staff if they do not follow through. • Receptive to peer advice. 3. Collaboration with physician • Seeks to be on physician rounds as possible. • Knows current medical plan. • Can intervene for patient when his or her goals conflict with medical goals.	1. Patient and family teaching • Provides patient education because of patient need or through delegation by the care plan. • Reinforces plan of primary nurse. • Advises primary nurse on changes. 2. Nursing care plan • Follows suggestions of primary nurse. • Changes plan when condition warrants. • When in conflict with controversial directives, discusses with primary nurse; may follow primary nurse's orders and then evaluate. 3. Collaboration with physician • Refers primary nurse's concerns to physician. • Answers physician's questions about daily status of patient. • Plans with physician when changes in patient care are necessary in the absence of primary nurse.

serious nursing shortage facing the nation, the distinction between levels of education may, of necessity, become blurred.

Partners in Practice

Similar to differentiated practice models, partners in practice team a professional nurse with licensed or unlicensed technicians, nurse aides, or nurse extenders. The "partners" work together to care for the patient caseload. Besides a difference in the composition of the work team, partners in practice ideally assign the professional partners to the same shift or hours.[26]

These models address the requirement to provide adequate care by distinguishing what tasks (or part of the job) are to be delivered by different levels of caregivers. Job design models are effective at a departmental level, but may have no impact on organizational structure, decision making, or working conditions for nurses.

System Redesign

The alternative to job design is system redesign, which considers the entire organization. This perspective is based on systems theory. Systems theory considers organizations to be open, interactive entities with an emphasis on an appropriate structure to allow work to be completed, while interacting with the boundaries of the environment and flexibly adapting to needed change. This theoretical perspective guides the design of nursing care delivery by increasing productivity while recognizing the interdependence of multiple competing goals. Case management and total quality management are examples of models based on system redesign.

Case Management

More recently, a new method of nursing care delivery, known as case management, has evolved. The ANA has defined case management to be a system of health assessment, planning, service procurement and delivery, coordination, and monitoring to meet the multiple service needs of clients.[27] Case management systems address the potential mismatch between client needs, services offered, and increasingly limited health care resources.[28] This system provides care that minimizes fragmentation and maximizes individualized care, as well as an all-inclusive and comprehensive model, not restricted to the hospital setting. The model may be operationalized in a variety of ways, but the usual approach involves a case manager in a matrix organizational structure who follows a caseload of patients according to a specialized plan. When a patient deviates from the usual expected course of recovery or health, consultation ensues to quickly correct the problem. This requires a great deal of systematic knowledge about a patient's problems and putting that knowledge into a type of nursing care plan (case management plans) with time lines to demonstrate progress or deviations from the critical paths. This particular system of care has been used for many years in the public health domain and recently has been introduced into the acute care institution. What is so exciting about this concept is that it builds on the primary nursing model and improves on its efficiency. It retains the accountability and responsibility of the professional nurse but creates a more orderly way of evaluating the patient's response to therapies. It goes without saying that in this age of financial concern, this system, with its built-in radar, prevents or recognizes complications and identifies costly problems for earlier treatment.

The organizational and structural configuration of case management involves the following:

- *Case manager*—a nurse responsible for evaluating the care of patients.
- *Care plan*—composed of (1) critical paths, (2) objectives of care, and (3) time lines.
- *Evaluation of variance*—if the patient varies from the critical path, a report is made to reduce the impact of the complication.

The nurse manager or unit leader, as the case manager, directs the actions of subordinates to provide managed care to a group of patients. The case manager functions are:

- Establish rapport and trust with the patient/family.
- Collect comprehensive assessment data including:
  - Physical status
  - Mental status
  - Emotional status
  - Family, community, and financial resources.
- Communicate problem statements to appropriate sources.
- Develop a plan of care in collaboration with patient, family, and other health care workers.
- Establish goals and objectives.
- Consider cost containment.
- Intervene/monitor delivery of care.
- Achieve case coordination.
- Make referrals/provide follow-up care.
- Assess/monitor patient outcomes.

The group of patients is subject to an ongoing and comprehensive evaluation involving multiple services known as a care plan. The care plan is based on accumulated data and is presented as critical paths that determine the ideal patient reaction. In addition to the nursing and medical services that are required for patients, other services are included, such as physical therapy and respiratory therapy. These services are identified according to what most patients experience at every critical point of their hospitalization, rehabilitation, or stage of illness. Since the care plan includes the usual reaction of patients to all interventions by all essential services according to critical paths with time lines, the staff nurse recognizes deviations quickly. The case manager is notified, and appropriate interventions are initiated. The comprehensive plan that is used as the source of evaluation is constructed by representatives from the various services. This particular system requires cooperation and teamwork from the practitioners and is capable of ensuring quality care and cost effectiveness. Using the individual practitioner's knowledge and skill is a way of building professional autonomy.[29, 30]

Total Quality Management

Another example of systems redesign is total quality management (TQM), a system which aims at using data (statistics, quality indicators, information from consumers and health care personnel) to continuously improve services. It has the capacity to take case management several steps further to integrated health care management. There is a requirement that all members of the organization be involved and committed to the philosophy of TQM. Top management shares authority with lower-level employees in the area of decision making while continuously gathering information to inform the decision-making process. The top-level executives provide the leadership for TQM by defining and reinforcing its values, managing a supportive culture, and creating a structure to create and support innovations. The value to nursing care delivery is that the core of innovation is at the unit level with the direct care providers. Management must set clear standards and expectations for staff nurse accountability.[31]

TQM proponents state examples of cost savings from identifying and correcting "system" problems. System redesign models are more complex, require the re-education of all personnel, and hold promise for an engaged and committed workforce. The system creates a context in which health professionals act autonomously with a defined framework of quality, cost savings, and productivity. Professionals are expected to participate in decision making, peer evaluation, and policy development, while their primary role is to deliver health services to clients.[32]

Nursing administration has several models to consider for the delivery of nursing care. In all the named systems for the delivery of nursing care, consideration for the quality of care and resource utilization remains the underlying motivation for the nurse manager.

Transition to Manager

The transition from a staff member to a manager requires the assumption of authority. There is inherent complexity in an authority role that is unique. By assuming authority, the manager is the custodian of the mission, traditions, rules, and responsibility associated with the organization. Thus, the manager is able to make decisions over subordinates' time, assignments, and all other aspects of work. Since there is a potential for confusion or conflict among the subordinates, the manager facilitates the individual and group toward meeting stated objectives. The manner in which the manager chooses to keep the group on track may vary from individual to individual and from situation to situation. This responsibility to maintain order differentiates the manager from the staff, and herein lies the real issue. The staff's reaction to the manager will reflect the staff's confidence that they will be able to control their decisions and work.

The new manager may face situations very differently from an experienced manager. The behavior of some staff members may be critical, protective, or hostile. New managers should avoid the tendency to take this as a personal assault; rather, they should understand this is defensive behavior aimed at maintaining personal control of the work or work-related activities.

MANAGEMENT ASSESSMENT GUIDE

Nursing models provide the nurse manager with a way of organizing the work of nursing, but the manager is still faced with the complexities of the modern health care institution. Despite uncertainties in the workplace, it is still possible to be an extremely effective manager. It requires taking into account the essential elements of the managerial situation and using the appropriate management function and skill. The managerial situation consists of relevant factors in the greater social and organizational environment as well as the immediate situation. Factors in the manager and employees that enhance or inhibit the achievement of goals must also be built into the equation. For the manager to be truly effective, information must be available to use the various resources properly. The Managerial Assessment Guide presented in Table 7-3 is offered to

TABLE 7-3. The Essential Elements a Manager Should Consider When Analyzing a Management Situation; These Elements Have Been Summarized In the Managerial Assessment Tool

- External environment: What factors impact the current situation?
- Identify regulatory bodies such as laws, professional standards, and government regulations.
- Identify stability or volatility in the external environment that may impact on the current situation.
- Identify relevant characteristics of the environment:
  Geographic and cultural considerations
  Population dynamics
  Political and financial dynamics.
- Internal organizational characteristics.
- Identify the boundaries of the unit of analysis.
- Identify the existing climate of the unit of analysis.
- Identify the nursing care system being used.
- Identify the staffing pattern for the organization and the specific area.
- Mission and goals.
  - Identify the general goal and structure of what is to be accomplished.
  - Manager and employee relationship.
  - Identify the participants, clients, or patients and personnel.
  - Identify formal and informal goals of the organization and the participants.
  - Identify the employees: education, experience, and level of performance.
- Resources.
  - Identify the necessary resources, both human and nonhuman.
- Barriers.
  - Identify possible barriers to the completion of the work: time, insufficient or inadequate resources, inadequate ratio of patient/personnel.

highlight those essential variables that will focus on meeting managerial goals. In conclusion, for a manager to manage work and adequacy of the personnel and resources to provide prepared employees in the proper ratio must be assessed. Once an assessment has been made, the proper managerial decision and plan can be made. The subsequent chapters will detail what the nursing manager does and will provide some suggestions to facilitate modern-day nursing management.

CASE STUDY

The New Manager

Mary Jones, the new clinical director of a coronary care step-down unit, has noticed that some of the staff members have been behaving in negative ways. Mrs. Green has been very sarcastic in interactions with Mary. Mrs. Green had competed for the role of clinical director and was very disappointed not to receive the promotion.

Mary has also noted that some of the older employees are acting strange. They are excluding her from social conversations, and suggesting "they hope things don't change around here."

In addition, Mary has overheard people compare her to the previous director, who had been in the position for 10 years and was well-liked and respected. Mary felt she was capable of fulfilling the new role but knew she had to deal with the individual reactions of the group.

- How should Mary deal with jealousy? Competition? Resentment? Managing older employees? Comparisons to a previous manager?

Suggestions to manage these problems include:

- Review communication techniques and conflict-resolution strategies. (*Remember*: ignore what isn't important, and that mature, disciplined behavior and emotional control will strengthen self-confidence. In situations where new leaders are being challenged simply because of their newness, temper any response with a non-answer and don't provoke further argument. This demonstrates emotional control and distance from the attack. Where possible, use the challenging person's experience, talent, or help, and follow-up with public praise.)

SUMMARY

This chapter has presented an overview of the management process. The management process is a specific form of problem solving that enables the manager to make wise decisions concerning the use of resources and to supervise staff for the purpose of meeting goals. Functions of management include planning, organizing, staffing, supervising, directing, coordinating, and controlling. Systems of nursing care are organizational frameworks to structure the work of nursing and are facilitated by the role of a nursing manager. To allow a thorough assessment of the managerial situation, a Managerial Assessment Guide (Table 7-3) is offered to focus on the essential factors providing information for a proper managerial decision.

LEARNER EXERCISES

1. Early in the chapter, nursing management was differentiated from professional management on the basis of a general philosophical position. Develop a position for nursing service. State simply, but clearly, why your nursing department exists.
2. Develop a managerial orientation including a course outline of what the nurse manager needs to know.
3. Divide the class into three groups. Have each group represent a different level of management. Give each group time to devise a plan that would reflect the type of planning expected at each level.
4. Observe a manager using the functions of management. Think about what it is the manager does while performing each of the following: (1) directing, (2) coordinating, and (3) controlling.
5. Take a real-life situation from your current clinical agency and apply the managerial assessment tool to identify relevant information. Select a management decision that you think would be best.

REFERENCES

1. Drucker, P.F. (1990). *Management, tasks, responses, practices*. New York: Harper & Row.
2. Kreither, R. (1995). *Management*. 6th ed. Boston, Toronto: Houghton Mifflin Co., pp. 5–7.
3. McGregor, D. (1960). *The human side of enterprise*. New York: McGraw-Hill.
4. Herzberg, F. (1987). One more time: How do you motivate employees? *Harvard Business Review, 65*, 109–120.
5. Argyris, C. (1964). *Integrating the individual and the organization*. New York: Wiley.
6. Likert, R. (1961). *New patterns of management*. New York: McGraw-Hill.
7. Volk, M.C., & Lucas, M.D. (1991, January-February). Relationship of management style and anticipated turnover. *Dimensions of Critical Care, 10*(1), 35–40.
8. Peters, T.J., & Waterman, R.H. (1982). *In search of excellence*. New York: Harper & Row.
9. Peters, T.J., & Waterman, R.H. (1982). *In search of excellence*. New York: Harper & Row, p. 13.
10. McClure, M. (1984, February). Managing the professional nurse. *Journal of Nursing Administration, 14*(2), 15–21.
11. Lynn, M., Layman, E., & Richard, S. (1999). The final chapter in the nursing administration research priorities stage. *Journal of Nursing Administration, 29*(5), 5–9.
12. Peterson, A.A. (1994). The changing management role: Autocratic doer to team facilitator. *Seminars for Nurse Managers, 2*(4), 209–212.
13. Peterson, A.A. (1994). The changing management role: Autocratic doer to team facilitator. *Seminars for Nurse Managers, 2*(4), 210.
14. Peterson, A.A. (1994). The changing management role: Autocratic doer to team facilitator. *Seminars for Nurse Managers, 2*(4), 210.
15. Adopted from Tannenbaum, R., & Schmidt, W. (1965). How to choose a leadership pattern. *Harvard Business Review*, 121.
16. Curtain, L. (1991). Strategic planning, asking the right questions. *Nursing Management, 22*(1), 7–8.
17. Sochalski, J., Estabrooks, C., & Humphrey, C.K. (1999). Nurse staffing and patient outcomes: Evolution of an international study. *Canadian Journal of Nursing Research, 31*(3), 69–88.
18. Jennings, E.E. (1961, Autumn). The anatomy of leadership. *Management of Personnel Quarterly, 1*(1), 213.

19. American Nurses Association Task Force for Organized Nursing Services Scope and Standards for Nurse Administrators. (1994–1995). Washington, D.C.: ANA.
20. Dienemann, J., & Gessner, T. (1992, July/August). Restructuring nursing care delivery systems. *Nursing Economics*, *10*, 253–258.
21. Dienemann, J., & Gessner, T. (1992, July/August). Restructuring nursing care delivery systems. *Nursing Economics*, *10*, 253.
22. Dienemann, J., & Gessner, T. (1992, July/August). Restructuring nursing care delivery systems. *Nursing Economics*, *10*, 253.
23. Dienemann, J., & Gessner, T. (1992, July/August). Restructuring nursing care delivery systems. *Nursing Economics*, *10*, 254.
24. Primm, P.L. (1986). Defining and differentiating ADN and BSN competencies. *Issues*, *7*(1), 1–6.
25. Rotkovich, R. (1986, June). ICON: A model of nursing practice for the future. *Nursing Management*, *17*(6), 54–56.
26. Matheny, M. (1989). Practice, partnerships: The newest concept in care delivery. *Journal of Nursing Administration*, *19*(2), 33–35.
27. American Nurses Association. (1988). *Case management*. Kansas City, MO: ANA.
28. Strong, A. (1992, April). Case management and the CNS. *Clinical Nurse Specialist*, 64.
29. Sterling, Y., Noto, E.C., & Bowen, M.R. (1994). Case management roles of clinicians: A research study. *Clinical Nurse Specialist*, *8*(4), 196–201.
30. Schmeidling, N.J. (1993). The complexity of an authority role. *Nursing Management*, *23*(11), 57–58.
31. Labouitz, G.H. (1991). Beyond the total quality management mystique. *Health Care Executive*. 6(2), 15–17.
32. Mansir, B.E., & Schacht, N.R. (1989). *An introduction to the continuous improvement process: Principles and practice*. Bethesda, MD: Logistic Management Institute.

8

Delegation

The Manager's Tool

"Never tell people how to do things. Tell them what to do and they will surprise you with their ingenuity."

George S. Patton

INTRODUCTION

In the past, effective delegation has not been an activity emphasized in nursing. As a result, many nurses do not value this skill. Educational programs have emphasized primary nursing as the dominant method of delivering nursing care which focuses on the skill of the individual nurse. In this era of restricted staff and teams of personnel (with different levels of education and experience), the ability to assign and supervise work is essential. Every organization's mission is expressed through its work, and coordinated and executed through the efforts of managers and employees. Delegation is the link that joins organizational concepts with the management process; it is that which allows a manager to manage. This chapter will explore the specialized management activity of delegation.

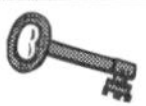

KEY CONCEPTS

Accountability is the process of furnishing a justifying analysis or explanation for the behavior/actions of self or subordinates.

Authority is the right to give orders and the power to exact obedience.

Decentralization is the delegation of authority away from the central office to the operating units.

Delegation is the process of entrusting or assigning responsibility and authority to members of the organization.

Responsibility is the inward obligation to perform so that the entire organization benefits.

Scalar Chain is the vertical line of authority within the organization from the chief executive to subordinates depicted in the organization chart.

DELEGATION

Delegation is the use of personnel to accomplish a desired objective through allocation of authority and responsibility (see Figure 8-1). Delegation is the process that facilitates complex organizations to accomplish work through the coordinated and differentiated efforts of others, and is extensively used by the manager. Delegation is pivotal to organizational dynamics because it is the direct outcome of planning and results in a system of differentiation of labor. Thus, it involves the assignment of work and the giving of orders, enabling the manager to operationalize the plan of the organization through the staff.[1]

Much of a manager's success depends on the efforts of the team, or how work is assigned and delegated. The most effective managers create an environment in which decisions about work are made by every member of the health care team, especially those involved in direct care. Delegation, in one sense, is a paradox: the manager who delegates and develops employees to make and take responsibility for decisions begins the process of eliminating the need for a manager. New managers can learn the art of skillful delegation. Experience has shown a remarkable capacity in people at all levels of the organization to shoulder responsibility and to get results. The best way to ensure organizational effectiveness is to delegate appropriate authority to the lowest level of employees. The proper use of delegation is an important tool for staff participation that will build morale.

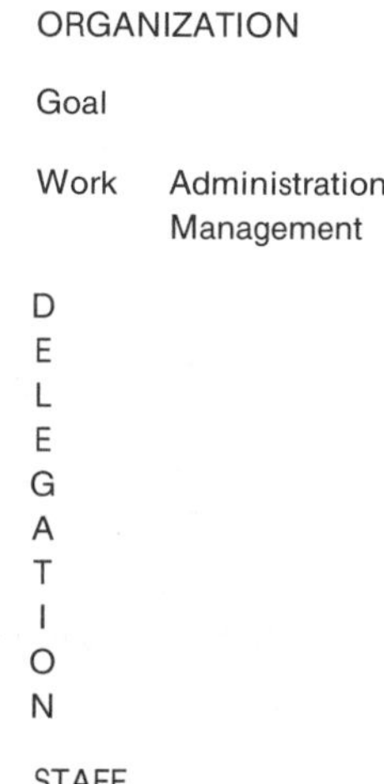

FIGURE 8-1. Graphic depiction of delegation as the process that links the organization with work and with the staff.

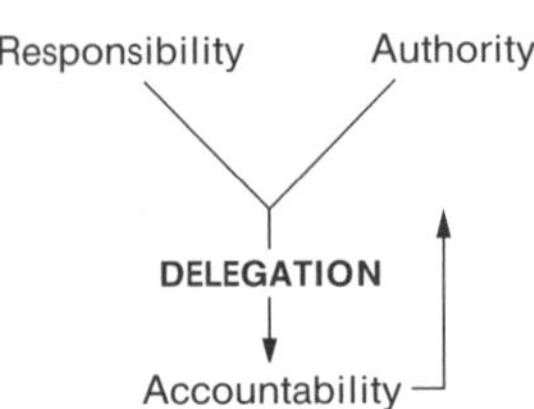

FIGURE 8-2. Graphic illustration of the relationship among responsibility, authority, delegation, and accountability by demonstrating the direction each takes in an organization.

Assignment of Work

The organizational structure is a formal plan for arranging people in order according to their authority and responsibility to achieve defined objectives. A closer look at responsibility will shed light on understanding the conceptual basis of delegation. **Responsibility** depends on three coexisting concepts: authority, delegation, and accountability (see Figure 8-2). For example, if a manager is given responsibility for a task, the manager will delegate the responsibility and the necessary **authority** to the appropriate employee. In turn, the employee is accountable to the delegator for completing the task satisfactorily. **Accountability** is the process of furnishing a justifying explanation for behavior of self or for others.

The delegator or manager, however, does not give up all responsibility but retains overall responsibility and authority consistent with the manager's position. What this means is that a manager at a higher level of the organization is willing to accept and to support the decisions and actions of others lower in the organization. The manager remains accountable for those below to superiors of the manager. Delegation is not a system to reduce responsibility but for making it meaningful. The process of delegation, based on the above-related concepts, forms the basis for the assignment of work throughout the entire organization.

Scope of Practice

The legal limits of what can be delegated involve the concept of scope of practice. There are limiting factors to what professional nurses are able to do. Individual state boards of nursing identify the legal boundaries of nursing practice through nurse practice acts (which differ among the states). Each nurse practice act defines the legal boundaries of nursing practice to safeguard the public. These same acts also prohibit unauthorized individuals from practicing nursing. Increasingly, there are more and more levels and types of health care personnel supervised by nurses. Just as it is incumbent on the nurse to know the legal limits of professional practice, it is just as important for the nurse to know what the certified and unlicensed personnel are able to do. Job descriptions help identify those activities each employee may perform. This information guides the delegation process and reduces the risk of liability for supervising the new configuration of employees. [2]

Liability

Liability, or being legally responsible for the actions of oneself or of those supervised, is a growing concern among professional nurses. Nurse managers have a legal duty to know what tasks are within the scope of their state's nurse practice act, the scope of practice of their staff members, and most important the competency of the staff member to complete the assigned task. In addition, if nurse managers breach the standard of care for either of those duties, the nurse may be held negligent if any harm results from the acts of the subordinate. If these standards are met, the nurse manager is not liable. However, nurse managers are gaining additional responsibilities in all types of health care institutions, and thus are facing a greater risk of liability. [3]

The legal principle of corporate liability involves an agency's legal duty to provide appropriate facilities, staffing, safety, and equipment in the delivery of a service offered to the public. The legal principle of *vicarious liability* or *respondent superior* holds the employer is legally responsible for the wrongful acts of its employees. Courts generally hold that when employees act within their scope of practice and perform a negligent act, the employer is responsible for the payment of claims. If a nurse acts outside of the appropriate scope of practice or performs an intentionally harmful or criminal act, the agency is not responsible. [4]

The nurse manager may be sued by patients for negligent hiring, negligent retention of incompetent or impaired employees, or for the provision of negligent references concerning employees. The organization's structure determines the degree of authority and responsibility the manager may exercise with employees.[5]

Scalar Chain

In classical management theory, the line of authority from the top on down is referred to as the **scalar chain**, illustrated on the organizational chart in the form of vertical lines that link the level of manager with subordinates and clearly shows the divisions of responsibility, from the broad total responsibility of the administrator to the specific responsibility of personnel in a given department. This also represents line authority, or the direct relationship of a superior to a subordinate. This is in contrast to staff relationships that are consultative or advisory. See Figure 8-3 to illustrate the scalar chain.

To exemplify, a nurse manager, who is responsible for all patient care on a particular unit, cannot possibly perform all that is required for the group of patients. Thus, the head nurse delegates responsibility to the appropriate caregivers to do what is necessary for the patients as well as the necessary authority to enforce the specialized functions. The head nurse, who has the legitimate right to give directives, provides an opportunity for professional nurses to give care. The caregiver now has an obligation to perform. The major rule of delegation is that authority and responsibility must be delegated equally. The staff nurse, who accepts the responsibility, is accountable to the head nurse not only for what has been accomplished but also for the methods used to deliver care. In the scalar chain, authority and responsibility flow downward and accountability moves upward.

Decentralization

When delegation occurs on the face-to-face manager-to-employee level, it is referred to as general supervision. When delegation occurs on the organizational level, it involves giving more autonomy to subunits and is called **decentralization.** The movement in health care toward decentralization has occurred because of the reduction of managers and the goal to empower professionals at the operative level. Authority is delegated as a way of increasing productivity and managing cost.

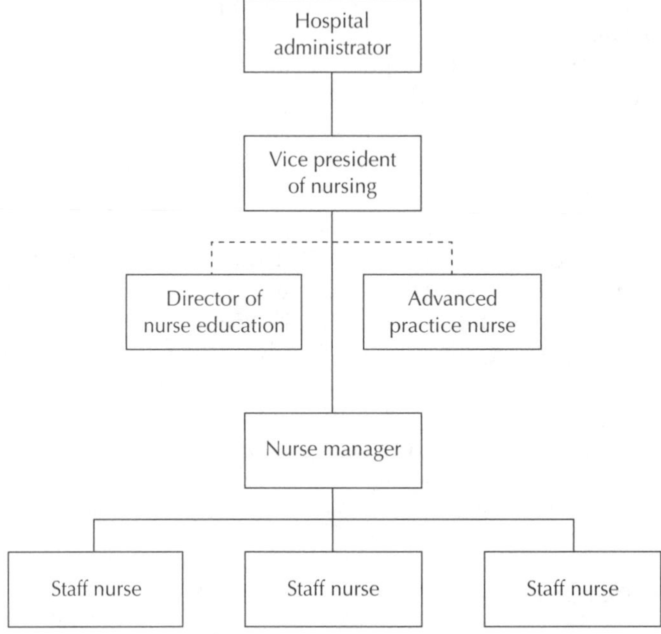

FIGURE 8-3. The scalar chain of authority depicted through the vertical lines on the organization chart.

Currently, decentralization is occurring downward and outward in health care organizations. Decentralization is often termed horizontal management because it aims to flatten the hierarchical organization structure and allows the staff nurse the opportunity to take more initiative and to become more autonomous. The practical result of this practice has been to eliminate or to reduce middle management and to give the front-line manager more authority and responsibility.

The Purpose of Delegation

The proper use of delegation, besides assigning work, serves a variety of purposes. Among them are a means for promoting internalized motivation and job enrichment by giving employees a sense of being their own boss through the opportunity to exercise control over his or her work. Some of the other reasons for the use of delegation include cost savings, time savings, professional growth for employees, and professional growth of the manager.

Cost Savings

Cost-saving strategies are being used by literally every health care organization today. The easiest and most efficient way to save on cost is to use resources properly, which ensures that the right person is doing the right work. This simply means that the manager should manage and the professional nurses should provide the nursing care. Managers are expected to increase the overall efficiency of their division. This cannot be accomplished if the manager is doing the work of the staff.

Time Savings

Time will be conserved if the manager allocates activities to the proper staff member. Different levels of personnel are able to perform work within their scope of practice. Time for professional staff will be best used when nonprofessional personnel assist them in completing some of the necessary tasks. Time is best used when tailored to meet the individual's workload requirements.

Professional Growth for Employees

Increasing the self-esteem of employees is an important reason to use the process of delegation. Personal and professional growth is expected as personnel experience the development of their talents and abilities by taking pride in the results of their efforts. This comes about in response to the decisions they have made. For the most part, it is difficult to expect people to take the risk of decision making without putting them in a position to make decisions. Delegation provides the opportunity to make decisions, and the employees' decisions are reflected in the outcome.

Delegation, by its very nature, allows the subordinate to make decisions that might result in mistakes. To minimize the possibility of serious error, the manager must use all aspects of the management process (in particular assessment of staff capability). Growth can occur in either case, however, and mistakes can sometimes lead to even greater professional change. Other advantages for the employees include the possibility that the subordinates' sense of responsibility and autonomy will grow, thereby enlarging the employees' sense of leadership, job satisfaction, and knowledge of organizational goals.

Professional Growth of the Manager

Effective and successful delegation centers around effective manager and staff relationships. The personal relationships that exist influence the work result. For example, the manager is accountable for certain results and gives permission to the staff members to perform part of the work and to take certain action. There are growing and shifting relationships between the manager and staff; the freedom and initiative exercised by the staff varies and cannot be spelled out in explicit detail. Thus, work habits and attitudes can be influenced by the interplay with the manager. In facilitating the staff's growth, the manager is truly fulfilling a major responsibility of the manager's role.

The Process of Delegation

The process of delegation is predominantly results-oriented. The delegator or nurse manager makes relatively few decisions alone but frames orders in broad, general terms, allowing the subordinate to work out the details of the work. The delegator or manager does the following:

- Sets goals.
- Tells subordinates what is to be accomplished.
- Fixes the limits within which the subordinate can work in accord with job descriptions and the job assignment.
- Allows employees to decide how to achieve goals.

The process of delegation allows the manager to assign responsibility, give authority, and create accountability within the subordinate. All three aspects of the process of delegation involve a degree of risk that necessitates the manager to know an employee's ability and to plan a program to increase his or her skill and knowledge levels. Successful managers systematically plan for delegation by determining what kinds of tasks can be delegated, who is ready to assume additional tasks, what assistance is needed, and what outcomes are expected. These managers view delegation as a means of helping their staff achieve their own objectives for growth and development.

Guidelines for Effective Delegation

For the beginning manager, some guidelines are offered to help when delegating to employees:

- Give a clear description of what it is you want the employee to do. Describe the overall scope and background of the current task. Give the reason for the assignment, and tell the employee if other departments or people are involved to achieve the desired outcome. If there are special problems, share this information with the employee.
- Share with the employee the outcome you expect and by when.
- Discuss the degree of responsibilities and authority that the employee will have.
- Ask the employee to summarize the main points of the delegated task.
- Know what cannot be delegated. This includes confidential matters, contractual responsibilities, discipline of the workforce, and ultimate responsibility for the work output.

As an example, assume you are the nurse manager of a busy step-down unit of cardiac surgery patients. Your division is well-staffed with registered nurses (RNs), and you feel it is time to give additional responsibility to your charge nurse. To use the appropriate guidelines, your conversation might go something like this:

> Tell the staff RN I need help with the orientation of our new staff members, and I would like you to take on this new responsibility. The orientation process is 1 month long, but if you could shorten that period, it would be very helpful. The new nurses need the information in the orientation manual, but feel free to use your own ingenuity to help them gain information. Their work will be evaluated at 2- and 4-week intervals. In addition, I think you would find it helpful to learn the orientation program that we are currently using. I will make arrangements for you to attend such sessions. You will have the authority to advise the employees of their positive performance and discuss with them areas of improvement. I feel confident that you will be able to do this very well, and I will be available for any questions you might have. Do you have any questions now? Would you please share with me your understanding of this new and important responsibility?

The delegator explains the task to an assistant by giving all the necessary information so that the task can be completed appropriately. In addition, the delegator delegates the necessary authority to accompany the responsibility. By delegating to the staff, the manager is helping them to develop their talents.

Barriers to Delegation

Often managers are reluctant to delegate. The common reasons for failure to adequately delegate vary from manager to manager. Some of these reasons are as follows:

- **"I can do it better myself" fallacy.**
  It has been found that nursing personnel with high standards of performance are naturally tempted to perform any activity that they feel they can do better themselves. A nurse manager must reconcile turning over the task to someone whose performance will be "good enough." The comparison is not between the quality of work, but the benefits to the total operation when the manager devotes attention to planning and supervision, which only the manager may do. Only after the manager accepts the idea that the work gets done through other people will the manager be able to make full use of delegation.

- **Lack of ability to direct.**
  The manager must be able to communicate to the staff, often in advance, what is to be done. This means that the manager must: (1) think ahead and visualize the work situation, (2) formulate objectives and general plans of action, and (3) communicate to the assistants. In essence, the manager must identify and communicate the essential features of the work plan. All too often administrative personnel have not cultivated this ability to direct.

- **Lack of confidence in staff.**
  To remedy this situation, either education through staff development or programs should be offered to help the employee to improve on the performance problem or to help the employee to find the proper role in the organization.

- **Absence of controls that warn of impending difficulties.**
  Care must be taken that the control system does not undermine the very essence of delegation. The nurse manager cannot completely delegate responsibility unless the manager has confidence in the controls.

- **Aversion to taking a risk.**
  The manager may be handicapped by a temperamental aversion to taking a risk. The greater the number of subordinates and the higher the degree of delegation, the more likely it is that sooner or later there will be trouble. The manager who delegates takes a calculated risk. Over a period of time the manager may expect that the gains from delegation will far offset the troubles that arise.

In addition to managers having problems with delegation, staff members may also have some difficulty accepting responsibility. Some of the more common reasons offered are as follows:

- **Easier to ask the "boss."**
  The staff may find it easier to ask the manager than to decide themselves how to deal with a problem. For some, making a wise decision may be hard work. Making one's own decision carries with it responsibility for the outcome. Asking the boss is one way of shifting or sharing this burden. This is known as upward delegation.

- **Fear of criticism.**
  The fear of criticism for mistakes keeps some people from accepting greater responsibilities. A great deal depends upon the nature of the criticism. Negative criticism may be resented, whereas a constructive review might be accepted.

- **Lack of necessary information and resources.**
  A belief that employees lack the necessary information and resources makes effective delegation difficult. The frustration that accompanies inadequate information and resources creates an attitude that might convince the staff person to reject further assignments.
- **May have more work than the employee can now do.**
  If the employee feels overburdened, he or she will probably shy away from new assignments that call for thinking and initiative.
- **Lack of self-confidence.**
  Lack of self-confidence stands in the way of some people accepting responsibility. A staff person who is unsure of his or her ability does not like to assume more responsibility. Self-confidence must be developed by carefully providing experience in increasingly difficult problems.
- **Positive incentives may be inadequate.**
  Accepting more responsibility requires more mental work and emotional pressure. Positive inducements for accepting delegated responsibilities include access to better personnel policies, opportunity for advancements, more desirable working conditions, prestigious title, recognized status in the organization, or other rewards.

Barriers to delegation can be overcome, but the first step is to understand the nature of the problem and how willing the manager or employee is to deal with the problem. The critical issue in delegation is decentralization of authority, and depending on the manager's attitude, delegation will be a productive activity or a frustrating experience. Effective management recognizes the strengths and capabilities of the staff and uses this talent appropriately. You, the new manager in this dynamic health care system, have the capability of transforming the workplace into an area where employees can be autonomous and challenged through effective delegation.

CASE STUDY

Delegation of Staff

Bob Jones is the 3-to-11 P.M. charge nurse at General Hospital's coronary care stepdown unit. A computer glitch has caused the staffing pattern for the institution became a nightmare: Not enough RNs were assigned to care for the patients in the ratio Bob preferred to provide quality care.

At the beginning of the shift, Bob called his coworkers and explained the staffing problem and the reason for it. Because of the computer problem, the float pool was also unavailable, so Bob proceeded to rearrange the usual assignments. He delegated functional tasks to the LPNs and reorganized the assignments for the RNs to maximize his staff and to provide quality of care.

Following the shift, Bob met with his coworkers for feedback. They were very positive and appreciated Bob's solution.

- What would you have done?
- Did Bob have the right to change the pattern of care delivery and to reorganize the work of the unit?

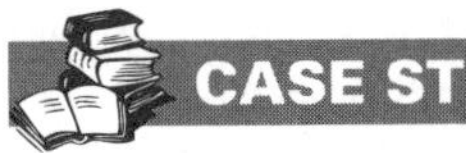

CASE STUDY

Improper Delegation

In all fields, different level employees have different tasks to do. For the nursing assistant, typical duties include giving bed baths, serving meal trays, checking vital signs, and completing a variety of other important tasks. Registered nurses, however, are expected to assess the patients, determine nursing care, delegate tasks to nonprofessional employees, and supervise their work. As in all cases, the nurse is ultimately responsible for the care received by patients.

With this in mind, consider the following situation: Jane James, RN, BSN, accepted a position in a skilled nursing facility and was expected to work with nursing assistants. On her first day, Mr. Williams, an experienced nursing assistant, and Jane were to work together. Jane began giving Mr. Williams a report when she was interrupted. Mr. Williams said that he would not complete his assignment because Jane, as a new nurse, needed to have experience. When Mr. Williams was sure Jane was proficient with the work, then and then only could he accept an assignment. In essence, Jane was told by the nursing assistant that she had to do the work of an RN and nursing assistant.

Jane was overcome with anger and confusion. She wasn't sure what to do. She replied, "I am ultimately responsible for the nursing care of your patients and mine. I would like to share the work with you. I cannot possibly comply with your suggestion. If you have concerns about my ability to provide nursing care, please feel free to discuss them with me, after you have completed the assignment I am delegating to you. Since we are going to work together, we need to understand each other."

- What is your analysis of this situation?
- What would you have done?
- How does understanding the process of delegation assist in conflict resolution?

SUMMARY

Delegation is an extremely important process that the effective manager must learn to skillfully handle. Delegation exists because the manager's personal responsibility exceeds the capacity to perform the necessary work. Ideally, the manager should concentrate on what is expected of a manager and delegate those activities that the staff is qualified to perform. Despite barriers to the process of delegation, guidelines are offered to facilitate the new manager's ability to delegate successfully.

LEARNER EXERCISES

1. Discuss some ways to implement effective delegation. What fundamental skills does the nurse manager require in order to delegate properly?
2. From your clinical practice, observe and identify how the nurse managers delegate. Note the process and techniques that an effective delegator uses. Notice the same when ineffective delegation is used.

3. List three tasks that you would consider easy to delegate and three that you would consider difficult. Would you use the same technique for both?
4. What legal issues are involved in the process of delegation? What information is required of the nurse manager to reduce the risk of legal problems?
5. Consider the following situations and determine whether or not the nurse manager is liable for the following actions:
   - When a nurse aide (allowed by policy) charts the care of a patient in the Nurse's Notes, and the RN cosigns the entries. (Remember the chart is a legal document and an RN is responsible for that which is charted in his/her name.) Is the RN liable if the aide injures the patient?

     Yes or No

     Yes, the RN signature indicates knowledge of the events which have been documented.
   - Are male nurses prohibited by law from performing certain tasks because of their gender?

     Yes or No

     No, a professional nurse has a scope of practice to determine limits of practice, not gender.
   - Is it appropriate for the RN on the day shift to pour or prepare medications for the RN on the next shift to provide to patients?

     Yes or No

     No, the nurse must be responsible for the entire activity of preparation and dispensing of medication.

REFERENCES

1. Kreitner, R. (1995). *Management*, 6th ed, Boston, Toronto: Houghton Mifflin Co., pp. 316–318.
2. Frohman, AL., & Johnson, L. (1993). *The middle management challenge: Moving from crisis to empowerment*. New York: McGraw-Hill.
3. Evans, M., & Aiken, T. (1998). In J. Catalano, *Nursing law and liability in nursing now, today's issues, tomorrow's trends* (pp. 173–206). Philadelphia: FA Davis.
4. Evans, M., & Aiken, T. (1998). In J. Catalano, *Nursing law and liability in nursing now, today's issues, tomorrow's trends* (pp. 189–196). Philadelphia: FA Davis.
5. Evans, M., & Aiken, T. (1998). In J. Catalano, *Nursing law and liability in nursing now, today's issues, tomorrow's trends* (pp. 189–193). Philadelphia: FA Davis.

SUGGESTED READING

Wick, J., Calhoun, L.U., & Stanton, L. (1993). *The learning edge: How smart managers and smart companies stay ahead*. New York: McGraw-Hill.

UNIT 3

Special Responsibilities of the Manager

9

Maintaining Standards

"The quality of a leader is reflected in the standards he/she sets for himself/herself."

Ray Croc

INTRODUCTION

Managers of patient care units are concerned with, and have the responsibility for, the delivery of comprehensive patient care. Today's managers are required to know the care contributions and the practice boundaries of each of the health care practitioners who come in contact with the patients. Most patient care units, especially those in long-term care and hospitals, are nursing labor-intensive (persons assigned to work are professional nurses, licensed practical nurses, patient care associates, or nurses' aides).

The boundaries of work for the different health care practitioners are established on the basis of an intricate framework composed of professional, societal, ethical, governmental, legal, and organizational inputs. At first glance, to act within such a complex set of norms, values, and regulations seems difficult; and to direct and guide others within this same framework is, at times, more difficult. Specifically, the integration of this framework exists for the maintenance of quality. The focus of this chapter is the professional and legal bases for the maintenance of standards that ensure quality nursing care. In addition, regulatory and licensing bodies are presented to show the forces that affect the boundaries of nursing practice.

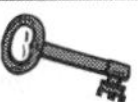

KEY CONCEPTS

Accreditation refers to the approval of an organization by an official review board after having met specific standards.

Answerability is a matter of legal or ethical responsibility.

Benchmarking is a tool that identifies best practices. It allows organizations to compare their performance within the organization and with other external organizations.

Certification is a process by which a nongovernmental agency or association certifies that an individual licensed to practice a profession has met certain predetermined standards specified by that profession for specialty practice. Its purpose is to assure the public that an individual has mastered a body of knowledge and acquired skills in a particular specialty.

Continuous Quality Improvement (CQI) a segment of quality management, is a systematic, organization-wide process to achieve ongoing improvement in the quality of services and operations and the elimination of waste.

Criteria refers to predetermined elements, qualities, or characteristics used to measure the extent to which a standard is met.

Disease Management is the provision of complete patient care for certain diseases (i.e., diabetes, transplants).

Incident Report is a written record of an event with possible or real untoward effects.

Indicator is an aspect of health care process or outcome that signals whether or not the appropriate interventions were provided.

Liability is the condition of legal risk due to the obligation of professional personnel obliged to provide reasonable care.

Malpractice refers to negligence, carelessness, or deviation from an accepted standard of practice by a professional.

Monitoring is observing and evaluating the degree to which a standard has been achieved.

Negligence is the carelessness or failure to act as a prudent person would ordinarily act under the same circumstances.

Outcomes Management is a management approach that focuses on the interrelatedness of clinical concerns of quality with cost effectiveness of care.

Performance Standards are specific written statements of nursing behaviors that further define what a nurse in a specific area of nursing should be doing; derived from standards of nursing care.

Practice Guidelines are standardized specifications developed through a process that uses the best scientific evidence and expert opinion for care of the typical patient in the typical situation.

Problems are questions or situations relating to patient care that are raised for inquiry, consideration, or resolution.

Quality is "the degree to which patient care services increase the probability of desired patient outcomes and reduce the probability of undesired outcomes given the current state of knowledge" (JCAHO).

Quality Management is a management approach that consists of systematic, ongoing monitoring and constructive actions to improve the quality of practice.

Registration is a process by which qualified individuals are listed on an official roster maintained by a governmental or nongovernmental agency. It enables such persons to use a particular title and attests to employing agencies and individuals that minimum qualifications have been met and maintained.

Risk Management is the function of planning, organizing, and directing a comprehensive program of activities to identify, evaluate, and take corrective action against risks that may lead to patient injury, employee injury, and property loss or damage with resulting financial loss.

Sentinel Events are unexpected occurrences involving death or serious physical, or psychological injury, or the risk thereof.

Standards are agreed-upon levels of excellence; established norms.

Standards of Nursing Practice are written statements of the expectations of the care the nurse should give; **process standards.**

Standards of Patient/Client Care are written statements of expectations of the care the patient should receive (or results of care received); **outcome standards.**

Structure Standards are written statements addressing the organization's culture (i.e., the mission, philosophy, goals, and policies).

Utilization Management is the process of integrating review and case management of services in a cooperative effort with other parties, including patients, employers, providers, and payers.

Utilization Review is the formal assessment of the medical necessity, efficiency, and/or appropriateness of health care services and treatment plans on a prospective, concurrent, or retrospective basis.

THE CLIMATE FOR NURSING PRACTICE

Each component of regulation adds a different dimension toward the maintenance of **quality** in nursing practice (see Figure 9-1). To begin, society recognizes the need for nursing's contribution, ultimately legitimizing nursing as a service profession and in turn requiring **answerability.** Professional standards guide appropriate nursing practice and to some extent are modified within specific organizations. A legal framework exists that grants nurses the right to practice through each state's nursing practice act. The government has a general responsibility for the health of its citizens and thus provides federal and state rules and regulations regarding health care delivery. The nursing profession is subject to these rules and regulations.

Perhaps the most influencial regulation was introduced in 1997 with the passage of the Balanced Budget Act (BBA), and amended by the Balanced Budget Act of 1999. These two acts have had the most impact on the delivery of health care in the United States by altering the reimbursement of patient care in acute care, skilled nursing, and rehabilitation facilities. Other forces impeding the delivery of quality nursing care are the regulations and oversight of care by managed care organizations.[1]

In order for the manager to formulate a personal approach to management, consideration must be given to the ethical standards rooted in professional, organizational, and

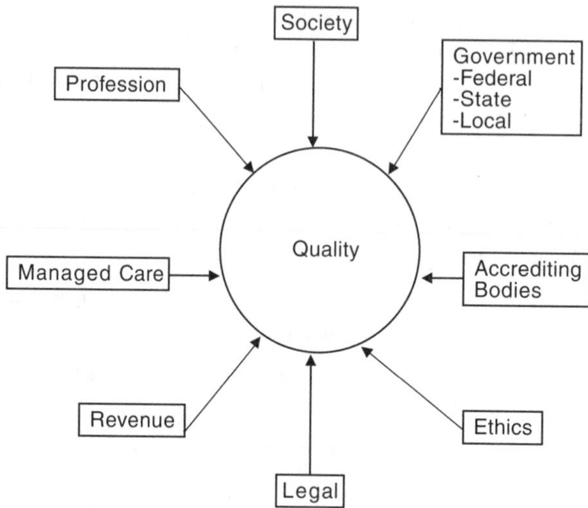

FIGURE 9-1. The variety of forces that create the climate for establishing standards of practice that ensure quality patient care.

personal values, as well as knowledge of the regulatory and accrediting bodies that impact the boundaries of professional practice. The nurse manager may also use **benchmarking** to evaluate nursing practice in his or her area of responsibility.

PROFESSIONAL BASIS FOR QUALITY ASSURANCE

Professional nurses possess responsibility and accountability, as well as answerability, for their professional actions. This necessitates establishing standards of practice to make an appropriate judgment as to what constitutes professional nursing practice. A **standard** is an agreed-upon level of excellence, or an established norm. In addition to a set of standards, **criteria** are also necessary. Criteria are predetermined elements, qualities, or characteristics used to measure the extent to which a standard is met. Criteria are needed to make the standard measurable. If the standards do not lend themselves to measurement, and specific criteria cannot be written, **indicators** are used to show that in all probability the standards were met. An indicator is an aspect of a health care process or outcome that signals whether or not the appropriate interventions were provided.

Standards of nursing are usually classified in one of three ways: structure standards, process standards, and outcome standards.

Structure standards address the environment, instrumentation, qualifications of personnel, job categorizations, number of staff, and committee configuration. Several structure standards usually address the integrative mechanisms of an organization (i.e., those that promote communication and decision making, such as committees and the divisions of work). Structure standards are influenced by regulatory bodies such as the federal government, as well as state and licensing agencies. For example, if an agency serves persons with Medicare (the federal insurance for the elderly) as the source of payment, the agency must meet the Medicare regulation that requires the services of a registered nurse for specific times and functions.

The Joint Commission on Accreditation of Healthcare Organizations (JCAHO) has an impressive, comprehensive set of standards that must be met to receive **accreditation.** This commission is a voluntary agency rather than an official government agency. The accreditation process of this body has traditionally focused its standards on quality concerns rather than fiscal or administrative concerns. The explicit mission of JCAHO is to improve the quality of care provided to the public.

Certification is another example of a structure standard. Certification reflects certain qualifications of an individual rather than an agency. In 1973 the American Nurses Association (ANA) created the ANA certification program to provide tangible recognition of professional achievement in a defined functional or clinical area of nursing. In 1991, the American Nurses Credentialing Center (ANCC) became its own corporation, a subsidiary of ANA. Although certification is voluntary for some specialties, it is required for nurse practitioners (i.e., nurses with master's degrees with a specialty in a certain field of practice) in all states. Certification is a credential that enhances one's professional status and is usually interpreted to indicate high competency in a specific area of practice. The American Nurses Association provides certification examinations in 37 specialized and advanced practice fields. Two new specialities were added in 2001: Advanced Clinical Diabetes Management and the Clinical Specialist in Pediatric Nursing. In 2000, ANCC re-conceptualized certification and created the Open Door 2000, a program that enables all qualified registered nurses, regardless of their educational preparation, to become certified in any of five specialty areas: Gerontology, Medical-Surgical, Pediatrics, Perinatal, and Psychiatric and Mental Health Nursing. Many specialty organizations are also participating in the certification processes. Certification requirements usually include at least three stipulations:

1. Written examination in a specific area of competence.
2. Active practice in the specialty.
3. Re-certification at specified periods.

The American Nurses Credentialing Center website can be found at http://www.nursingworld.org/ancc/.

Process standards address nursing activities that nurses perform. These written statements include nursing actions of assessment, diagnosis, interventions, and evaluation. These **standards of nursing practice** emanate from patient needs and are captured in guiding documents such as the American Nurses Association's (ANA) specialized group of standards, the medical-surgical standards, or cardiovascular nursing standards.[2] Many of the specialty nursing organizations, such as the emergency nurses, have published standards of practice for their specialty.[3]

These standards are available on most of the websites of the organizations:

- American Association of Colleges of Nursing: http://www.aacn.nche.edu
- American Association of Critical Care nurses: http://www.aacn.org
- American Cancer Society: http://www.cancer.org

- American College of Nurse Midwives: http://www.acnm.org
- American Diabetes Association: http://www.diabetes.org
- American Heart Association: http://www.amhrt.org
- American Nurses Association: http://www.ana.org
- American Psychiatric Nurses Association: http://www.apna.org
- Association of Operating Room Nurses, Inc.: http://www.aorn.org
- Emergency Nurses Association: http://www.ena.org
- Joint Commission on Accreditation of Health Care Organizations: http://www.jcaho.org
- National Association of Neonatal Nurses: http://www.nann.org
- National Council of State Boards of Nursing, Inc.: http://www.ncsbn.org.
- National Student Nurses Association: http://www.nsna.org
- Oncology Nursing Society: http://www.ons.org

In addition to the ANA standards and the specialty organizations' standards, nurses have the Agency for Healthcare Research and Quality (AHRQ), formerly the Agency for Health Care Policy and Research (AHCPR), as a resource.[4] This agency, a component of the Department of Health and Human Services, commissioned the Institute of Medicine of the National Institutes for Health to create a framework for analyzing health care processes. The work of developing clinical practice guidelines intended to assist practitioners in the prevention, diagnosis, treatment, and management of clinical conditions began in 1989. The development of guidelines is now carried out by the specialty organizations following the format of the practice guidelines of AHRQ. The guidelines are used for evaluating the quality of care and for implementing strategies for improvement. The clinical **practice guidelines** are also used for care management to reduce the cost of care by decreasing inappropriate diagnostic and therapeutic procedures. The intent of the guidelines is to present the best patterns of practice for a particular condition. For example, the American Association of Clinical Endocrinologists has developed nine sets of clinical practice guidelines. These guidelines are based upon the latest research and practice patterns available and are inclusive so that they represent a multidisciplinary focus and thus serve all practitioners. The guidelines may be accessed through the Website of the association: http://www.aace.com

Outcome standards address the end results of patient care. These groups of standards are patient centered and are usually identified along with the process standards. In other words, to what end are the nursing activities directed? How do nurses evaluate their work? These **standards of patient/client care** are frequently written in terms of the behaviors of patients (for example, regular cardiac rhythm). An indicator would be the strip of the electrocardiogram that shows normal sinus rhythm.

PRACTICE FRAMEWORK

If standards are indeed agreed-upon levels of excellence or established norms, then it seems reasonable that the organizational structure should be based on these agreed-upon levels of excellence or established norms. To this end, the following model has been developed to demonstrate the interrelatedness of all standards: structure, process, and outcome.

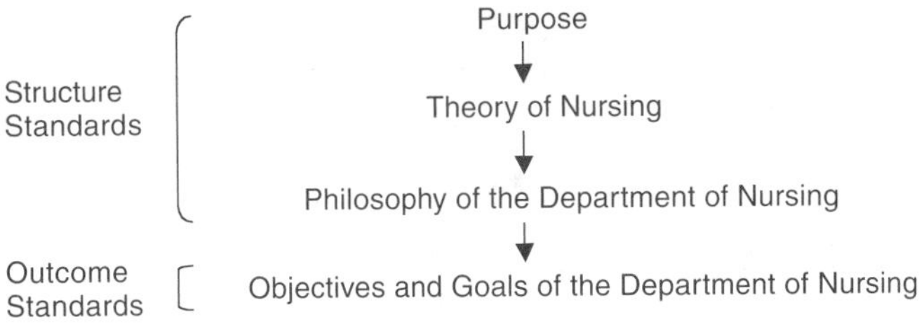

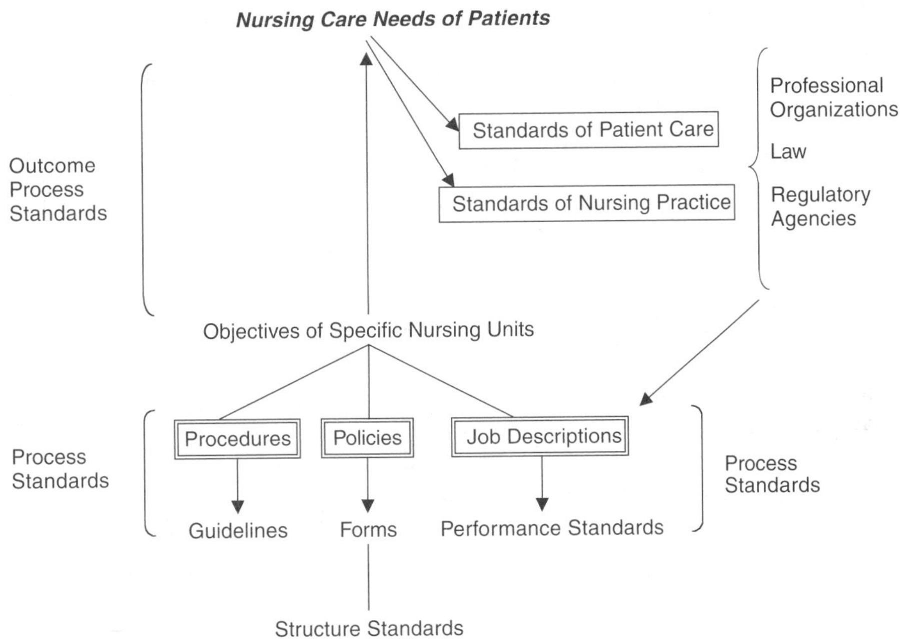

FIGURE 9-2. A graphic of a quality assurance model.

The standards framework model shows the various types of standards that are derived from the definitions of structure, process, and outcome (see Figure 9-2). At the heart of the model are the nursing care needs of patients. These needs directly influence all standards of the model. The standards of patient care and the standards of nursing practice are developed from the identified patient care needs. From these standards, which create the direct work of nursing, the additional process standards of procedures and job descriptions/**performance standards** flow. In addition, the structure standards (i.e., policies) should flow from the patient care needs. Policies should be developed to facilitate the implementation of care and process standards.

Moving upward on the model, it is noted that the objectives of the department of nursing are considered outcome standards, whereas purpose, theory of nursing, and philosophy are considered structure standards. This model and the definitions are shown to demonstrate that the many different terms used in most organizations are really variations of standards. There are different levels of abstraction used in the formulation of statements in that a philosophy statement is usually broader in scope and less definitive than a procedure. The standards framework model allows one to see the interconnectedness of various standards.

LEGAL BASIS OF NURSING

A nursing practice act is a legal statement that defines nursing and what nurses may do. Nursing practice acts differ from state to state, but generally represent that which the ANA has set forth. All professional nurses have a responsibility to be aware of their individual state's nursing practice act. Most organizations establish guidelines for nursing practice within the organization; however, these guidelines cannot exceed the boundaries of the nursing practice act of the state in which the nurse is practicing.

The nurse manager is responsible for understanding these guidelines as well as for the compliance of those working under her management. The wording of each nursing practice act is by design general, since this allows growth within the profession without enacting new legislation for every minor change.

Typically, nursing practice acts address definitions of practice and practitioners, allowable titles, licensure requirements, and qualifications/appointments of the board of nursing. Licensure allows a nurse to use the title of "registered nurse." Licensure is given after successful completion of the State Board of Nursing examination. **Registration**, which is tied to licensure, means that a qualified individual's name is listed on an official roster maintained by a government agency. Nursing practice acts also spell out the duties of the State Board of Nursing.

The interpretation of the act occurs at a state and organizational level for the purpose of creating policies to guide professional activities. For example, the profession of nursing is generating new and useful knowledge for patient care, and this explosion of knowledge has the potential for changing the work of nursing. A process known as research utilization is attempting to develop operational models that will incorporate clinical research findings into the usual and expected care of patients. Nurses must be allowed flexibility in practice based on sound research while at the same time be assured of freedom from legal sanction.

Ethical and Societal Concerns

Ethical and societal values influence health care legislation. This legislation often deals with particular populations and, accordingly, can be a powerful determinant of who and how we care for individuals. The growing number of elderly in the United States and the moral conflict surrounding legalized abortion are but two complex concerns for health care. The rationing of health care is another ethical and societal concern exemplified by the State of Oregon's plan to limit services.[5] Rationing deals with the distribution of resources and is currently used in health care practice. For example, triage and even some health insurances are forms of rationing. Active congressional legislation is attempting to correct some of the existing problems in insurance coverage, but enactment of law is a slow process, and those who lack insurance coverage experience a form of rationing. Literature is sparse on the rationing of nursing care. However, a manager does indeed ration when he or she makes assignments, places patients in rooms, moves patients, and delegates.

Ethical analysis can be used to examine health care rationing. Ethics provides the tools (principles, such as justice and beneficence) and the framework (theories, such as utilitarianism) to address both substantive and procedural questions (see Chapter 5 for additional information on ethical analysis). Thus, this complex network has the power to influence the profession's work, requiring the nursing practice act to be broad enough to allow for the active growth and change that is mandated by issues from society.

GOVERNMENTAL REGULATIONS

In 1965 an amendment to the Social Security Act of 1935 established the federal program known as Medicare, a health insurance program for older persons. The Medicare program is the largest single payer in the United States. The rising costs of health care soon became a concern with the inflation of the 1970s and the federal government's extended involvement with health care insurance.

The public concern, as well as the concern of government officials, toward these social conditions led Congress to enact two pieces of legislation. These acts tried to enforce self-regulation in the health care industry. The first act was the passage of the Bennett Amendment in 1972, which established professional standards review organizations.[6] This legislation provided for a review of medical care at those institutions or at those programs receiving federal monies such as Medicare reimbursement. There were two purposes in this legislative act: **utilization review** and quality review. The focus of utilization review, now referred to as **utilization management**, was the appropriate site for care, while the focus of quality review was the effectiveness of care. This legislation had little effect on either medical effectiveness or control of costs. Hospitals were reimbursed on a retrospective fee-for-service basis and the incentive to change was not present or demanded.

The second piece of legislation Congress passed was the National Health Planning and Resource Development Act of 1974 (amended in 1979). The purpose of this act was to correct the poor distribution of health care facilities and health care personnel.[7] Health systems agencies were established. Both of these acts focused on the maintenance of quality health care through government and professional regulation.

The most significant impact of government regulation was the enactment of the Social Security Act Amendments of 1983 (HR 1900, SI), Prospective Payment for Medicare Inpatient Hospital Services, which changed the way hospitals were reimbursed for Medicare patients.[8] The payment changed from a fee-for-service reimbursement to a prospective payment system. The basic thrust of this legislation involved the reorganization of the Medicare Trust Fund and the introduction of diagnosis-related groups (DRGs).[9] In essence, this involved the formation of DRGs, which represent a homogeneous grouping of variables for the purpose of consistent payment and to prospectively pay institutions a preset amount for each of the DRG categories. This was an attempt to limit the increases in the costs of hospital health care.

Under the DRG system, utilization review and quality assessment have taken on new and important meanings, which are to ensure that the most effective and efficient health care is being delivered. The appropriate use of resources became a critical issue. New meanings demanded new approaches to utilization review and quality assessment.

The administration for the Medicare program is handled by the *Health Care Finance Administration* (HCFA), now known as the Center for Medicare and Medicaid Services (CMS). The name change became effective in 2001. This program oversees the conditions of participation for all entities with the program. In many cases, the federal government delegates the oversight responsibility for Medicare conditions of participation to state agencies.

The term *quality assurance* was used in the 1981 JCAHO hospital standards to convey attempts to formalize the issues of quality-assessment programs in hospitals.[10] Currently, the terms quality management, **disease management**, **continuous quality improvement**, outcomes management, or care management are used to denote the approach to quality care.[11] **Quality management** is considered a pervasive, constant **monitoring** of actions to improve the quality of care. It was popularized by the late W. Edwards Deming.[12]

Outcomes management has been popularized through the demands of third-party payers for evidence of quality. It was also called for as part of the Omnibus Budget Reconciliation Act of 1986. As a result of this act, the Institute of Medicine (IOM) carried out a comprehensive review. The report of the IOM called for an emphasis on outcomes. Following the IOM report, Congress supported a number of new health care research initiatives through the Omnibus Reconciliation Act of 1989 (Public Law 101-239). Legislation was signed in March 1990 creating the eighth agency of the Public Health Service, the Agency for Health Care Policy and Research (AHCPR). The major thrusts of AHCPR are appropriateness of care and outcomes effectiveness.[13]

RISK MANAGEMENT

Another aspect of managing quality is the concept of **problems** or risk. **Risk management** is the function of planning, organizing, and directing a comprehensive program of activities to identify, evaluate, and take corrective action against risks that may lead to patient injury, employee injury, and property loss or damage with resulting financial loss.[14] It is apparent from the definition that implied in a program of risk management are concerns for medical and nursing malpractice as well as negligence and the issue of professional **liability. Malpractice** is a legal term that implies improper action on the part of a professional resulting in some form of injury to the patient as a direct result of care from the professional.[15] Malpractice involves deviation from a standard of usual professional conduct or interventions and results in injury. **Negligence** is the carelessness or failure to act as a prudent person would ordinarily act under the same circumstances. Professional personnel are obligated to provide reasonable care to patients. If this care is not provided, the professional is said to be liable or at risk for legal action. For the plaintiff (the individual who claims injury) to bring about a lawsuit, certain conditions must be met. The conditions include:

- Proof that the nurse owed a duty to the patient.
- Proof that failure to act properly would cause harm to the patient.
- Proof that the prevailing standard was not met.
- Proof that the injury directly resulted from the nurse's actions.

In our current social climate, lawsuits are not uncommon and risk management is necessary as a hospital manager attempts to resolve the problem. Management of lawsuits involving malpractice and negligence fall under the purview of the risk management department, as does concern for product liability, worker's compensation, and director's and officer's liability.

Accrediting and regulatory bodies require substantial attention to patient and personnel safety. For example, JCAHO has a standard that requires an organization to collect data to monitor the performance of processes that involve risks or may result in **sentinel events.**

Model of Risk Management

One way of conceptualizing risk management is through a model that identifies the essential components of a risk management system. These components are financial management, risk transfer, risk identification, risk analysis, risk treatment, and risk evaluation (see Table 9-1).

Financial Management

This is by no means a simple concept, but provision has to be made in the overall budget to deal with the problem of financial loss through a crisis, lawsuit, or settlement of an unanticipated natural event, such as a tornado. Insurance through a variety of companies may be the best way of managing potential emergencies. What this is doing is transferring the risk either to a self-contained fund or to insurance carriers. The individual professional is also in a position to transfer the risk of financial loss to insurance carriers. Liability insurance is available for the practicing nurse, but adherence to hospital policy and the standards of nursing care are the best insurance.

Risk Identification

Risk identification involves finding, through the process of auditing charts or reviewing incident reports or in conversation with staff, those problems with financial and legal risk to the institution.

TABLE 9-1. The Major Elements of A Risk-Management Program

Financial management
- Self-insurance program
- Property insurance coverages
- Casualty insurance coverages
- Education: Patient education
  - Employee education
  - Visitor education
- Risk transfer
- Risk identification
- Risk analysis
- Risk treatment
- Risk evaluation

Risk Analysis

To a great extent, the analysis process of determining the risk is a mathematical or statistical maneuver. Information exists to determine the probability of a particular event occurring in a particular institution, and how the risk to the agency can be calculated. For example, a medical center may incur more risk because of the nature of the care provided, such as experimental treatments and very ill patients. This may, according to the laws of probability, produce opportunities for a mistake or mismanagement of patient care. The analysis process identifies this and produces data to plan for these events. As part of the process to produce data, the analysis usually reviews a problem in light of several factors:

- The probability of the occurrence of the loss.
- The probable severity of the loss.
- The possible severity of the loss.
- The effects the potential loss would have on the organization clinically as well as financially.

Risk Treatment

Risk treatment involves dealing with the situation in such a way as to reduce the risk to the organization's resources, whether they be financial, human, or intangible. The programs available to reduce the risk depend entirely on the problem. For example, an educational program may be necessary to prevent patients from falling, or perhaps a human relations program is necessary to preserve and to reward staff for their contributions. Another tool that might be employed is to maintain an active public relations department so that the relationship with the community served is always positive.

Risk Evaluation

As in any problem-solving method, the evaluation of the interventions establishes the effectiveness of the interventions and methods used to gain information about the potential problem. Evaluation usually centers around basis issues, such as the impact on: (1) the organization's assets, (2) the future credit standing of the institution and its capital worth, and (3) the relationship with the community depending on the outcome of the problem.

Impact on Nursing Management

The impact on nursing management is significant. The nurse manager is in a position to control the activities of the staff to prevent problems and facilitate the goals of the organization. Risk management and nursing management are interdependent in meeting this end. Many institutions today employ nurse attorneys to oversee the risk management functions. These nurses are invaluable for the nurse managers and serve in an advisory capacity for many issues.

One tool that is available to the nurse manager is the **incident report**. This serves a very important function in identifying problems of a high-risk nature and allows for documenting the corrective action taken to deal with the problem. Incident reports are also referred to as occurrence reports, which is more descriptive of the function they serve because they alert the risk manager of potential problems that may require the intervention of members of the risk-management committee.

The success of this tool is directly related to administrators' attitudes and their use of the information. A punitive use could dissuade its intended use. As a nurse manager, you will want to encourage the reporting of every occurrence that could escalate into an incident. Doing this may control unexpected problems.

CASE STUDY

An Incident Report

Mary Reynolds, a staff nurse on a postoperative neurosurgical division, had been assigned five extremely dependent nursing care patients. Mary was also working with one nursing assistant. She realized this was a very heavy assignment, but she nonetheless decided to do her best. One of her patients, Mr. Morrow, a postoperative craniotomy patient who had also suffered a stroke, needed to get up in a chair. Mary and the nursing assistant got him up and restrained him in a chair since he remained listless and unresponsive. Mary checked him at 12:30, and all was fine. At 12:45, the neurosurgical resident found Mr. Morrow slumped on the floor. The resident immediately started shouting. Mary walked in the room and tried to explain that Mr. Morrow was fine 15 minutes earlier. The resident accused Mary of negligence and continued an angry diatribe. The head nurse walked in at this point, and immediately agreed with the doctor. The arguing continued, ending by the doctor leaving the area in midsentence, the head nurse retreating to her office, and Mary crying.

- What are the appropriate steps to take when an accident has occurred?
- Is an incident report required?
- What could Mary have done differently?
- Was Mary's practice consistent with the institution's policy on restraints?
- What could the head nurse have done differently?

SUMMARY

This chapter has addressed the maintenance of quality through the process of quality management. The professional and legal bases for nursing practice are presented as the foundations for monitoring quality. Quality management as a process is a systematic, ongoing function with explicit standards and criteria. The process is highly influenced by governmental, legal, and professional bodies. To some extent, society and ethics give direction to both the government and the profession. An associated process known as risk management deals with serious problems associated with financial loss, professional and staff problems, and intangible problems such as the agency's status in the community. Quality management and outcomes management are vital activities in the current health care system. Major third-party payers are demanding data that shows quality care.

LEARNER EXERCISES

1. Review your nurse practice act. Discuss in class what this act means to you as a professional.
2. Select a patient's chart, and review it to see what DRG is selected for the patient's condition. Find out how much the hospital will be reimbursed for the care depending on the category. Make a judgment as to how you, as a manager, could shorten the patient's stay.
3. Review the written standards of your agency. Are the standards monitored? How?
4. You are a case manager, and one of the patient care associates working with you spilled a basin of hot water on himself or herself. Complete the incident/occurrence report. What information should be included?
5. Define "nursing malpractice." What constitutes a legal transgression? What can you do to protect yourself from a malpractice suit?

REFERENCES

1. Finkelmann, A. W. (2001). *Managed care: A nursing perspective.* Englewood Cliffs, NJ: Prentice Hall.
2. American Nurses Association. (1991). *Standards of clinical nursing practice.* Washington, D.C.: Author.
3. Emergency Nurses Association. (1994). *Emergency nurse core curriculum.* Philadelphia: Saunders.
4. U.S. Department of Health and Human Services. (1995). *Using clinical practice guidelines to evaluate quality of care.* Rockville, MD: Agency for Health Care Policy and Research.
5. Weiner, J. M. (1992). Oregon's plan for health care rationing. *The Brookings Review, 10*(1), 26–31.
6. 92nd Congress of the United States. (1972). *Social security amendments of 1972* (publication No. PL92–603). Washington, D.C: U.S. Government Printing Office.
7. 93rd Congress of the United States. (1974). *Health planning act of 1974* (Publication No. PL 93–641). Washington, D.C.: U.S. Government Printing Office.
8. 98th Congress of the United States. *Social security amendments of 1983* (Publication No. PL 98–21). Washington D.C.: U.S. Government Printing Office.
9. Curtin, L., & Zurlage, C. (1984). *DRGs: The reorganization of health.* Chicago: S-N Publications.
10. Joint Commission on Accreditation of Healthcare Organizations. (2001). *Comprehensive accreditation manual for hospitals: The official handbook.* Chicago: JCAHO.
11. Lighter, D. E., & Fair, D. C. (2000). *Principles and methods of quality management in health care.* Gaithersburg, MD: Aspen.
12. Walton, M. (1986). *The Deming management method.* New York: Putnum Publishing Group.
13. U.S. Department of Health and Human Services. (1996). *Information dissemination to health care practitioners and policymakers.* Rockville, MD: Agency for Health Care Policy and Research.
14. Solomon, S. (1985). *Handbook of health care risk management, risk management process and functions.* Rockville, MD: Aspen.
15. Cushing, M. (1988). *Nursing jurisprudence.* Norwalk, CN: Appleton & Lange, pp. 26–27.

10

Motivation in the Work Setting

> "A leader's success is largely determined by the ability to motivate others."
>
> Author Unknown

INTRODUCTION

Of the multiple, interacting forces influencing people's performance in work settings, **motivation** is among the most complex. The theme of motivating factors that affect an individual nurse's performance will be carried throughout the chapter. Time-related factors, work climate that springs from a mix of worker backgrounds, plus a wide variety of other factors affecting motivation are described. All have had, and continue to make, a significant impact on the practice of nursing. Selected theories of motivation are described along with how motivational climate affects groups and individuals. Finally, common problems that interfere with productivity in work settings are discussed.

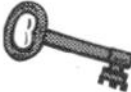

KEY CONCEPTS

Climate is a systems concept described as the human environment in which people work.

Dissatisfiers in Herzberg's theory are factors of motivation that are extrinsic to work content. Examples are salary, pleasantness of surroundings, and policies; also known as hygiene factors and maintenance factors.

Expectancy is a term used in Vroom's theory of motivation, meaning effort-performance association.

Intentionally Disinviting is the level in Purkey's Intentional Model of Motivation in which the individual is dissuaded and rejected.

Intentionally Inviting is the level in Purkey's Intentional Model of Motivation in which the individual is respected and encouraged.

Macromotivation describes the expectation that personal-needs satisfaction be a part of the employment situation; also known as type B motivation.

Micromotivation describes the expectation that only work-related needs be met through employment; also known as type A motivation.

Motivation is caused behavior; a psychological process that gives behavior purpose and direction.

Satisfiers in Herzberg's theory are factors that relate to work content. Examples are responsibility, autonomy, and achievement; also known as motivation factors.

Valence from Vroom's expectancy theory means one's feeling of satisfaction/ dissatisfaction about an outcome.

X Characteristics in McGregor's theory are those characteristics that cause a person to dislike work and to be productive only through coercion.

Y Characteristics in McGregor's theory are those characteristics that cause a person to enjoy work and to seek responsibility and challenges.

DEFINITIONS AND SOURCES OF MOTIVATION

Motivation is defined by Kreitner[1] as a psychological process that gives behavior purpose and direction, and by Davis[2] as caused behavior, the switch that turns the motor on. Motivation is sparked by internal and external interacting forces that modify one's perception of, and commitment to, goals. Motivation is a phenomenon internal to the individual but can be influenced by a variety of circumstances, including other people (coworkers and managers) and overall conditions in a setting. When managers take time to acknowledge employees' contributions, one-on-one or in teams, the personal satisfaction experienced by employees produces dividends for the overall organization. Bass cites Combs and Snygg's self-concept theory in which they assert that the most basic human drive is to maintain, protect, and enhance the perceived self, and Purkey and Schmidt's belief that the perceived self constitutes one's self-concept.[3] Along with these considerations is the assertion that self-concept is learned and modifiable. What is learned about self-concept is partially determined by time.

McBurney and Filoromo[4] remind us that in nursing, the Nightingale pledge continues to motivate and give direction to nurses today; it is not a Victorian ideology. Written in 1893, it still "serves as a professional mission statement, one that truly reflects the deep-seated vision and values of nursing. A modern analysis of this classic work creates a frame of reference to measure nursing practice." In it, one can recognize the source of many of today's nursing standards of practice statements.

THEORIES OF MOTIVATION

Overall, motivation theories are generalizations about the "why" and "how" of purposeful behavior. Motivation theories provide managers with a knowledge base for encouraging individuals to willingly pursue organizational objectives.[5] Nelson[6] quotes Harris on the importance of "connections" between workers and managers. When managers take time to connect with individuals and groups, the workers feel free to speak up because they know their opinions matter. Listening is highly motivating; the more "high tech" the environment, the more important it is and the more "high touch" managers need to be. The result can be the mutual development of high quality goals and service. Goal setting is one way in which managers attempt to influence motivation. Participation in goal setting gives the individual personal ownership of them, and triggers the motivational process that directs behavior toward a common goal. In order to be effective as motivators, goals must be specific, difficult, and participative.[7] Without some degree of difficulty, a goal does not generate motivation.

Needs Theorists

In 1943, Maslow described the propositions upon which he developed his theory of human motivation, popularly known as the hierarchy of human needs theory.[8] The propositions Maslow described include the following:

1. The human organism should be treated as a whole.
2. Somatically based drives are atypical in human motivation.
3. Basic goals of an unconscious nature are more fundamental in motivation theory than conscious goals.
4. Behavior must be understood as a channel through which many basic needs are simultaneously expressed or satisfied.
5. Human needs arrange themselves in a hierarchy of prepotency.
6. Classifications are based upon goals.
7. The total situation in which behavior occurs must be taken into account.
8. Both integrated and isolated reactions explain motivation.

Motivation theory is not synonymous with behavior theory, but rather motivation is only one class of behavior determinants, including biological, cultural, and situational determinants. Maslow formulated his theory of motivation on these theoretical demands and presented it as a framework for research through which his theory would be tested and either stand or fail. Today, we are familiar with his arrangement of prepotent needs into a five-classification hierarchy from lowest to highest: *physiologic needs*—the need for air, water, food; *safety needs*—the need to be secure from harm; *belongingness*—the need for friendship, affection, and love; *esteem*—the need for feelings of self-worth and for respect from others; and *self-actualization*—the need to make the most of one's life.[9] Lower-level needs must be partially satisfied before higher needs are activated and become the motivating force for behavior. Whether there is support or criticism of Maslow's work, the important consideration is the contribution he has made to the emerging body of knowledge about motivation. An important lesson learned from Maslow's work is that fulfilled needs do not serve as motivators.[10]

Over the years some have claimed that Maslow's theory has not stood the test of empirical assessment relative to distinct classifications or to an absolute, five-level, ascending hierarchy.[11] McClelland and Atkinson offer a modification of Maslow's hierarchy by stressing the influence of changing priorities in determining the relative importance of needs to individuals.[12] In the 1960s, McClelland described the following trichotomy of needs: affiliation, power, and achievement.[13] According to McClelland, individuals possess high, moderate, or low levels of each as a function of personality traits. Similarly, Alderfer, cited in Aldag, suggests a less-rigid arrangement of needs than what is defined by Maslow by presenting them as a no-set hierarchy.[14] Alderfer arranges needs into three categories: existence, relatedness, and growth. When frustrated in one area, an individual concentrates on another.

Personality Type and Motivation

A well-known theory of motivation in the work setting is Herzberg's two-factor theory.[15] Herzberg postulates that there are two separate sets of factors that influence motivation, each having a high-through-low value on a continuum. He labeled his two sets as motivation factors and maintenance factors. Maintenance factors are also known as **dissatisfiers**, or hygiene factors. Dissatisfiers are extrinsic influences that do not relate to job content. Instead, they relate to pay; job security; working conditions, such as lighting and pleasantness of surrounding; agency policy; and interpersonal relations with peers and supervisors. Poor quality or negative perceptions about these factors greatly dissatisfy some workers, who are referred to as maintenance seekers. Improvement in the factors, even in the perception of the workers, results in a neutral state and not in improved motivation. In other words, these factors are potent dissatisfiers but not strong motivators. Motivation factors are also known as **satisfiers.** Satisfiers come from intrinsic influences, relate to work content, and, when workers have opportunities to realize them, serve as strong motivators. These workers are referred to as motivation seekers. Some examples of satisfiers are the nature of the work itself, a sense of achievement, recognition, advancement, responsibility, and autonomy.

No factor from either set is wholly one-dimensional. Individuals are affected to some degree by each. At any given point in time, each person can be identified as predominantly a maintenance seeker or a motivation seeker. A significant difference separates those who are primarily maintenance seekers (i.e., while motivation seekers desire and appreciate improved dissatisfiers, maintenance seekers tend to purposefully avoid satisfiers). This phenomenon is partially explained by the fact that innate potential limits motivation. Situational variables influence how a person acts relative to job-related factors. In times of scarce job opportunities, different motivators influence people as opposed to when such a condition does not exist. Herzberg has contributed to motivation theory by emphasizing the potential of enriched work.[16]

An example of how Herzberg's theory is demonstrated in nursing practice is the development of nursing care patterns that fit situations. Ideally, when and how to utilize services of nonprofessionals in the delivery of nursing care belongs to nursing. Nurses who work toward this goal are motivation seekers. Without the return of decision making that affects meeting professional standards, health care will not be optimized and the current nursing shortage will continue. Herzberg counseled, "If you want to motivate the worker, don't put in another water fountain, provide a bigger share of the job itself."[17]

When nursing practice was restructured by administrators in the 1990s, professional autonomy was taken from nurses and they responded in a variety of ways. Most became frustrated when their numbers were greatly reduced and they were replaced by nurse assistants. The nurses who kept their positions were expected to supervise the nurse assistants and were therefore unable to fulfill their professional roles in the same way as before the change. In addition, the nurses felt unprepared and uncompensated for managerial roles. It has been reported by Blythe, Baumann, and Giovannetti[18] that the restructuring of nursing practice caused problems for individuals, teams, and organizations. Problems for nurses were felt at work and eventually confounded relationships and functioning at home. Relationships became less integrated, work activities became less controllable, and the ability to deliver effective care was compromised. Uncertainty became a daily concern for them as they often reported to non-nurse supervisors. One result was that the avenue for reporting nurse concerns to upper administration was lost. Nurse leaders in all domains (practice, education, research, and management) must demonstrate to administrators and economists the critical importance of professional autonomy that optimizes professional practice.

McGregor's theory X and theory Y present two contrasting sets of assumptions about human beings and work.[19] The assumptions are labeled **X characteristics** and **Y characteristics.** X-type individuals dislike work and avoid it when possible; have little ambition; need control, direction, and coercion; and respond when threatened with punishment. Their primary concern is security. Reasons for X-type behaviors vary with individuals and might be persistent or temporary.

Y-type individuals are self-directed, self-controlled, like work, seek challenges and responsibilities, and are inspired to increased commitment with success. As with individuals' preferences in Herzberg's two-factor theory, the total situation accounts for a departure from one's usual characteristics. One who typically performed at peak levels might suddenly begin to behave more like an X-type person. Factors internal or external to nursing might be the cause of such a change. Ironically, an event intended as a reward, such as the practice of "promoting" an excellent bedside nurse to the role of first-level manager, can produce a negative change in the individual's performance. If the promotion places the nurse outside her or his field of expertise, the move can produce widespread problems for the organization, as when newly promoted nurses begin to avoid situations and responsibilities they are not prepared to meet. At one time, promoting practitioners into management positions was more commonly seen when there was no other form of reward for nurses. McGregor suggests arranging conditions and methods so that the worker can attain his or her own goals within the organizational goals.[20] Programs to prepare nurses for new roles have made a significant difference in how nurses can be rewarded today.

Motivation as Rational Decision Making

Vroom's expectancy theory, cited in Aldag, views motivation as a rational decision-making process involving **expectancy**, defined as effort-performance association;

valence, defined as one's feelings of satisfaction/dissatisfaction about an outcome; and *instrumentality*, defined as one's perceived performance-outcome association.[21] Porter and Lawler, cited in Aldag, designed a model of Vroom's theory in which valence is the strength of one's desire for something, expectancy is the probability of getting it with a certain action, and motivation is the strength of drive toward the action.[22] The formula is as follows:

$$[\text{Expectancy} \times \text{sum of } (\text{Valence} + \text{Instrumentality})] = \text{Effort}$$

Motivation is high when an individual has a good chance of getting personally satisfying rewards through his or her efforts. Expectancy theory might be seen in nursing when a nurse initiates a request to be considered for more responsibility on the unit. Perhaps the nurse sees a need for an experienced staff member, other than the head nurse, to coordinate orientation activities and functions for new graduates beginning their professional careers. Once the nurse manager approves the idea, together they agree on what new competencies the nurse will need to develop to serve in the new role. They establish a time frame for readiness, and the expectancy–valence instrumentality connection is put into motion. If the unit budget permits an increase in salary for the added responsibility of the role, the nurse's valence will undoubtedly go up in the direction of satisfaction, even though salary was not the original motivating force. In this example, the nurse engaged in participative management by being instrumental in decisions, problem solving, and organizational change.

The nurse in the above example can also be viewed as operating at a high-need level in Maslow's hierarchy, a motivation seeker in Herzberg's theory, and as a McGregor's Y-type individual. The same can be said about nurses who are instrumental in designing nursing care patterns that meet specific organizational and patient needs.

Motivation theorists present different perceptions on the same theme, and they suggest different explanations of what influences performance. They are the postulates upon which theoretical demands are satisfied. While the theories presented in this chapter continue to undergo the scrutiny of empirical assessment, they provide a framework for greater understanding of the complex phenomenon of motivation. A question of motivational differences based on gender arises as the number of male nurses increases. Henderson found, however, that when correlating the need for power, risk taking, and influence, no gender differences were found.[23] Sharpening understanding of the many different internal and external forces that influence performance in the work setting remains an ongoing challenge to practitioners in striving for excellence in nursing care delivery.

ORGANIZATIONAL CLIMATE AND MOTIVATION

A person's interest, ability, and will to accomplish, while essential for success, are not sufficient to ensure the kind of performance needed to accomplish goals. Work-related goals are formulated and carried out in complex organizations where the worker is affected by numerous changing events over which he or she has little control. The collective events operating simultaneously create a climate described by Davis as the human environment in which people work.[24] It surrounds and affects everything that happens and in turn is affected by everything that occurs in the setting. **Climate** influences the quality of performance that can take place in a given situation. High-quality performance is more likely to take place in settings where the climate is predominantly positive relative to both the organization and its goals and to individual workers and their needs. Climate can be the result of chance or design. Climate by design in the work setting aims to improve motivation for the purpose of improving performance. Arranging work relationships within and between departments is one way the organization can maintain some control over its internal climate. It is an important way to promote organizational goal attainment. Having an understanding of how workers and groups are alike and different from one another is critical in planning a positive work climate. The effectiveness, then, of an organization's structure partially depends on the participation of representatives of all major work groups employed.

Nelson,[25] in the introduction of his book, writes about energizing workers as individuals, team members, and as employees of an organization. He believes the quality of one-on-one relationships between workers and managers is at the core of energized workers. One-on-one relationships:

- Build morale.
- Empower and foster independence and autonomy.
- Strengthen communication chains.
- Encourage suggestions.
- Encourage creativity.
- Encourage use of training and development opportunities.
- Energize enthusiasm for challenging work.

Strong teams are an effective and efficient way to accomplish goals. Nelson states "none of us is as smart as all of us." [26] Productive teams have:

- A clear purpose and well-defined goals.
- Team spirit (described in the following acronym developed by Singer)[27]
    - **T**ogether
    - **E**veryone
    - **A**chieves
    - **M**ore
    - **W**ith
    - **O**rganization
    - **R**ecognition
    - **K**nowledge
- Productive meetings.
- Team initiative.
- Team suggestions.
- Creative teams.
- Self-managed teams.

Managers reawaken in workers the spirit that makes an organization great. Organizations thrive when workers use initiative and creativity. Innovative companies energize individuals through organizational practices[28] by:

- Designing less-restrictive policies and procedures.
- Fostering independence and autonomy.

- Facilitating organizational communication.
- Using suggestion programs.
- Creating employee development programs.
- Creating and maintaining a rewarding environment and benefits.
- Allowing community involvement on company time.

The effectiveness of nurse leaders in organizations greatly influences the climate in which nurses at all levels function. Important skills include communication, group dynamics, decision making, and conflict management. Climate is a strong determinant of opportunities afforded nurses in the organization, which results in high or low motivation. There is an increasing mix of nurses from more and more different backgrounds in practice. Some of the differences include ethnic background, age (those who enter nursing for the first time as a second career or after having raised a family, and those who have delayed their education for a variety of other reasons). Age differences of new practitioners and the kinds of responsibilities individuals in the mix bring to the practice situation differ, and they influence motivation, sometimes in a profound way. Mature individuals find themselves being mentored by much younger, but more experienced, nurses, and these situations call for high levels of mutual regard for each other.

Individuals working together in a work setting affect the work climate. Nurses in practice can represent distinctly different orientations to the profession, each having been groomed by different times. As a consequence, they frequently hold different values and attitudes relative to expectations in the work setting. An interesting analogy of this is presented by Toffler in his book *The Third Wave*, cited in Buchholz.[29] Toffler describes three revolutionary eras in the history of humankind dating from primitive man to the present. The first two eras proceeded at a slow and placid pace, gradually introducing changes that persisted over long periods of time. The first era began when primitive, roving hunters settled into permanent communities and began to farm the land. It is the longest of the eras, lasting until the Industrial Revolution ushered in the second era. With the advent of mechanization, men flocked to cities for employment in factories where machines took over tasks previously done by hand. While short in comparison to the first era, industrialization produced changes in society that dominated the thinking, values, and attitudes of several generations, roughly for a 100-year period. Lastly, the development of cybernetics and the introduction of computers in the marketplace marked the beginning of the third era, characterized by rapidly occurring changes and shifts in individuals' expectations relative to all aspects of living, including the work setting.

Toffler refers to individuals from the second and third eras as second wavers and third wavers, respectively.[30] The terms come from the comparison of the third era to *tsunami*, the giant Pacific tidal wave set off by an underwater earthquake that caused sudden, dramatic, and permanent changes in land masses. For several decades, second- and third-wave nurses who had experienced vastly different life experiences worked side-by-side with their different expectations from employers. Simon subdivides goals into personal goals and role-defined goals.[31] Second-wave nurses tended more toward role-defined goals relative to their work, while third-wave nurses expected both categories to be satisfied in the work setting. The differences produced conflict when not managed well.

The profession was, for a time, strongly influenced by nurses who lived through the Depression with the concomitant fear of being out of work, followed immediately by World War II with its demand for ongoing sacrifices from civilians in their daily lives. They can be thought of as second wavers whose experiences equipped them to conform to established management-dominated work situations. The generation that came after them can be thought of as third wavers who were strongly influenced by attitudes that came about as a result of the many societal changes during the 1960s. They tended to question established practices, such as standard 8-hour shifts, and expected to participate actively in decisions that affected them. Using Toffler's analogy, Buchholz suggested that it was to the advantage of second wavers to use the power of the third wave—to ride it rather than try to turn it back to sea.[32] The task was a reciprocal one requiring effort from both groups. Similar differences continued to separate groups of nurses over time, based on their backgrounds. Nurses in practice today have similar differences, with some entering the profession for the first time during midlife while others are beginning their careers just out of high school. Each brings different degrees of maturity, responsibilities, and life experiences to his or her work. Retirement and retirement issues are more of an issue for older nurses, making them more likely to stay in their employment situations, while younger nurses seek more variety within the profession, including pursuing higher degrees while working part time.

Understanding what motivates each other can bridge the gap that separates people. Focusing joint efforts on criteria that remain constant in the face of changes holds the most promise in finding a common ground that can enable the two groups to work effectively together. In nursing, the criteria are the standards of professional nursing practice. Agreement on standards is the stabilizing force that enables individuals with different approaches to the practice of nursing to work together in harmony. Each generation must respect the fact that, unavoidably, different forces produce one's motivation. Skillful managers can predict under what conditions second wavers and third wavers will complement each other and therefore work well together, and when they are serious antagonists who need to be separated. Keeping standards of nursing practice the focal issue for all nurses requires that conflicts be managed so that they do not predominate to the point of becoming the focal issue. Maintaining positive relationships, high-quality standards, and attainment of organizational goals depends on a purposefully designed pattern of people relationships. Relationships are established through organizational design and are depicted graphically in organizational charts.

Micromotivation and Macromotivation

When second wavers were the only practitioners in nursing, motivational efforts in the work setting were directed toward the work to be done within organizational conditions. Davis refers to this approach as type A, or **micromotivation.**[33] There were few problems with this system because second wavers had known, or had been directly affected by, unemployment. Being gainfully employed was highly self-fulfilling for them. When third wavers entered practice, work-related goals alone no longer sufficed for their felt sense of self-fulfillment. They had not been directly affected by unemployment as their predecessors had been. The experiences of third wavers permit them to think of themselves in broad terms, not only in terms of what they do for a living (e.g., a nurse or a banker). They perceive themselves more holistically and seek broader considerations in their workplace. The shift in organizations is therefore toward type B, or **macromotivation,** which includes outside environmental considerations that influence performance.

The shift from micromotivation to macromotivation can be seen in lengthening lists of employee benefits in organizations today. Fringe benefits have implications for motivation. They are tangible rewards, relatively easy to provide, and have the potential to produce high levels of satisfaction in workers. While fringe benefits influence climate, they are extrinsic to work and tend to add to satisfaction but do not improve performance. For example, a worker can experience heightened commitment to a disliked job because of the company's comprehensive fringe benefits. The worker does not feel a need to improve his or her performance because the benefits are not contingent on performance.[34] This example demonstrates the real dichotomy between extrinsic and intrinsic sources of motivation. There can be serious problems in organizations where the fringe benefit package is the dominant mechanism for satisfying workers.

Aldag reminds us that one cannot generally assume that making an employee happy will in turn make him or her more productive.[35] Fringe benefits, such as sick leave, salary, and vacation time are examples of extrinsic sources of motivation that are not related to the work that one does. Teachers who continue to teach primarily because having summers off suits their lifestyle are extrinsically motivated. Intrinsic sources of motivation, however, are derived from the work itself because it is self-fulfilling to the individual. Teachers who enjoy teaching because their work helps develop minds remain committed to their profession despite average-to-mediocre benefits. They are intrinsically motivated in the same way that nurses who worked long hours to develop the system of primary nursing care were intrinsically motivated.

Because intrinsic sources of motivation hold more promise for improving performance, organizations must design work that will increase performance-related satisfaction. Recall what Herzberg had to say about additional water fountains versus a greater share of the work itself. In nursing, this can be done by designing a climate that will allow nurses to realize their true professional potential. Academic preparation of baccalaureate nurses equips them to move forward from an initial state of task and relationship concerns, described in the Hersey-Blanchard model in Chapter 2, to the mature level of independence relative to autonomous decision making in health matters that fall within the realm of nursing practice. Climates dominated by rigid bureaucratic policies and procedures that are primarily concerned with efficiency frequently frustrate the potential that professional nurses bring to their places of practice. The unfortunate consequence all too often is a willingness of many nurses to remain in the prevailing dependent role perpetuated by administrative paternalism that characterizes some health care organizations.

MOTIVATIONAL PROBLEMS

There is no formula to improve motivation that would apply to all situations, or to take what has been successful in one situation and apply it to another. Differences exist between individuals and within groups that spring from ability, experience, preference, values, culture, ideals, time, place, and beliefs. Such wide variations make uniformity impossible. Davis points out that primary physiological needs differ in intensity from person to person, and in the same person from time to time, and that secondary psychosocial needs are vague and change with one's level of maturity.[36] These facts complicate efforts to improve motivation. Experience shows that the same factor can exist as opposites in two different people, such as submission and aggressiveness. At times, several factors in combination act as a single factor to influence people, such as hunger. When victims of a disaster, such as a fire or earthquake, suffer from a variety of losses, hunger becomes a primary need. A behavior can be produced by several different factors. Take, for example, absenteeism that can be due to a lack of interest, conflict with coworkers, or an attempt to avoid an unpleasant or feared task.

Simon describes the responses of three bricklayers to the question: "What are you doing?" One said, "Laying a brick"; another said, "Building a wall"; and the third said, "Helping to build a cathedral."[37] Obviously, each was motivated by very different perceptions of his task.

A Situational Approach

Bassett discusses the Japanese spinoff on the concept of participative management, originated in but never implemented in the United States.[38] The Japanese used the concept successfully in industry to foster motivation that improved performance. It was felt at the time that the United States should learn from Japan how to implement participative management. There were, however, vast differences between people of these two countries. There was little in common between the two regarding societal factors and major historic events. Historically, the Japanese lived in an ancient, single-culture, imperialistic society, whereas Americans lived in a young, multicultural, democratic society. The outcome of World War II left Japan's cities war-torn and their country defeated, whereas Americans experienced neither event. A consequence of the widespread destruction in Japan resulted in modern factories being built during its reconstruction with newer, more modern equipment, whereas the United States continued to operate with outdated factory buildings and equipment designed early in the Industrial Age. Participative management filled a need for the Japanese to demonstrate unity and to restore some of the pride lost as a result of their loss from the war. The differences between the two situations made it unlikely that the outcomes could be duplicated. This example demonstrates that what works in one situation does not necessarily work in another.

What, then, is necessary to improve motivation? The answer is clear that careful analysis of all situational factors is necessary to know how to begin. Experienced, skilled managers understand that they have a first-line major responsibility to provide their staff with a climate that is conducive to the actualization of each individual's needs. Bass featured a description of Purkey's Intentional Model that depicts two different ways to influence motivation, one positive and one negative.[39] Introduced in 1978, it and has been utilized by several disciplines. Nurse managers are encouraged to make use of it as a strategy for influencing positive motivation within nursing. One level of functioning in the model is **intentionally inviting** and consists of four elements:

1. Optimism
2. Respect
3. Trust
4. Intentionality

In the intentionally inviting level, people are viewed as being valuable and capable of being self-directed. Their uniqueness is acknowledged through courtesy, they are trusted to choose what is best for the overall good, and actions are designed to accomplish a beneficial end.

Another level, by contrast, is **intentionally disinviting**, which consists of actions designed to:

1. Dissuade
2. Discourage
3. Defeat
4. Destroy

People are insulted, criticized, and ignored, usually through the manner in which policies are formulated and/or implemented. Naisbitt, cited in Bassett, says that "ordinary people are dying to make a commitment," and managers pave the way for them to be internally motivated to do so.[40] The most promising approach managers can adopt to influence motivation in a positive direction is to concentrate on what is central to a group's existence and develop skill in the use of strategies to accomplish that end.

Issues Central to Nursing

As stated earlier in this chapter, values central to nursing are found in practice standards of the profession. Nurses in formal management positions must, while hand-in-hand with practitioners, design plans that can foster staff participation and shared decision making in carrying out professional standards.

Managers must shift from being order givers to being facilitators. Individuals participating in ongoing staff involvement in matters that pertain to practice are rewarded through improved performance, increased responsibility, increased independence, improved knowledge of the overall organization, and improved capacity to change.

Benefits to the organization that can result from the shift in managers' functions are the combined strength of several competent individuals, sharpened and refined ideas, incorrect ideas that go unnoticed by one person which can be picked up by the group, competition replaced with cooperation, increased morale and motivation among group members, gained knowledge which alters opinions and attitudes, clearer understanding of the nature and feasibility of goals, and goals that are congruent with group-perceived values.[41]

Barriers to sharing responsibility with the staff include fear of losing control by management, risk of not knowing what the staff will do, a felt threat to authority and position, and feeling the staff is not mature enough, smart enough, or motivated enough. Realizing professional standards in practice is a result of participation and cooperation on the part of management and staff who respect and trust each other.

CASE STUDY

Motivation

The nurse manager's seemingly diminishing interest in, and knowledge about, issues that directly affect patient care and staff nurse satisfaction is creating a serious morale problem. Committed and enthusiastic nurses feel extremely frustrated that their efforts to maintain high standards on the unit are being negatively affected by the lack of involvement on the part of the head nurse.

The nurses decide that the best course of action is to approach the head nurse with their perception of what is happening. They know that if nothing is done, their motivation to continue to invest their energy on that particular unit will suffer and that many requests for transfer to other units in the hospital will result. As a representative of the staff, you are asked to meet with the head nurse to present a planned program for turning the situation around. The planned program has been designed by the group of staff nurses, not only by yourself.

Analyze the problem relative to the needs of the unit. Your goals are to be effectively assertive as you:

- Attempt to solve the problem at the unit level.
- Offer support, rather than blame, to the nurse manager by acknowledging her responsibilities that take her away from the unit.
- Maintain the high-level motivation of the staff that everyone had become accustomed to.

CASE STUDY

Charge Nurse Shows Favoritism

Lately a competent charge nurse on a busy medical unit has been showing an unusual degree of favoritism toward one particular nurse for time off and special requests for care assignments. The other staff members are given equal opportunity for work-related requests. The unit as a whole has had a history of high morale and *esprit de corps*, but as expected the recent behavior of the charge nurse threatens the cohesiveness of the staff. The nurse manager has become aware of the problem and plans a conference with the charge nurse because she knows what poor morale can do to motivated staff.

- What approach should the nurse manager use with the charge nurse?
- What elements are essential in the work setting for keeping motivation high?
- What are the likely consequences to the overall group if the nurse manager fails to stem the unfair practices of the charge nurse?
- What would you do if you were one of the staff on this unit?

SUMMARY

Early on in this chapter, the influence of Florence Nightingale was presented as the force that focuses attention on the need for cooperative efforts to maintain standards of practice as a unifying force in nursing. The importance of nurse managers in fostering motivation was stressed. Motivation was defined as caused behavior, and four theories of motivation were reviewed to provide a basis for understanding the propositions from which motivation comes. Examples were cited of how nurses have demonstrated high levels of motivation to meet their personal standards of excellence, as well as those of the profession. Climate was looked at relative to its influence on group and individual motivation, and the shift from micromotivation to macromotivation in organizations was traced back to its cause. Finally, problems with motivation were explored, misconceptions of how to improve motivation in unique situations were described, and the responsibilities of nurses to improve the quality of practice by taking responsibility for their own level of motivation were defined. The role of nurse management was specified for designing a climate conducive to improving motivation along with the personal rewards and organizational benefits that accompany growth. Barriers to constructive climates were identified as a reminder of inadvertent behaviors that stand in the way of advancing professional practice.

LEARNER EXERCISES

1. Think of a time during clinical practice when situational factors in your life prevented you from performing as a McGregor Y person or a Herzberg motivation seeker. To what degree did situational factors influence your professional responsibilities to your patients and the operation of the unit where you were assigned? How did you handle the situation? How did the instructor and staff respond to your performance? What did you learn from the experience? How will you handle a similar situation in the future?
2. You have an idea that you feel will encourage daily updating of patient care plans. You are a senior student and your instructor tells you to present your idea to the charge nurse. How will you go about this, considering your level of experience compared to that of the charge nurse? What motivational factors should you stress?
3. Older nurses on a unit continually refer to younger nurses and students as being less committed to patients than their generation of nurses. This is causing a gulf between older and younger nurses, as well as a morale problem. Based on Toffler's description of the reasons for generational differences, propose an approach for stabilizing the conflict.
4. You overhear a group of nurses, who recently returned from a conference on improving performance, discussing their reactions to the program. Opinions vary relative to the practicality of what was presented. Reactions include:
   - "We should do what nurses in agency X did to improve performance."
   - "It is impossible to improve performance here because our benefits provide no incentives."
   - "Even though we have an outdated building and old equipment, we should be able to identify ways to improve meeting basic standards of practice."
   - "It's such a big problem, and I feel frustrated trying to balance my nursing practice responsibilities along with all the other expectations placed on me outside of work."
   - "Attending the conference was a waste of time. I went to find out how to make the changes needed on our unit, and no one told us that."
   - "It was a nice day away, with pay, from the confusion of the unit."

Respond to each reaction, giving your reasons for agreement or disagreement based on content from this chapter. Your instructor thinks it would be a good assignment for you, individually or as a group, to propose a strategy to bring some commonality to these diffuse reactions. Using content from Chapters 1 through 10, propose a theoretical approach to the situation.

REFERENCES

1. Kreitner, R. (1995). *Management*, 6th ed. Boston, Toronto: Houghton Mifflin Co., p. 398.
2. Davis, K. (1981). *Human behavior at work: Organizational behavior*. New York: McGraw-Hill, p. 42.
3. Bass, L.S. (1991). Motivation strategies: A new twist. *Nursing Management*. 22(2), 24.
4. McBurney, B.H., & Filoromo, T. (1994, February). The Nightingale pledge: 100 years later. *Nursing Management*, 25(2), 72–74.
5. Kreitner, R. (1995). *Management*, 6th ed. Boston, Toronto: Houghton Mifflin Co., p. 398.
6. Nelson, B. (1998). *1001 ways to energize employees*. New York: Workman Publishing, p. 4.
7. Kreitner, R. (1995). *Management*, 6th ed. Boston, Toronto: Houghton Mifflin Co., pp. 405–406.
8. Shafritz, J.M., & Hyde, A.C. (editors). (1987). *Classics of public administration*, 2nd ed. Chicago: Dorsey Press, p. 135.
9. Aldag, R.J., & Brief, A.P. (1979). *Task design and employee motivation*. Palo Alto, CA: Scott Foresman, pp. 9–10.
10. Kreitner, R. (1995). *Management*, 6th ed. Boston, Toronto: Houghton Mifflin Co., p. 402.
11. Aldag, R.J., & Brief, A.P. (1979). *Task design and employee motivation*. Palo Alto, CA: Scott Foresman, pp. 9–10.
12. McClelland, D.C., & Atkinson, J.W. (1975). *Power: The inner experience*. New York: Ewington Publishers, p. 585.
13. Henderson, M.C. (1995, April). Nurse executives: Leadership motivation and leadership effectiveness. *Journal of Nursing Administration*, 25(4), 45–51.
14. Aldag, R.J., & Brief, A.P. (1979). *Task design and employee motivation*. Palo Alto, CA: Scott Foresman, p. 11.
15. Davis, K. (1981). *Human behavior at work: Organizational behavior*. New York: McGraw-Hill, p. 56.
16. Kreitner, R. (1995). *Management*, 6th ed. Boston, Toronto: Houghton Miffin Co., p. 404.
17. Bassett, L.C. & Metzger, N. (1986). *Achieving excellence*. Rockville, MD: Aspen, p. 86.
18. Blythe, J., Baumann, A., & Giovannetti, P. (2001). Nurses experiences of restructuring in three Ontario hospitals. *Journal of Nursing Scholarship, First Quarter*, 33(1), 61–68.
19. Claus, K.E., & Bailey, J.T. (1977). *Power and influence in health care*. St. Louis: Mosby, p. 128.
20. Bassett, L.C., & Metzger, N. (1986). *Achieving excellence*. Rockville, MD: Aspen, p. 86.
21. Aldag, R.J., & Brief, A.P., (1979). *Task design and employee motivation*. Palo Alto, CA: Scott Foresman, p. 18.
22. Aldag, R.J., & Brief, A.P. (1979). *Task design and employee motivation*. Palo Alto, CA: Scott Foresman, p. 18.
23. Henderson, M. C. (1995, April). Nurse executives: Leadership motivation and leadership effectiveness. *Journal of Nursing Administration*, 25(4), 45–51.
24. Davis K, (1981). *Human behavior at work: Organizational behavior.* New York: McGraw-Hill, p. 104.
25. Nelson, B. (1998). *1001 ways to energize employees*. New York: Workman Publishing, pp. ix–x.

26. Nelson, B. (1998). *1001 ways to energize employees*. New York: Workman Publishing, p. 23.
27. Nelson, B. (1998). *1001 ways to energize employees*. New York: Workman Publishing, p. 86.
28. Nelson, B. (1998). *1001 ways to energize employees*. New York: Workman Publishing, pp. 125–206.
29. Buchholz, S. (1985). *The positive manager.* New York: Wiley, p. 5.
30. Buchholz, S. (1985). *The positive manager.* New York: Wiley, p. 5.
31. Simon, H.A. (1976). *Administrative behavior: A study of decision-making processes in administrative organizations*, 3rd ed. New York: The Free Press, p. 265.
32. Buchholz, S. (1985). *The positive manager*. New York: Wiley, p. 9.
33. Davis, K. (1981). *Human behavior at work: Organizational behavior.* New York: McGraw-Hill, p. 77.
34. Aldag, R.J., & Brief, A.P. (1979). *Task design and employee motivation*. Palo Alto, CA: Scott Foresman, p. 24.
35. Aldag, R.J., & Brief, A.P. (1979). *Task design and employee motivation*. Palo Alto, CA: Scott Foresman, p. 23.
36. Davis, K. (1981). *Human behavior at work: Organizational behavior*. New York: McGraw-Hill, p. 42.
37. Simon, H.A. (1976). *Administrative behavior: A study of decision-making processes in administrative organizations*, 3rd ed. New York: The Free Press, p. 27.
38. Bassett, L.C., & Metzger, N. (1986). *Achieving excellence*. Rockville, MD: Aspen, p. 86.
39. Bass, L.S. (1991). Motivation strategies: A new twist. *Nursing Management, 22*(2), 24.
40. Bassett, L.C., & Metzger, N. (1986). *Achieving excellence*. Rockville, MD: Aspen, p. 83.
41. Bassett, L.C., & Metzger, N. (1986). *Achieving excellence*. Rockville, MD: Aspen, p. 83.

11

Monitoring and Improving Performance

"To avoid criticism, do nothing, say nothing, be nothing."

Elbert Hubbard

INTRODUCTION

During the formal educational experience, course objectives serve as the basis for evaluating one's level of academic success. Each set of course objectives contains statements of expectations and criteria for acceptable knowledge attainment and performance. The content of course evaluation forms are based on course objectives. Students are familiar with this system of evaluation and therefore have some preparation for taking an active role in judging their own performance as practitioners. In this chapter, the focus is on monitoring performance in the work setting by stressing performance appraisal as important to the profession, to organizations, and to individuals[1] and to encourage students to become familiar with all aspects of the process in order to advance their careers, to contribute to organizations, and to advance the profession. Study of performance appraisal as a system is therefore important.

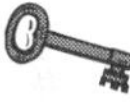

KEY CONCEPTS

Career Ladder is a design of a concept to select a career path beyond the basic functional level. In nursing, career paths include practitioner, educator, and manager. Master's and doctoral degrees are required as the individual progresses.

Clinical Ladder is a design of a concept to permit progression within a position category (e.g., the staff nurse level).

Disciplinary Action refers to corrective measures designed to improve the performance of workers. The focus is on improvement for the future rather than punishment of the past.

Evaluation Interview is the formal evaluation meeting of a supervisor and an individual employee during which the employee's performance is reviewed relative to his or her position responsibilities.

Grievance is a real or imagined feeling of personal injustice that an employee has about the employment relationship. The feeling of injustice is not necessarily true or correct.

Management by Objectives is the evaluation method based on attainment of predetermined goals that have been set by mutual agreement between a supervisor and an employee. A specified time frame for achieving a goal or set of goals is part of management by objectives. It is a method that fosters active participation in evaluation and self-determination in career development.

Performance Appraisal is the process in use in an organization by which the performance appraisal system is implemented. It is the means of redefining and improving work performance.

Performance Appraisal System is an integral function of an organization to monitor employee performance.

Reliability is a characteristic of measurement in which an instrument consistently assigns scores to an attribute.

Validity is a characteristic of measurement in which an instrument measures the attributes it is intended to measure.

THE PERFORMANCE APPRAISAL SYSTEM

Performance appraisal is one element in a broader organizational system of quality assurance. It is itself a system having several interdependent parts and is designed to serve organizations and individuals. Developing an effective system is an expensive endeavor for organizations, requiring time, space allocation, and qualified personnel. The system in nursing departments is designed to protect patients by insuring competent practitioners who meet professional standards, nurses' rights and autonomy, and the interests of the organization.

There is a strong legal obligation in being employed as a professional nurse. The beginning nurse enters a highly complex organization and immediately becomes an active participant in the mission of the whole organization, not simply an assigned nursing unit. The **performance appraisal system** is an effective avenue that measures the obligations of the employment agreement for both the organization and individuals.

Departments within organizations develop written plans to objectively and systematically oversee the effectiveness of the program, with monitoring done by individuals and their supervisors. When understood and used appropriately, the system benefits patients, nurses, organizations, and the profession by providing opportunities for improvement, resolving identified problems, and identifying individuals' readiness for advancement. It is a very important process for career development.

Design of a Performance Appraisal System

Good performance appraisal provides a systematic, orderly source of information not available to the organization in any other way. Performance appraisal systems, in order to be effective, must be suited to the philosophy, goals, and objectives of an organization, understood by all personnel, and enacted and operationalized by qualified managers and staff. Queen gives the following purposes of performance appraisal: (1) to maintain safe competent care, (2) to meet organizational goals, (3) to foster professional development, and (4) to develop ideas for clinical nursing research.[2]

In many health care organizations today, a matrix structure is common. The performance appraisal program in any organization must allow for a design that permits each department within the matrix to produce the kind of information that identifies its primary contribution to the overall mission. The business office clearly contributes differently to the organization than does the nursing service department. It is important, however, that issues in a matrix structure be understood by everyone. Departments having essentially different responsibilities must work together to allow organizational survival in the volatile environment of the changing health care delivery system. The linkages between departments in organizations were discussed in Chapter 6, *Organization and Management Theory*.

Performance appraisal is multifaceted, dynamic, and a managerial tool designed to evaluate performance, identify staff development and training needs, identify unrecognized talent and ability, influence motivation, assign rewards, take disciplinary action, and encourage career goal planning.

Beck describes the development and piloting of a performance appraisal tool for use when primary nursing, as a patient care delivery pattern, is used.[3] The framework for developing the standards of performance are 24-hour accountability, case method of assignment, communication among caregivers, and change in the role of the nurse manager. The tool, while specific to primary nursing, is valuable to other patterns of care such as case management.

Generally speaking, the hallmarks of modern performance appraisal systems are performance orientation of everyone in the organization, focus on goals, and mutual goal setting between managers and staff.

Career Planning

Early involvement in functions designed to meet organizational goals can permit earlier advancement in personal career goals. Opportunities for growth and advancement are more readily perceived by those who are informed and involved. The knowledgeable individual also influences a system and makes it serve the organization better. Well-formulated and thoughtfully stated questions and comments that reflect expectations about the system can serve as a spark to turn an ineffective process toward greater effectiveness.

Nursing has entered a global sphere through sharing information by way of the Internet. *Sigma Theta Tau*, the international honor society of nursing, has established Internet sites (log onto http://www.nursingsociety.org) on a wide variety of professional nursing topics that are available to both members and non-members.[4] Increasing numbers of nurses are logging on for information that is vital to their careers and practices. The career planning page, "8 Skills for a Healthy Career," lists the following skills:

- Personal self-development.
- Locate and use special resources.
- Learn financial principles.
- Think futuristically by keeping abreast of professional organizations.
- Develop leadership skills—make use of mentors; learn a second language.
- Develop technological know-how.
- Position yourself for recognition via professional, political, and community organizations.
- (plan to) Remain professionally active during retirement.

Source: International Leadership Institute, Sigma Theta Tau International, "Eight skills for a healthy career," Reflections on Nursing Leadership, *First Quarter 2000: 20–21.*

Students are referred to the previously mentioned website for complete coverage of the career page. It is not too early for students to develop skills that will advance their careers. See the "Learner Exercises" at the end of this chapter for some ideas in getting started.

The experience of health care workers worldwide contributes to the store of knowledge available on all health care topics. Hern et al.[5] note that through the web the world of nursing education has become a village. In practice, through the use of interactive video, innovative ideas enhance nursing practice and performance appraisal. Lewis[6] cites peer review as an area that contributes to quality performance in direct care as well as increased collaboration and open communication with patients and families. Delaney[7] describes an intrahospital design that disseminates staff awareness of issues facing practice in-house as well as the computer linkage between the hospice clinic and hospital. Nurses in Iceland use information from the web to make recommendations for policy changes to authority. While the possibilities of the Internet seem limitless, only time will clarify the extent of its usefulness to the profession.

Interdisciplinary collaboration is becoming more common in health care. The aim of interdisciplinary teams is to increase the quality and efficiency in health care delivery.[8] In such a milieu, maintaining professional integrity is complex. Differing values, boundary questions, and power affect success. Medicine has traditionally used a pathophysiological paradigm, social work an individualistic paradigm, and nursing a holistic paradigm. It requires understanding, communication, mutual respect, and creative thinking to maximize health care delivery, and for professionals to grow in their thinking and understanding of each other's contributions to comprehensive care. In collaboration, team members share the planning, action, and responsibility for outcomes. Joint coursework and practice can support collaborative care. All team members come together in courses, and in the practical component students "shadow" members of different disciplines to provide care and discuss issues.

Interdisciplinary care differs from multidisciplinary care in that shared decision making in planning care becomes the hallmark of interdisciplinary care models that promote a unified approach. Nurses who practice in interdisciplinary teams are professionally obligated to model and articulate nursing's core values and principles.

CRITERIA FOR NURSING STANDARDS

Professional standards of nursing practice constitute the basic framework and serve as a criteria for evaluating nurses' performance in the work setting in the same way that course objectives do in the classroom. Different standards serve as the criteria for performance of personnel in each department of an organization. At times, standards of some departments can appear to conflict with the standards of other departments. When nursing standards are threatened, the concept of tailoring preserves professional standards in the face of other demands. Tailoring differs from abandoning because it preserves attitudes and values, such as caring and compassion, that are essential to the nursing profession. They are values that must not be jeopardized in the delivery of patient care due to economic constraints.

Professional standards and money do, however, frequently become competing forces in today's health care delivery. A classic example is the early discharge of patients from acute care settings as a cost-containment measure. Nurses are frequently caught in economy/quality conflicts and cost-containment/compassion conflicts. They are frequently reminded of the ethics of resource allocation in today's practical world. The economic advantage of early discharge is easily understood, whereas research on the effects it has on care outcomes for patients is new. While professional standards must dominate decision making relative to patient care, nurses must remember that the effective use of resources and prevention of waste is included in professional values. It is important that there be communication, collaboration, and cooperation between departments. Gropper and Skarzynski discuss interdepartmental differences in the performance appraisal system.[9] In an effort to integrate and unify the system, each department's high-risk, high-cost, and problem-prone issues are identified. Outcomes are shared, thereby giving each department a new appreciation of the role others play in the care of the patient.

Expectations and criteria for nurses' performance, as defined by the organization, can be found in position descriptions. The nursing service department is charged with the responsibility to formulate position descriptions for nurses that reflect professional standards of practice. They are frequently presented in the format familiar to all nurses (i.e., the nursing process). Gregory stresses the importance of including attitudinal data into the performance appraisal tool to be a link between the quantitative requirements and qualitative environmental factors.[10] Concern for output information from the performance appraisal system is an indication of the growing appreciation for using evaluation results in maintaining standards in all departments of organizations. Knowing what is included in the position description is the first step in being prepared to participate in performance appraisal.

In the sections that follow, performance appraisal will be considered as a comprehensive process that demands interaction between supervisors and staff. All the content from earlier chapters in the text is integral to a quality performance appraisal system. Ideally, supervisors and staff understand and continue to improve their skills in communication, group dynamics, decision making, understanding of motivating forces that influence people, valuing ethical principles, and management of conflict. Furthermore, they have an organizational orientation and a professional commitment to nursing practice. The evaluation conference is viewed comprehensively as an interactive process that takes place between a supervisor and a staff member. Planning for, and participating in, the conference are seen as key activities of effective evaluation.

ACTIVE PARTICIPATION IN PERFORMANCE APPRAISAL

Performance appraisal must be interactive to be effective. One-way evaluation results when supervisors, staff, or both lack the knowledge or the skills needed to use the process or when they ignore the process. In one instance, evaluation can be something done to staff by supervisors. This happens when the staff nurse does not actively participate in the process. In another instance, objective evaluation of performance remains an expectation of the staff nurse because the supervisor does not appropriately enact the process. Either can be the result of a variety of factors that require analysis to arrive at a cause and solution to the problem.

Two-way participation in evaluation is important from a societal and a professional perspective. Society expects professionals to maintain high standards of performance. This expectation is indeed challenging in light of today's rapidly changing knowledge and technology advances. Toffler's depiction of the third-wave generation takes on new meaning when applied to accountability in nursing today. There is the real possibility that supervisors, who are the evaluators, are significantly influenced by second-wave norms (see Chapter 10 for a review of these generational differences), making active participation by the nurse in evaluation highly desirable.

A developing professional person assumes responsibility and accountability for personal growth in the ability to assess, plan, and evaluate values, skills, and interests relative to professional state-of-the-art changes. The performance appraisal program provides the opportunity for formal participation in evaluation. It is there that latitude is accorded professionals for self-determination by enactment of internal motivation. Conscious awareness of strengths and weaknesses in oneself and in the organization can be identified there. Through self-inspection, incongruencies between ideal and actual behavior become apparent.

Active participation in evaluation then lies at the core of professional effectiveness. For a staff nurse to participate well in the process, adequate knowledge about performance appraisal is needed. Essential elements of a performance appraisal program are presented next because effectiveness begins there.

ESSENTIAL ELEMENTS

Queen identifies the elements of the performance appraisal system as:

- Position description.
- Evaluation tool in harmony with the position.
- Planning.[11]

Documents and activities of an effective performance appraisal system in any organization will:

- Reflect its philosophy, mission, and objectives.
- Have a clear statement of purpose.
- Contain tools that produce desired information.

Philosophy, Mission, and Objectives

Each health care organization has a philosophy that states beliefs about health care, the nature of clients, and how it serves a defined population. State-sponsored agencies differ philosophically from privately supported agencies. While the organizational philosophy is a mandate for all departments, each fashions its performance appraisal on those aspects for which it has major responsibility. For example, the nursing department incorporates professional standards of nursing practice as guiding principles for performance but also considers the need for economy. The business department incorporates practices of sound money management as a predominant responsibility but also considers the service mission of the agency. The overall performance of the organization is contingent on mutuality between departments.

Mission statements further distinguish the primary responsibilities of departments and individuals. The mission of a neighborhood clinic differs from that of an acute care facility. The mission of general acute care facilities differs from the mission of specialty acute care facilities. The mission is a determinant of the clinical credentials of the staff and specifies the proficiency expectations in performance appraisal statements.

Ways in which an organization plans to carry out its mission are found in its objectives. One objective is to implement a comprehensive performance appraisal system that reflects its philosophy and mission through the performance of competent and effective managers at all levels. Position descriptions specify the competencies of personnel and the expected quality of performance. The format of departmental performance appraisal tools might differ, but each remains congruent with the total management system designed to support the organization.

Well-Defined Purpose

The purpose of performance appraisal should be clearly stated and understood by all in the organization, and it is the supervisor's responsibility to clarify this information to the staff (see Table 11-1). The effective supervisor has a staff that is informed about performance appraisal and holds them accountable for knowing the following:

1. The importance of evaluations.
2. What is on the evaluation form.
3. What the priorities are.
4. What role they play in evaluation.
5. How much autonomy and accountability they have.
6. How to influence success.
7. What the rewards are and when disciplinary action is enforced.[12]

The desired outcomes of performance appraisal are a wise allocation of resources, motivated employees who improve performance, fair distribution of rewards and use of discipline, employee growth, and non-discrimination.[13] Non-discrimination regulations protect against unfair employment practices. It is one of the areas in the system having serious legal implications. Regulations require employers to have written records of evaluations, clearly stated position descriptions, evaluations based on job-related criteria,

TABLE 11-1. In column 1, the supervisor's responsibilities to the staff relative to the organization's performance appraisal program are listed. In column 2, the corresponding staff nurse areas of accountability are listed. The information in this figure should be reviewed periodically at staff meetings to encourage skillful implementation of the program.

Supervisor Responsibilities	Corresponding Staff Nurse Responses
Informs and interprets for staff the organizational performance appraisal program, to include:	Being appropriately informed about the performance appraisal program, the nurse is accountable for:
• Its purpose.	• Viewing evaluation as important.
• What is valued by management.	• Acting on defined priorities.
• What results to expect.	• Awareness of rewards and disciplinary action.
• What methods are used.	• Familiarity with the evaluation form.
• What resources are available for goal attainment.	• Using resources to influence personal success.
• Whether active participation is expected.	• Being appropriately active in evaluation interviews.
• How much self-determination is encouraged.	• Exercising appropriate autonomy and being accountable for own decisions.

evidence of tool validity and reliability, and trained, qualified raters. Non-discrimination, along with other legal issues, are discussed in detail in Chapter 12.

See Figure 11-1 for an illustration depicting the ongoing, interactive nature of performance appraisal and the individuals involved.

Evaluation Tools that Produce Desired Information

The selection of an evaluation tool is based on what information is desired. The format should permit systematic collection and analysis of objective data. The tool should have both **validity** and **reliability**.[14]

Validity refers to the extent to which a tool measures the attributes it is intended to measure (i.e., does it measure a target attribute?). Validity is the correlation between a tool result and a criterion (a professional standard) against which performance is measured. For example, if a standard requirement is individualized care based on cultural considerations and the tool does not measure assessment for cultural differences, then it is not valid for that target standard.

Reliability refers to how consistently the tool assigns scores to an attribute. An automobile odometer that does not consistently measure actual miles traveled is not reliable. Tools that are not reliable cannot be valid. Validity and reliability are essential characteristics of measurement and are part of the measurement theory used by managers. For staff nurses, the tool must make sense and evaluate what it is supposed to relative to position descriptions. Experience with evaluating tools provides practical reinforcement of information about measurement for the practitioner. Since the mid-1980s, computer technology has become a part of the performance appraisal system in terms of collecting and storing data and analyzing the results. Stalker et al.[15] list the following ways in which a computerized system improves evaluation. Computers:

- Articulate and promote professional standards.
- Integrate philosophy and practice.

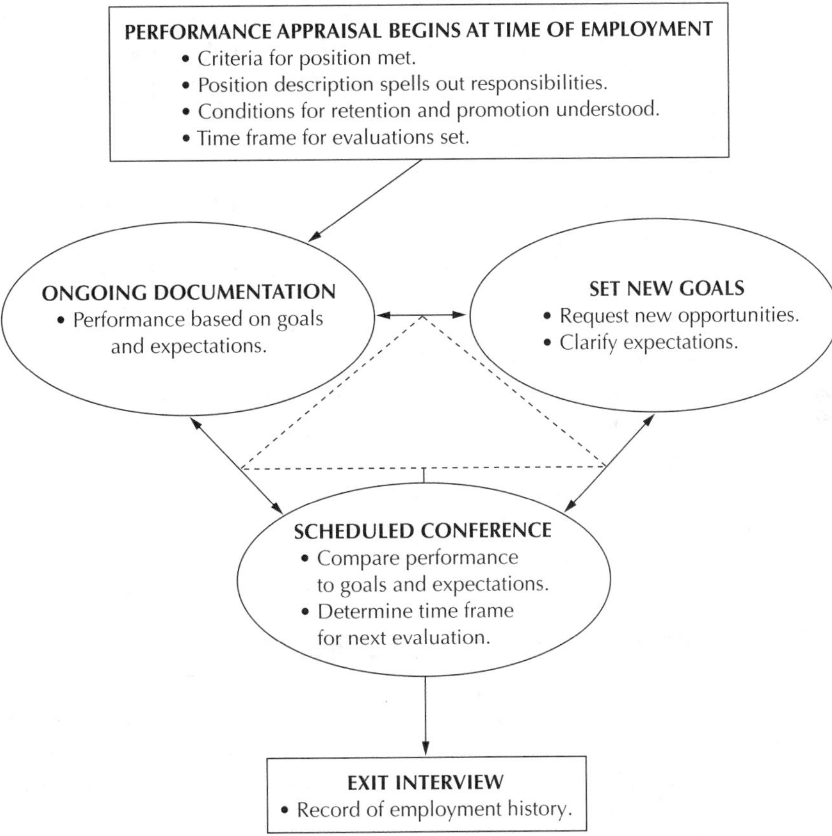

FIGURE 11-1. The performance appraisal process is continuous and interactive.

- Replace a long, redundant, confusing, and expensive system.
- Improve staff confidence in the managers as evaluators of their performance.
- Provide ease when weighting categories being evaluated.
- Define meritorious performance.
- Identify issues for staff development.
- Identify the need for counseling.
- Predict nurses who will be promoted in the future.

Adoption of a system that yields results similar to the above could benefit nurses who wish to remain in, and be promoted within, the caregiver role rather than into a management role. While technology is expensive and requires training time, it holds promise for several other positive changes in nursing in the area of personnel management. Another factor to consider in tool selection is whether individuals are being evaluated comparatively relative to the performance of others in their category (normative–referenced approach) or relative to the accomplishment of predetermined goals (criterion–referenced approach). Both can be useful depending on what information is sought. Professionals are frequently evaluated using the criterion–referenced approach. A popular method of the approach is called **management by objectives**, a concept introduced by Drucker in 1954 and used in nursing since 1970.[16] The approach allows staff nurses the opportunity for active participation in their evaluation by increasing individuals' autonomy and accountability for their own growth. The concept forces ongoing involvement of the staff in performance appraisal through goal setting, selecting methods to meet goals, and evaluating success. Therefore, performance appraisal is not an isolated, passive experience that occurs annually; instead, it is a process that becomes an integral part of everyday performance.

The normative-referenced approach is useful in situations when more than one person competes for a single position. It is competitive in nature and ranks individuals on attributes from high to low. Through normative-referenced evaluation, the best applicant can be selected for a position.

In summary, the way in which performance appraisal systems are structured is important because the system can fail if it is not part of a total management system. It must reflect formal organizational documents—philosophy, mission, and objectives. Its purpose must be understood by all, and the tool selected must measure performance relative to each category of position description. Furthermore, the system must be sensitive to legal and ethical issues as described in equal opportunity regulations.

PERFORMANCE APPRAISAL PROCESS

The three main phases of the performance appraisal process are: planning, interviewing, and utilization of outcomes. Success of the process can be determined by indicators about performance in employees' files and quality care indices in unit records, such as the incidence of errors, accidents, and operational expenses.[17] Outcome indicators serve as targets for future goals, and the process is put into motion. A performance appraisal program is only as good as the process by which it is operationalized and the people who use it. A one-on-one **evaluation interview** is where the process is operationalized. The immediate supervisor and one staff nurse come together in a formal way to review past performance and to plan for the future. Each have responsibilities to make the program successful. Careful attention to each phase of the process is the key to productivity.

Planning for the Interview

Preparing for the evaluation interview is important. A period of reflective inspection of past performance by the nurse helps identify his or her strengths and weaknesses. It is a time to revitalize ideals and commitments and to target an area for improvement. A positive approach to improving performance is better than a list of "don'ts" that are quickly forgotten. For example, a nurse might share a success through presenting an informative series of staff development sessions. In this way, leadership skills are developed while others profit from his or her experience.

Supervisors also need to prepare for evaluation interviews. A record of firsthand observations of the nurse's performance over time and a review of the previous evaluation report are necessary to focus on the individual. Judgment about performance must be

TABLE 11-2. Column 1 is a list of recommended supervisor behaviors preparatory to the evaluation interview. Column 2 lists recommended staff nurse behaviors preparatory to the evaluation interview. The behaviors are designed to facilitate a productive interview.

Supervisor Behaviors	Staff Nurse Behaviors
• Records spaced, periodic observations of the nurse's performance relative to position and standards in a variety of situations. • Validates interpretation of important incidents in which the nurse is involved. • Offers counsel and support as needed, citing position and standard expectations. • As the time for a formal evaluation interview approaches, plans a date and time collaboratively with the nurse. • Confirms the interview in writing. • Reviews nurse's past evaluation record. • Completes the written evaluation form.	• Utilizes position and standard expectations daily. • Documents specific patient outcomes that reflect planned nursing interventions. • Asks for clarification of expectations when there is doubt, citing position responsibilities and professional standards. • Summarizes accomplishments during the evaluation period. • Prepares a list of activities that could advance career to the next level, and negotiates for opportunities. • Collaborates with the supervisor relative to date, time, and expected preparation for the evaluation interview.

related to position description expectations. Logistically, the supervisor selects a place that provides uninterrupted privacy and adequate time. The date and time are planned collaboratively with the nurse whenever possible. A reminder of the scheduled interview is sent in writing to the nurse. See Table 11-2 for a checklist for planning the evaluation interview.

Questions to include and avoid during interviews are regulated by the laws affecting employment. Questions to include should address position requirements, solicit information about the skills and qualities that are sought, seek examples of the applicant's experiences, and determine the applicant's willingness and motivation to do the work called for. Questions to avoid include those regarding age, date of birth, race, religion, and national origin.

Participating in the Evaluation Interview

Participating in the interview is the second phase of the process. The interview allows the supervisor to evaluate an individual staff member. It is never appropriate to discuss anyone else or allow the interview to deteriorate into a charge-countercharge situation during which the staff member becomes the evaluator. It is generally agreed that a review of successes be the first topic for discussion to set a positive climate for the rest of the interview. It is important that an attitude of importance about evaluations prevail throughout the interview. Joking and idle chitchat are out of place, as are discussions of mutual social interests. Whether such events occur through nervousness or as deliberate, time-consuming distractions to avoid addressing critical issues, they interfere with accomplishing the task at hand. Either party can and should assume the role of "gatekeeper" so that the interview can proceed in an orderly fashion.

The supervisor and the staff nurse have different roles and responsibilities in making the evaluation interview productive. **Disciplinary action** is covered in more detail in Chapter 12, but some comments about it as it relates to the evaluation interview are included here. Disciplinary action is warranted by documented evidence of inferior performance that relates to position standards. When disciplinary action is invoked, it requires due process to protect the rights of the staff member. Due process assumes innocence until proof of wrongdoing, ensures the individual's right to be heard, and assigns discipline that is reasonable relative to the wrongdoing. Disciplinary action should be instructive, be corrective, and aim to improve performance in the future rather than punish the past. Counseling is a positive approach to discipline based on fact finding and guidance. Counseling encourages desirable behavior instead of punishing undesirable behavior. Effective counseling preserves workers' self-image and dignity and keeps working relationships cooperative and constructive.[18]

Ways in which managers can maintain a positive climate when disciplinary action is necessary include identifying resources to help the individual, expressing confidence in his or her ability and willingness to improve, and making a sincere offer of help and support whenever needed. Offering to schedule a follow-up interview when improvement is demonstrated lifts the staff member's stigma of being disciplined. Even with the best of efforts, however, the potential for a grievance action exists whenever disciplinary action is used. When the nurse's best efforts fail to solve a serious misunderstanding, a true grievance can exist. **Grievance** is defined as any real or imagined feeling of personal injustice that an employee has about the employment relationship.[19] The staff nurse should be aware that a grievance can be filed by anyone and does not depend on having a collective bargaining mechanism in place.

Having a grievance system is a requirement of equal employment regulations. It benefits organizations as well as individuals by bringing problems into the open so that corrective action can be attempted. Problems can then be caught early and solved before they become serious. When a grievance system exists, everyone in the organization knows their actions are subject to scrutiny, and they are therefore put on guard to make decisions carefully. Disciplinary action, the grievance process, and discrimination are covered in detail in Chapter 12.

The staff nurse's role during the evaluation interview is active participation facilitated through planning. The informed, constructively assertive nurse can gain more from the interview than the unprepared nurse. Interviews can boost morale or can be a source of dissatisfaction. Skillful and effective participation in the evaluation interview is important and should be a stated expectation for everyone in the organization. See Table 11-3 for a checklist of supervisor and staff nurse roles and responsibilities relative to evaluation interviews.

Using Evaluation Results

Making use of interview results is the third, and ongoing, phase of the performance appraisal process. Careful attention must be given to how the results will be used if they are to be of optimal value. Brookfield cautions that blindly rushing into action in the excitement of new insights and opportunities can lead to bad decisions.[20] Time is needed

TABLE 11-3. Column 1 is a list of supervisor responsibilities for conducting the evaluation interview. Column 2 is a list of staff nurse responsibilities for active participation in the evaluation interview. All activities listed in both columns are essential if the interview is to benefit the nurse and the organization.

Supervisor Responsibilities	Staff Nurse Responsibilities
• Conducts the interview. • States judgments about the nurse's performance relative to position and standard expectations beginning with positive accomplishments. • Provides justification for rewards or disciplinary action based on criteria. • Encourages the nurse to new challenges. • Specifies time period for next formal evaluation interview. • Secures from the nurse specific goals to be accomplished during the next evaluation period.	• Shares documented evidence of main accomplishments since the last evaluation interview relative to position and standard expectations. • Clarifies circumstances of situations as necessary. • States goals for the immediate future. • Requests opportunities for specific activities that will promote progression. • Expects guidance and direction from the supervisor. • Adds comments to the evaluation form in writing, stating degree of satisfaction with the interview. Attaches any documentation needed.

to consider alternative courses of action. All planning for, and active participation in, evaluations will have no long-range effects if results remain in the personnel office file. It is necessary, therefore, that a structured plan for using the evaluation outcomes be formulated and used.

Scheduled interim review of evaluation reports by supervisors and staff nurses permit improvements to occur in increments as each stage of improvement solidifies. The substance of an interim review could come from thinking about how much closer one is to a goal, and how much farther one has to go. Motivation is strengthened as short-range goals are accomplished on the way to reaching the long-range goal.

REWARDS

Rewards in nursing have become an issue in recent years and a concern of management. Recall the reorganization of patient care standards discussed in Chapter 1 and the different expectations among nurses because of their different orientations to the profession discussed in the chapter on motivation (Chapter 10). Satisfying expectations of staff nurses and meeting the needs of higher acuity-level patients as a result of DRGs forced management to reconsider the traditional single-track reward system for nurses. For decades, the only way a staff nurse could advance was vertically into an entirely different role. Staff nurses, proficient at the bedside, were "promoted" to a management or teaching position. Few management and teaching positions were available, however, and most nurses remained in staff nurse positions throughout their careers with the concomitant salary compression and shift change schedules.

Attempts on the part of nurse managers to satisfy the different needs of individuals included experimenting with variable scheduling to replace the traditional 5 days a week, 8-hour shifts. Several alternatives have emerged that provide attractive incentives for some nurses to remain in nursing. Various patterns provide for:

- Four 10-hour shifts a week.
- Three 12-hour shifts a week.
- Two 12-hour weekend shifts every week.

In some acute care settings, the latter provides a salary greater than that of a 40-hour-a-week schedule.

The "menu" of schedules has been met with varying degrees of enthusiasm and success. The hours can be ideal for students who need to be free during the week to attend classes. Parents of young children might find the hours attractive in that they can avoid costly child care expenses. Variable scheduling has the potential to reduce the dissatisfaction of nurses in patient care settings and to improve staff nurse satisfaction because it fits their lifestyles.

However, there are also problems with variable scheduling. Coordinating the schedule when nurses work different time patterns can be difficult. Confusion about patient care responsibilities during overlap hours can cause conflicts. Finally, there has been no systematic evaluation of the effect of long working hours on the ability to perform quality patient care.

Another strategy for improving rewards for nurses has been the introduction of **clinical ladders** (see Figure 11-2). The concept of a clinical ladder permits horizontal advancement, keeping excellent clinicians in their chosen role. Nurses advance through a determined number of levels within a position category (e.g., staff nurse) based on predetermined criteria. At each level there are additional advantages for the nurse (e.g., fewer rotating shifts, higher salary, or fewer weekends on duty). Once the highest level in the category has been reached, advancement requires additional education, usually a master's degree in nursing.

Sometimes vertical progression is referred to as moving into a **career ladder** (see Figure 11-3). Nurses move out of the basic practice levels and pursue advanced education as preparation for their roles as managers, educators, or clinical specialists.

Clinical and career ladders have met with considerable success but are not totally without problems. Confusion over authority and responsibility between clinical specialists and head nurses on the same unit can cause conflicts. While the organizational chart shows what their relation is to each other, no document can clarify how to handle day-to-day events.

A menu of benefits is another way an organization can attempt to satisfy individuals with different interests and needs (see Figure 11-4). Nurses with bachelor's degrees have no use for the tuition remission benefit to complete the bachelor's degree. Not all agencies support graduate education, meaning a lost benefit to nurses with bachelor's degrees. A married nurse whose spouse's employer provides comprehensive family health insurance coverage has little use for health insurance.

Some organizations elect to offer variable benefits that can be selected from a menu. Employees select from the menu up to a specified monetary allowance that is the same for all. In this way, the cost of the benefit package remains the same for the organization, and employees have the opportunity to meet their own individual needs. Young nurses with small children can choose more life insurance rather than retirement benefits.

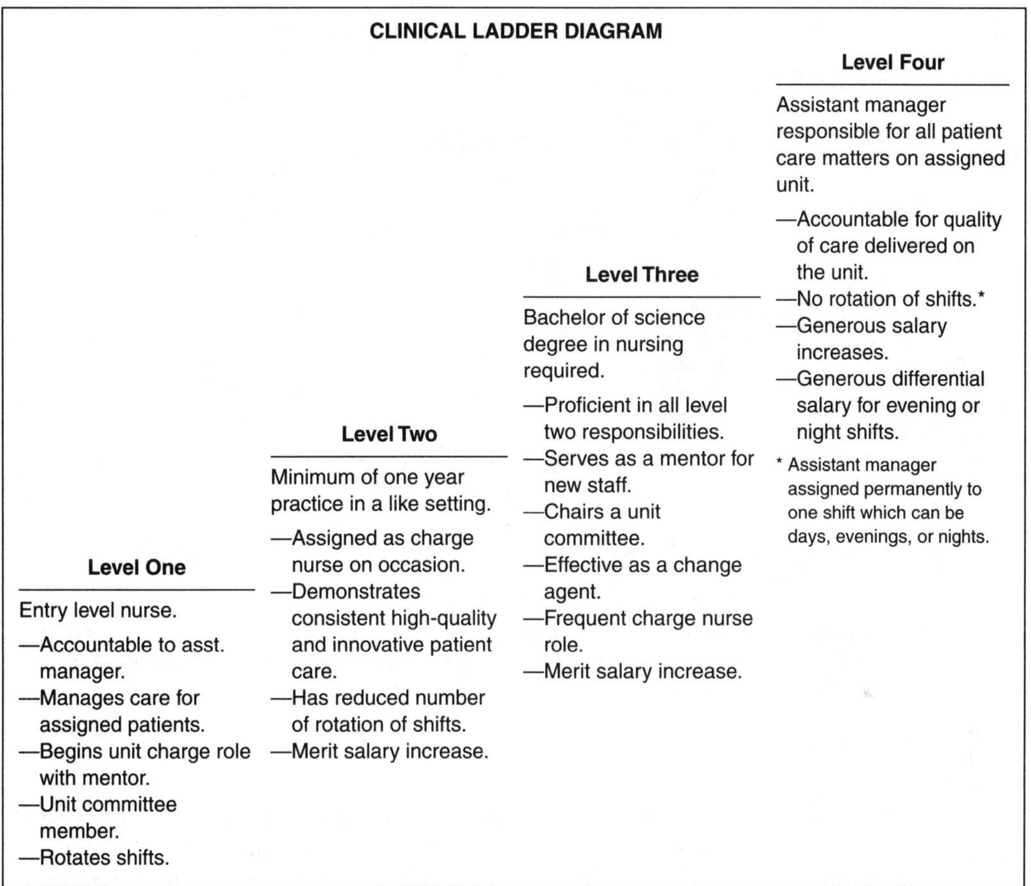

FIGURE 11-2. A diagram of levels within the staff nurse category allowing for progression without having to leave the patient care role. The levels with benefits and responsibilities depicted *are examples.* The assistant nurse manager position at Level Four is considered a clinical role rather than a formal management role.

Nurses close to retirement can choose additional retirement benefits in place of life insurance or vacation time. Nurses with bachelor's degrees can choose additional vacation time or additional retirement benefits in place of tuition remission. The use of variable benefits is an example of how organizations change to meet volatile internal and external environmental demands.

OBSTACLES TO PERFORMANCE IMPROVEMENT

The obvious obstacles to performance improvement are a program that does not address performance requirements, vagueness of purpose, unqualified raters, a tool that does not provide desired information, poor record keeping, and failure to use results. The obstacles come about for a variety of reasons, which might include any or all of the

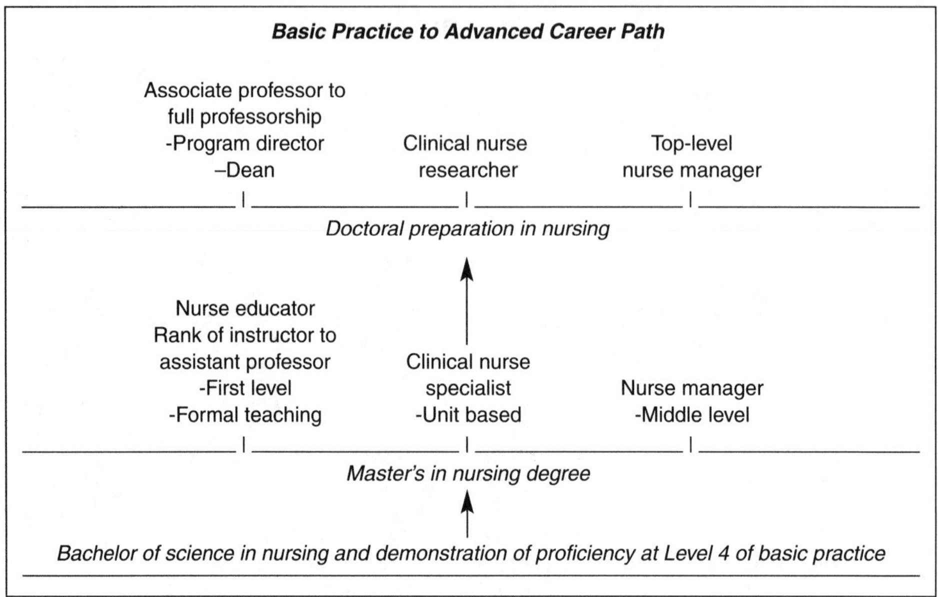

FIGURE 11-3. The path from basic clinical practice to advanced career levels in nursing. The academic preparation represents recent changes in recommended preparation for professional nurse roles.

following: lack of support from administration; resistance on the part of raters because of the time involved; rater biases and rating errors that result in unreliable and invalid information; lack of clear, objective standards of performance; failure to communicate the purposes and results of evaluation to staff; and failure to monitor the process effectively. Queen summarizes these problems into three categories: time, paperwork, and incongruent judgments.[21]

Rater biases and errors have been listed as commonly occurring distortions in performance appraisal by Stevens.[22] They first appeared in print in 1976, but readers might still find some of them familiar in their own experiences. Labels applied to the errors and distortions help explain them.

The *halo effect* is a distortion that occurs when the rater assumes that the individual who performs well in some areas must therefore perform well in other areas that have not been observed. Instead of acknowledging that there was no opportunity to observe a particular behavior, the rater assigns a high score to the behavior.

In the *recency effect*, the rater weighs recent events more heavily than other events that occurred throughout the evaluation period. Observations and record keeping can facilitate a more accurate assignment of value to performance that occurred since the last evaluation interview.

Problem distortion occurs when a single, poorly observed performance weighs more than good performances that went unobserved. Conferring with the staff nurse about the circumstances of the problem when it happens can reduce the distortion.

Menu of Employment Benefits

General Hospital
Liberty City, USA

All full-time employees are entitled to the following schedule of benefits.

Everyone receives:

- Two weeks paid vacation.
- Paid holidays established by the hospital.
- Participation in the retirement plan.

During the first five (5) years of employment, each employee may select thirteen (13) additional benefit points from the following list:

- 5 pts - Full family-health insurance coverage.
- 3 pts - Individual health insurance coverage.
- 2 pts - Individual dental insurance coverage.
- 5 pts - Tuition remission for a baccalaureate degree.
- 2 pts - Additional two (2) weeks paid vacation.
- 3 pts - Paid life insurance equal to 3 times basic salary.
- 3 pts - Increased retirement program contributions by the hospital.
- 8 pts - Remission of child care costs during work hours.
- 5 pts - Free meals during work hours.
- 2 pts - Free parking on hospital lot during work hours.

After five (5) years of full-time, consecutive employment, an additional five (5) points may be selected.

FIGURE 11-4. An example of what a menu of employment benefits might look like. The point system shown is a rough guesstimation of value of each benefit and has no basis in fact. A reduced benefit package can be developed for permanent, part-time employees.

The *sunflower effect* occurs when the rater grades everyone on the unit the same based on the overall group performance. There is failure to focus attention on the individual. Assets go unrewarded, and weaknesses are not corrected.

Central tendency errors are the result of rating the staff nurse "average" when in fact his or her real performance is unknown. Raters should not hesitate to record that certain behaviors were not observed during the evaluation period. Since evaluation is interactive, the rater might ask the nurse to bring to the conference self-evaluation statements about behaviors not observed by the rater.

Rater temperament effect reflects variances in the degree of importance different raters assign to the same attribute. Prioritizing performance based on total situational factors reduces the incidence of making judgments based on predetermined expectations of a person who sees performance out of context.

The *guessing error* occurs when the rater guesses about performance rather than recording that it is unknown. All distortions and errors described are caused by some flaw in the system. Rater incompetence or low priority of evaluations as an organizational attitude are some possible causes.

CASE STUDY

The First Evaluation

Kim Jackson, a new graduate, recently accepted her first position as a graduate nurse. When she interviewed for the position, she was given a packet of materials that described all aspects of her staff nurse position. As a part of her orientation, she was expected to become familiar with the information in the packet. A portion of the orientation period was spent in discussion and clarification of the materials.

By the time orientation was over, Kim felt confident about her preparation to function as an informed nurse in the organization. Everything seemed designed to unify the various aspects of employment to focus on the delivery of high-quality nursing care throughout the nursing department. She was glad she had decided to practice in such a well-organized and high-quality organization.

After 6 months as a staff nurse, Kim remembered that she was due for her first evaluation as a bona fide professional. She decided to review the materials she had received at the time of her employment to be prepared for the interview with her nurse manager. Two weeks went by, during which she heard nothing from the nurse manager about an evaluation. She decided to ask about it. In response, the nurse manager said, "Oh yes, your evaluation form has been completed and is ready for your signature. You are doing fine. Don't forget to stop by my office soon to sign the form, or you won't get a raise."

Based on the purpose and process of performance appraisal information that was presented in this chapter, recommend a course of action for Kim.

CASE STUDY

Change in Performance Level

Melanie Jamieson has a several-year history of receiving excellent evaluations. Her nurse manager has appropriately used the evaluation system in describing Melanie's progression as a staff nurse, providing documentation of her behaviors as called for. Shortly after her last evaluation conference, Melanie found herself in a situation where personal responsibilities were competing for her time, attention, and energy. She knew that the quality of her nursing performance suffered as a result and was certainly not up to her personal standards or the standards of her manager. Consequently, she was prepared to explore with the manager ways in which she could resolve the problems inherent in her situation. She definitely did not expect a raise because her recent performance did not warrant one. To her surprise, the manager was unrealistically high in her rating of Melanie's performance and recommended a raise. It was as if she were totally unaware of the changes in Melanie's performance.

There are several possible reasons for the manager's behavior. One possibility is that she felt justified in "carrying" Melanie because of her earlier history, thinking she would "snap back." Another possibility is that the manager had no experience or skill in delivering a difficult message.

- What is your response to the first possibility?
- What are the problems created when the second possibility exists?
- How difficult would it be for you to deliver a difficult message?
- What would you do if you were Melanie?

CASE STUDY

Evaluations and Morale

The morale of staff nurses on a particular unit is very low. According to the staff, the reason is due to the outcomes of their evaluation conferences. Comments by the nurse manager seem "out of the blue." A single event that happened months ago became the focus of the manager's evaluation of the nurses. Nurses feel they enter the evaluation conference without any idea that the manager attached so much importance to a one-time behavior. The performances the nurses feel good about are discounted in the written report. The result is that the staff nurses feel that they are being scrutinized for errors. There is an increasing level of stress and anxiety among them. Communication is guarded, adding to the strife and poor working relationships.

- Apply principles from this chapter to analyze the problem.
- Recommend an approach to this deteriorating situation.
- List as many causes as you can think of for the head nurse's behavior. Keep in mind that there are two sides to every story

---

SUMMARY

In this chapter, performance appraisal is viewed as a highly valuable system designed to improve performance. While it is an expensive endeavor for the organization, it is worthy of the time and expense. The program must reflect the organization's philosophy, mission, and objectives, and a process must be developed that produces the desired results. The process is interactive, consisting of three phases: planning, the interview, and using results. It should be a clearly stated expectation, understood by everyone in the organization, that all participate actively in the program. Because of complexities in organizational settings, performance appraisal must be studied in order to be understood by its participants. Use of results is a frequently neglected phase. Failure to act on results negates the other two phases, because results are essentially the "evaluation of evaluations." Individuals and organizations benefit from effective performance appraisal programs: Individuals more readily advance in their careers, and organizations make better use of personnel strengths. Early identification of problems allows corrective action in an economic way. Problems with performance appraisal programs are described.

Throughout the chapter, the focus is on active participation in the program by informed nurses. The ultimate goal is to keep professional standards of nursing practice pivotal to an evaluation of nurses' performance. Economic constraints must not significantly interfere with professional standards since standards and economic efficiency are not mutually incompatible, and adherence to professional standards is the only way to preserve the values of the profession.

LEARNER EXERCISES

1. A staff nurse is told by her supervisor to remain in the conference room after the change-of-shift report so that the supervisor can review her evaluation. It is the first time the supervisor has communicated to the nurse about the evaluation. Outline the major problems with the manner in which the supervisor is handling evaluations. Propose solutions.
2. During a floor meeting, the head nurse on a unit explains to the staff that evaluations are going to be late because she had to fill in for the unit secretary, who was on vacation for a week, and then had to take a full-patient assignment because of staff vacations and nurses who called in sick. She seems to take the situation in stride even though expected salary increases and evaluation interviews will be delayed. What principles of management are being violated? As a staff nurse whose salary increase will be delayed, respond to her announcement.
3. You overhear a fellow staff nurse say that professional nursing standards of care can no longer be met because of budgetary cuts. From what you understand about professional standards of practice, respond to the nurse's comment.
4. As a student, you have rich opportunities at your disposal for learning, not only from your instructors, but also from experienced nurses. In clinical practice agencies, nurses in a variety of positions can be helpful. Check with your instructor about approaching nurse administrators, practitioners, researchers, and educators for an interview about their careers and how they prepared for them. A formal note from your instructor to an agency nurse explaining the assignment will usually open the door for you in seeking an interview. Request such a communication. Plan the interview using all the skills covered in earlier chapters in this text. On the day of the interview, dress as you would when applying for a position. Invite your interviewee to attend the class session when you will be reporting on your project. If your school has resources for class events, plan to serve light refreshments—note that you are responsible for organizing this aspect of your presentation. Organize a committee of your classmates to help with this.

REFERENCES

1. The Joint Commission on Accreditation of Health Care Organizations. (1988). *Monitoring and evaluation of quality and appropriateness of care*, pp. 1–13.
2. Queen, V.A. (1995, September). Performance evaluation. *Nursing Management*, *26*(9), 52–55.
3. Beck, S. (1990, January). Developing a primary nursing performance appraisal tool. *Nursing Management*, *21*(1), 36–42.
4. Fledderjohann, S. (2001). Connecting nurses worldwide *www.nursingsociety.org*. *Sigma Theta Tau, International Honor Society of Nursing—Excellence in Clinical Practice, 1st Quarter,* 2(1), 2.
5. Hern, M., Chung H.S., Lindell, A., & Kim, C.J. (2000). Linking hands on line: The Korean connection. *Reflections on Nursing Leadership, 4th Quarter,* 16–19.
6. Lewis, D. (2000). Direct to consumers. *Reflections on Nursing Leadership, 4th Quarter,* 24–26.
7. Delaney, C., Thoroddsen, A., Ruland, C., & Ehnfors, M. (2000). Linking hands on line: The Scandinavian connection. *Reflections on Nursing Leadership, 4th Quarter,* 20–26.

8. Lindeke, L., & Block, D. (1998). Maintaining professional integrity in the midst of interdisciplinary collaboration. *Nursing Outlook*, 46(5), 213–217.
9. Gropper, E.I., & Skarzynski, J.J. (1995, March). Integrating quality assessment and improvement. *Nursing Management*, 26(3), 22–23.
10. Gregory, G.D. (1995, July). Using a performance information system. *Nursing Management*, 26(7), 74–77.
11. Queen, V.A. (1995, September). Performance evaluation. *Nursing Management*, 26(9), 52–55.
12. Bassett, L.C., & Metzger, N. (1986). *Achieving excellence*. Rockville, MD: Aspen, p. 31.
13. Davis, K. (1981). *Human behavior at work—Organizational behavior.* New York: McGraw-Hill, p. 457.
14. Stamps, P. (1986). *Nurses and work satisfaction: An index for measurement.* Ann Arbor, MI: Health Administration Press, p. 66.
15. Stalker, M.Z., Kornblith, A.B., Lewis, P.M., & Parker, R. (1986, April). Measurement technology applications in performance appraisal. *Journal of Nursing Administration*, 12–17.
16. Spitzer, R. (1986). *Nursing productivity—The hospital's key to survival and profit.* Chicago: S-N Publication, p. 101.
17. Spitzer, R. (1986). *Nursing productivity—The hospital's key to survival and profit.* Chicago: S-N Publication, p. 101.
18. Davis, K. (1981). *Human behavior at work—Organizational behavior.* New York: McGraw-Hill, p. 321.
19. Davis, K. (1981). *Human behavior at work—Organizational behavior.* New York: McGraw-Hill, p. 361.
20. Brookfield, S.D. (1987). *Developing critical thinkers.* San Francisco: Jossey-Bass, p. 79.
21. Queen, V.A. (1995, September). Performance evaluation. *Nursing Management*, 26(9), 52–55.
22. Stevens, B.J. (1976, October). Performance appraisal: What the nurse executive expects from it. *Journal of Nursing Administration*, 6(10), 26–31.

12

Legal Issues in the Workplace

"We cannot expect people to do the right thing unless they know the right thing to do."

Author Unknown

INTRODUCTION

Nurse administrators and managers need to be familiar with the laws and legislation related to nursing practice, administration, labor management, and employment. Both federal and state laws influence how health care is given and reimbursed and, therefore, have an impact on nursing practice. Nurse administrators and managers also need to be cognizant of not only their own rights and responsibilities, but also those of their employees, particularly professional nurses, since it is the practice and welfare of this group of workers to whom and for whom they are most often accountable. Awareness and understanding of legal issues is imperative for a number of reasons. One, these are times of considerable change and increasing complexity in the health care environment. Runaway health care costs have resulted in integrated health systems or networks. Two, work redesign has been a consequence of such restructuring. The impact on the workforce, changes in work hours, and/or a change in job descriptions have led to anxious and, in several cases, dissatisfied workers, especially RNs. Yet, in times of change, organizations depend on committed workers for their success.[1] Three, health care institutions and agencies employ racially and ethnically diverse workers, as well as large numbers of women workers. Several laws/legislation have been instituted to protect women and minority workers from discrimination. Four, litigious tendencies of the American public are widespread and have been particularly acute in the health care field, with multimillion dollar awards to not only patients and families for malpractice or negligence by employees but also to employees as a result of employers' insensitivity to, ignorance of, or flagrant violation of legal rules and regulations.

Consequently, it is imperative that nurse managers know the kinds of situations that can lead to **litigation** and take steps to avoid being sued. A first step is gaining knowledge about legal regulations that apply to workers and the work environment. Nurse administrators could be held liable for violations of these laws. There are many legal issues and **legal constraints** involved in hiring and employment. Few aspects of the employer–employee relationship are free from regulation by either state or federal law.[2] Many of these relate to specific aspects of personnel management and will be the focus of this chapter.

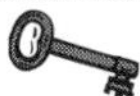

KEY CONCEPTS

Affirmative Action refers to the active legislative attempt to ensure that minorities (or others so deemed discriminated against) are provided set-aside positions in the workplace. These laws were enacted to right historical wrongs.

Collective Bargaining is an attempt by a formal group to negotiate terms of a contract.

Discrimination is an illegal act that prohibits an individual from working on the basis of gender, age, ethnic, racial, or disability status.

Equal Employment Opportunity (EEO) laws refer to those legislative acts that ensure fair hiring and conduct in the workplace.

Equal Employment Opportunity Commission (EEOC) refers to the enforcing agency for EEO laws.

Legal Constraints refer to the structural limitations imposed by existing law.

Litigation refers to the acts of bringing a lawsuit.

Sexual Harassment is a special case of EEO law that prohibits unwanted sexual advances from those who directly influence the work. May be of two types: (1) *quid pro quo*—sexual requests for privileges in the workplace; and (2) *hostile environment* (blatantly offensive)—creation of a workplace setting that interferes with or intimidates an individual's ability to work.

Strike is an organized action and work stoppage by a formal group who uses this methodology to negotiate terms of a contract. This is usually a last resort when negotiating fails.

Strikebreaker ("scab") is a temporary worker (RN) hired to replace striking workers (RNs).

EQUAL EMPLOYMENT OPPORTUNITY (EEO) LAWS

Equal Employment Opportunity laws were the first legislation in the area of employment hiring practices; they resulted from years of **discrimination** toward persons of color. The federal government has enacted several laws to expand equal employment opportunities by prohibiting discrimination not only on the basis of race but also on the basis of sex, age, religion, physical impairment, pregnancy, or national origin. There are also state laws addressing equal employment opportunities. The nurse manager should be familiar with, and abide by, the following equal employment opportunity laws when hiring and assigning nursing personnel.

Title VII of the Civil Rights Act of 1964 (Amended in 1972)

Title VII of the 1964 Civil Rights Act protects people from discrimination for reasons of race, color, national origin, sex, and religion. It prohibits discrimination based on factors unrelated to job qualifications and promotes employment based on ability and merit. Executive orders by President Lyndon Johnson in 1965 and 1967 strengthened the Civil Rights Act. Because some groups had a long history of being discriminated against, the government sought to assist those groups in catching up with the rest of the workforce. Therefore, the executive order created an **affirmative action** component. In most states, affirmative action plans are voluntary unless government contracts are involved. Affirmative action isn't the same as equal opportunity. EEO laws are aimed at preventing discrimination, whereas affirmative action plans are aimed at activity seeking to fill job vacancies with groups who are underemployed and have had a history of being discriminated against.

The Act also created the **Equal Employment Opportunity Commission** (EEOC), which is responsible for enforcing Title VII.[3,4]

Civil Rights Act of 1991

This act expanded the scope of civil rights statutes to provide remedies for intentional workplace discrimination and harassment and established punitive damages for malice in discriminatory practices.

Civil Rights Act, Amended 1993

This amendment ensured that all persons have equal rights under the law and outlined damages available to complainants in actions brought against employers under Title VII, the ADA—see below—(and the Rehabilitation Act of 1973).[5]

Age Discrimination in Employment Act

In 1967, Congress enacted the Age Discrimination in Employment Act to prohibit job discrimination solely because of age (discrimination against people aged 40 to 70). This act applies to employers of 20 or more persons. An amendment in 1978 prohibited mandatory retirement for persons under 70 years of age. A second amendment in 1987 removed even this restriction, except in certain job categories.[6]

Pregnancy Discrimination Act

The Pregnancy Discrimination Act of 1978 prohibits sex discrimination against women who are or might become pregnant. Women unable to work for pregnancy-related reasons are entitled to disability benefits and sick leave on the same basis as employees unable to work for medical reasons. Under the protection of this act, neither potential legal liability nor protecting the woman's fetus is sufficient reason to practice sex discrimination.[7]

Americans with Disabilities Act (ADA)

Passed in 1990, the ADA mandates that people with physical or mental disabilities be integrated into the mainstream of the workforce. It states:

> No qualified individual with a disability shall, by reason of such disability, be excluded from participation in or be denied the benefits of the services, programs, or activities of a public entity, or be subjected to discrimination by any such entity. One who is disabled is defined as anyone who has a record of or is perceived as having a mental or physical impairment that substantially limits at least one major life activity.[8]

The act went into effect in 1992 and not only prohibits discrimination but also delineates enforceable standards. It prohibits inquiries and medical examinations intended to gain information about an applicant's disabilities before a conditional job offer.

Immigration Reform and Control Act

The Immigration and Control Act of 1986 mandates that employers verify the identity of employees and sanctions employers who knowingly hire an unauthorized alien.[9]

Consolidated Omnibus Budget Reconciliation Act (COBRA)

Effective 1986, this act requires employers in the private sector to make available to terminated or retired employees and their families continued health benefits for a specified period. The time period depends on the size of the business organization.[10]

Occupational Safety and Health Act (OSHA)

The Occupational Safety and Health Act of 1970 requires employers to provide job safety and health protection. It provides regulations for unsafe work practices, hazardous conditions, and exposure to hazardous chemicals and other agents. Inspectors may issue citations for violations. In 1996, OSHA created guidelines to define and describe the scope of workplace violence; however, the guidelines do not carry any regulatory force.[11]

Sexual Harassment: A Special Case of Discrimination

Although **sexual harassment** has become a newsworthy topic since such highly publicized events as the Anita Hill–Clarence Thomas Supreme Court hearing and the Navy Tailhook scandal, the sexual exploitation of women at work is not a new problem. Bularzik and Seagrave cite records dating as far back as colonial times.[12,13] Further, sexual harassment was not named or made a household word until the mid-1970s.[14,15] However, approximately 40 to 50 percent of working women experience sexual harassment.[16-18]

In her influential book, MacKinnon, a feminist legal scholar, argued that sexual harassment was primarily a women's problem and should be considered a form of sex discrimination under Title VII of the Civil Rights Act .[19] Consistent with her position, the EEOC established its now well-known guidelines in 1980. Although the guidelines per se do not have the force of law, the courts generally rely on them. According to the EEOC, sexual harassment is defined as follows:

> Unwelcome sexual advances, requests for sexual favors, and other verbal or physical conduct of a sexual nature constitute sexual harassment when: (a) submission to such conduct is made either explicitly or implicitly a term or condition of employment, (b) submission to or rejection of such conduct is used as the basis for employment decisions affecting the individual, or (c) such conduct has the purpose of reasonably interfering with an individual's work performance or creating an intimidating, hostile, or offensive work environment.[20]

Most of the early cases were quid pro quo in nature ("this for that") in which there was an overt demand for sex in exchange for job privileges or promotions ([a] and [b] in the above definition). However, these cases soon gave way to hostile environment harassment [(c) in the definition above], which is more widespread and more difficult to prove.[21] In 1986, the landmark case *Meritor Savings Bank v. Vinson* set the precedent for deferring guidelines to the EEOC when the U.S. Supreme Court concurred with the D.C. Court of Appeals' decision that sexual harassment that creates a hostile environment is just as discriminatory as quid pro quo harassment.[22,23] Therefore, actionable sexual harassment can include unsolicited nonreciprocal verbal and physical sexual advances; other sexual contact, such as leering, gestures, touching, and pinching; and pejorative behaviors and remarks directed at women (e.g., sexist jokes or pin-up calenders). According to the EEOC, the greatest number of legal complaints about sexual harassment have occurred in the service industry, which includes health care.[24]

Later, the EEOC calculated that 6.7 percent of reported claims (114,480) from 1992 to 1999 came from the health care industry.[25] Sexual harassment is clearly a problem in health care—and pervasive in nursing because it is predominantly female and because of the physical nature of nurses' work.[26]

Employers can be held liable for acts by coworkers, supervisors, and managerial staff if the employer knew of the conduct and didn't address it. Although cases are still being decided that will give more guidance in determining the type of evidence necessary for holding the employer accountable, it is clear that employers have a responsibility for fostering a "no tolerance" environment.[27] Even if an employer has a well-written sexual harassment policy, the facility may be held liable if the policy is incomplete, not followed, or contains promises that were not kept.[28] Employer liability may be minimized by taking immediate and appropriate corrective action in instances of sexual harassment.

Costs of sexual harassment are high, not only for the harassed individual, but also for the organization, and include not only litigation costs but also other direct and indirect costs.[29-32] The financial impact of sexual harassment was assessed by the federal government in a large-scale survey of federal workers: Sexual harassment cost the federal government an estimated $267 million over a 2-year period. In another survey of Fortune 500 companies, harassment cost a typical company approximately $6.7 million per year.[33] Costs included replacing employees who left their jobs, paying employees sick leave, reduced individual and group productivity, and costs of internal complaint handling. In addition, these studies found that there were indirect costs; for example, lower confidence in management in general, reduced job satisfaction, diminished commitment to the organization, and a less-positive view of the organization's communication practice.

Prevention programs are the best way to avoid or reduce costs.[34,35] To treat employees fairly and to avoid such costs, the administrator needs to develop a clear policy statement opposing sexual harassment; establish grievance procedures and processes for reporting harassment; take prompt and appropriate action in response to reported incidents; develop training programs for managers to increase awareness and sensitivity; and develop educational programs or workshops for all employees regarding reactions and behaviors on the part of victims that are likely to resolve or reduce harassment, reporting procedures, and disciplinary action for perpetrators.[36] Education must be specific and deliberate. Content needs to be based on structural impediments to a positive workplace environment and include interactive information conveyed by those who have experienced harassment. Both a purposeful approach and listening to the perspectives and experiences of informants are necessary.[37]

The emergent change in the social context of gender issues in the workplace is challenging nurse administrators as organizational leaders. This means that they need a clear understanding of the complex issues surrounding sexual harassment, must voice opposition to it, initiate appropriate actions within their organizations, and get the message down through the ranks to the non-administrative nurses. [38-40]

Hiring and Interviewing

When interviewing a job applicant, questions posed to the applicant should be based on the goals for hiring, the job description, and the information the applicant has provided on the application and/or resume. Pose questions that address job requirements, information about the skills and qualities desired, and examples of the applicant's experiences. Avoid questions that can be considered discriminatory and, therefore, illegal. For example, age (date of birth), race, religion, marital status, and national origin can be volunteered by the applicant but cannot be asked by the interviewer. It is permissible to do background checks and to ask for proof of legal eligibility for employment.

FAMILY AND MEDICAL LEAVE ACT (FMLA) OF 1993

The Family and Medical Leave Act was the first major initiative of the Clinton administration.[41] However, it does not preempt state or local laws with more generous provisions.[42] The original concept was directed at pregnancy and maternal leave but eventually became very broad and extended to cover the entire family.[43] The act requires employers with 50 or more workers to provide up to 12 weeks per year of unpaid, job-protected leave. Eligible employees must have been employed for at least 12 months and completed 1,250 hours of service during the 12-month period immediately preceding the leave.[44]

An eligible employee is entitled to a leave under the following four circumstances: (1) upon the birth of the employee's child, (2) upon adoption or foster placement of a child with the employee, (3) to care for a child, spouse, or parent with a serious health condition, and (4) when the employee is unable to perform functions of the job position because of a serious health condition.

Both the employee and the employer have rights and responsibilities. The nurse administrator needs to be aware of both parties' obligations. The employee has the right to: (1) return from leave to the same or an equivalent position with equivalent benefits, compensation, and conditions of employment, and (2) take leave on an intermittent or reduced-time strategy if medically necessary for a serious health condition of the employee or child, spouse, or parent. However, the employee also has an obligation to provide the employer with a 30-day advance notice if the need for the leave is foreseeable.

Employers have both the right to require the employee to provide medical certification for a claim for leave associated with a personal serious medical condition or to care for a seriously ill child, spouse, or parent and the right to require certification that the employee is eligible to return to work if leave was taken for a personal illness. The employer can also require that the employee's accrued paid vacation time or sick leave be used in lieu of part of the 12 weeks of unpaid leave. However, the employer must maintain the employee's health benefits coverage for the duration of the leave. Records must be made, kept, and preserved. In addition, the employee's medical information must be kept confidential and in separate files from the employee's usual personnel file.

LABOR-MANAGEMENT LAWS

Some observers feel that employment and labor-management laws are too prescriptive and, therefore, prevent creativity. They view them with resentment and hostility. More recently, progressive managers have taken a proactive stance, adopting an attitude of acceptance and tolerance and starting to forge newer models of work structures and relationships between labor and management.

Unions and Collective Bargaining

Labor organizations have become a significant factor in hospital–employee relations. Nurse administrators must understand the impact of unionization on the health care industry and the legislation regarding employment practice. Since they may be dealing with employees represented by unions and working under collective bargaining agreements, they need to be familiar with the provisions and protections offered by law and the basic tenets of these labor relations laws.

The National Labor Relations Act (Wagner Act) of 1935 governs collective bargaining between employee groups (unions) and their managers or employers.[45] **Collective bargaining** includes the activities occurring between labor and management that concern employee relations, such as negotiation of formal labor agreements and day-to-day interactions. The NLRA is administered by the National Labor Relations Board (NLRB), which determines an employee's union representation status and resolves labor-management disputes.

Since its initial passage, several amendments have changed the provisions of the act. In 1947, the Taft-Hartley Amendment excluded not-for-profit hospitals from the definition of "employer" in the National Labor Relations Act. Consequently, unionization of workers in health care institutions was illegal until 1962 when President Kennedy amended the act by executive order to allow public employees to join unions. As a result, the first collective bargaining by nurses employed by city, county, and state hospitals and agencies began. Congress amended the act further in 1974 to allow employees of not-for-profit hospitals and organizations to form or join unions.[46]

The initial NLRA recognized only three bargaining units: all professionals, all nonprofessionals, and guards. However, in 1991, in a major case involving the American Hospital Association, the U.S. Supreme Court upheld the rule of the NLRB that allowed recognition of up to eight categories, including a separate one for registered nurses (RNs). This issue had an enormous impact for the American Nurses Association (ANA) and its state affiliates, which act as collective bargaining units or agents for RNs. Both the ANA and other unions began targeting hospitals and RNs for organizing when the new NLRB rules were instituted.[47] In 1999, the ANA created a national labor committee—the United American Nurses (UAN)—to strengthen and support state nurses associations' collective bargaining efforts and to advise the ANA board of directors on the labor implications of proposed association policy.[48]

Still, many RNs have been reluctant to unionize. At the center of such reluctance are concerns that collective bargaining and strike clauses are contrary to professionalism and patient safety.[49,50] Yet, other RNs see collective bargaining and unionization as an opportunity to improve relations with management; raise the status of the profession; resolve staffing and mandatory overtime issues which affect patient safety; and improve health care delivery.[51-53]

According to Moylan, the nurse manager must be thoroughly versed in four parts of the NLRA: Section 7, Section 8A, the definition of supervisor, and the definition of employer.[54] Section 7 guarantees employees the right to organize while protecting the rights of those who refrain. Section 8A identifies five categories of unfair labor practices that restrict employee rights: (1) interference with the right to organize, (2) domination (for example, the nurse administrator supports one collective bargaining agent over another), (3) encouraging or discouraging membership in a union by preferential treatment of union or non-union employees, (4) discharging an employee for giving testimony or filing a charge with the NLRB, and (5) refusal to bargain collectively (for example, negotiate salaries or working conditions).

According to the terms of the NLRA, supervisors are excluded from coverage (that is, they have no right to organize or engage in collective bargaining). The NLRA defines "supervisor" as:

> Any individual having authority, in the interest of the employer, to hire, transfer, suspend, lay off, recall, promote, discharge, assign, reward, or discipline other employees, or responsibly to direct them, or to adjust their grievances, or effectively to recommend such action, if in connection with the foregoing the exercise of authority is not merely a routine or clerical nature, but requires the use of independent judgment (29 U.S.C.142,11).

It also states that anyone acting in a supervisory capacity, regardless of job title, is acting as the "employer." It is this issue of the definition of supervisor that has implications for all RNs.

For several years, the NLRB maintained that staff nurses who direct the work of less-skilled employees in the exercise of professional judgment do so with a focus on the "well-being of the patient" and are not exercising their authority "in the interest of the employer." Therefore, they were not considered supervisors by the NLRB.[55] However, this argument was rejected in 1994 when the U.S. Supreme Court upheld a decision by an appellate court in the case of *National Labor Relations Board v. Health Care Retirement Corporation of America*, and again in 2001, in the case of *National Labor Relations Board v. Kentucky River Community Care*, Inc., which ruled that nurses who exercise supervisory authority are excluded from the coverage of the NLRA.[56,57] In the former case, the appellate court held that licensed practical nurses (LPNs) at an Ohio nursing home, who directed the work of nurses' aides, acted as supervisors and, therefore, were not protected from firing when they took action to improve working conditions.[58] In the latter case, the appeals court held that duties of registered nurses working at a nonprofit mental-health facility in Kentucky made them supervisors, and that the supervisory test of "independent judgment" was ambiguous and not supportable in the NLRA.[59,60] The confusion for nursing management is which definition is binding: the Supreme Court's definition of supervisor, which includes some staff nurse responsibilities (thus eliminating the right of staff nurses to unionize), or the NLRB's more restrictive definition of nonstatutory supervisor (thus staff nurses can unionize).

Some observers feel that the former interpretation may open the door for employers seeking to exclude RNs from bargaining units since they could argue that RNs have supervisory status when directing the work of less-skilled employees, especially since one facet of the mid-1990's work redesign and restructuring in hospitals was to downgrade the number of professional nurses and increase the number of unlicensed assistive personnel.[61-64] In fact, a Montana hospital attempted to eject the collective bargaining unit that represented its RNs based on the Supreme Court's ruling on nurses' supervisory status. The hospital's Board of Trustees voted not to recognize the union after expiration of the contract ("Hospital uses top court issues," 1994). In similar situations in hospitals in Michigan and New York, the state nurses' associations have filed unfair labor practice charges.[65,66] Although the Supreme Court's recent ruling could dampen nurses' willingness to speak out when they have concerns about safety in the workplace, labor union leaders hope that the NLRB will reinterpret certain provisions of the NLRA's definition of supervisor.

While this seems to be an era of uncertainty for labor leaders and formation of new collective bargaining units, several observers note that the uncertainty is part of an era of transition and change in health care that necessitates new models for labor-management relations. They advocate a model for professional collaboration for labor relations, working together to establish mutual agreements of language interpretation, and forging win-win approaches to the grievance process. The need to decrease costs is forcing employers to change the way they do business. More progressive employers are adopting more cooperative and collaborative approaches to labor management relations, such as flattening hierarchical organizations, creating self-directed work teams, and forging new partnerships with workers, which increase their ownership and participation in outcomes. "Magnet" facilities, known for their success in creating environments without recruitment and retention problems, have common characteristics: reduced morbidity and mortality rates, increased patient satisfaction levels, improved nurse-patient ratios, significantly lower rates of nurse burnout, lower incidence of needle-stick injuries, nurse perceptions of adequate support services and enough RNs, and high education of nursing staff.[67]

Strikes

Strikes are not a common tactic used by nurses. However, nurses have used strikes as last-resort efforts to improve care and working conditions.[68,69] Over the past few years, strikes by RNs in the United States have noticeably increased. In 1995, RNs were involved in only four work stoppages; in 2000, there were four times as many strikes, involving thousands of nurses in Massachusetts, New York, Washington D.C., Ohio, Michigan, and California. Nurses across the country are concerned about the shortage of hospital nurses, inadequate staffing, use of unlicensed assistive personnel, and mandatory overtime, and feel such conditions put themselves and patients at risk. A national survey of RNs in 2000 showed that there were enough RNs to deliver care. The difficulty is that the current work environment is so stressful—particularly in hospitals—that it has become almost impossible to recruit and retain a sufficient supply of RNs.[70] In cities or states where the shortage is severe, some ERs "divert" ambulances to other facilities; others temporarily close units—occasionally housewide—to new admits. For example, on two separate occasions, five hospitals in St. Paul and Minneapolis shut their doors to all admissions—with the exception of patients who came in through the emergency department. Hospitals attributed this to a lack of staff.[71] Facing tremendous workplace pressures and unable to negotiate contract agreements, some nurses feel they have no recourse but to strike.

The law requires that there must be a 10-day notice given before a strike takes place in order to give the hospital a chance to prepare for the strike.[72] The U.S. Supreme Court gave employers the right to permanently replace striking workers. However, this practice did not become common until 1981 when President Reagan fired striking air traffic controllers and hired replacements. Legislation that prohibits employers from permanently replacing strikers has been rejected by the Senate twice, most recently in 1993.[73] Still, some employers hire temporary **strikebreakers**, commonly known as "scabs," to staff their facility. Having a supply of temporary workers, employers are less inclined to negotiate an agreement or use alternative dispute resolution to address the problems that lead to strikes.[74]

In essence, strikes are often detrimental to both labor and management. In the few instances where nurses have gone on strike, patient safety and well-being have not been jeopardized. However, nurses who have participated in strikes have suffered retaliation, including losing gains made by seniority, being denied opportunities afforded others, being given difficult assignments and heavy patient loads, losing full-time jobs, or being permanently replaced.[75]

Some collective bargaining units have developed alternatives to strikes for achieving their goals: (1) launching nationwide campaigns to mobilize nurses around crisis issues[76] and (2) calling on state and federal legislators to enact legislation that requires facilities to provide appropriate staffing levels, restrict mandatory overtime, mandate the collection of nursing-sensitive patient indicators (make public the staffing level and mix and related patient outcomes), provide protection for whistle-blowers (protect nurses from retribution when they voice concern about unsafe patient conditions) and hold health care administrators accountable for management decisions that affect the quality of patient care.[77-80] For example, Kentucky and Virginia passed legislation in 1998 to set appropriate staffing methods.[81] In 1999, California passed legislation that required minimum nurse-patient ratios in acute care hospitals, prohibited the use of unlicensed personnel to perform procedures normally done by RNs, and restricted unsafe "float" assignments[82]; New Hampshire approved data collection on the rates of RNs per bed.[83] In the 2000 legislative sessions, 34 such bills were introduced in 16 states. In addition, nurses annually gain protection by successfully negotiating hundreds of collective bargaining agreements or contracts that address their workplace concerns.[84,85]

Nurses have many concerns about collective bargaining and strikes. However, most problems plaguing nurses are only ameliorated from time to time; therefore, they remain longstanding and unresolved. If employers collaborate with nurses to initiate a means for them to practice professionally on a long-term basis, nurses will probably be less likely to form collective bargaining units or join unions. It is only when they are dissatisfied with several issues and feel like pawns in the work environment that joining or organizing a union is considered.

Just as the interpretation and tenets of the NLRA keep changing and evolving, the union—management relationship must evolve and change. The old polarized approach to the resolution of differences will need to give way to outcomes that benefit both. Both have a chance to be proactive as health care workplaces are continually restructured. The need to control costs depends on empowered workers who feel connected and invested in the workplace which means labor and management have to reconsider the character of their relationship and join together in constructing new models of relationship.

CASE STUDY

Sexual Harassment

A female staff nurse was assigned to care for a middle-aged male patient with a pulmonary diagnosis of a chronic nature. The patient has a history of frequent admissions and is often admitted to the same nursing unit. Throughout his admission, he consistently tells the nurse dirty jokes, makes intimate comments about her physical appearance and sex life, and the wall in his room sports a nude poster. The climate created by this patient makes the nurse want to avoid going into the patient's room.[86]

CASE STUDY

Physical Abuse

A nurse executive recounts an incident reported to her by the manager in the operating room. A physician, who stated he was "just having fun," attached a vaginal clamp to the abdominal area of a staff nurse's scrub attire. The clamp pinched and broke the staff nurse's skin.[87]

CASE STUDY

Hostile Environment

A staff nurse found a "sexual harassment consent form" posted in the women's bathroom, shortly after a legitimate notice about sexual harassment had been posted in the hospital. She called the personnel director to report it. He not only verified it but stated it originated at a department head meeting as a joke. The nurse told him she didn't think it was funny at all.[88]

- If these cases had been reported to you as the nurse manager, how would you handle each of them?

SUMMARY

The legal system is just one part of the whole health care system. Some laws relative to health care organizations are made to protect workers and promote peaceful and productive interactions between employers and employees, as well as between coworkers. Both the health care environment and legislation are constantly changing and, therefore, constantly challenging the nurse administrator to stay abreast of these changes. Effective nurse administrators must develop an understanding of the basic principles and processes of current legislation and its implications for both themselves and the nursing staff for whom they are responsible and to whom they are accountable. Developing a working knowledge of laws and legal rules and regulations related to health care organizations and their relationship to their workers has the potential to increase the quality of the work environment and, therefore, the quality of care the nurse delivers.

LEARNER EXERCISES

1. List questions that cannot be included in a hiring interview.
2. If you were asked any of the questions just named, how would you answer?
3. If you were in a situation in which you felt you were being sexually harassed, what would your responsibility be? (Remember assertive communication, sharing your discomfort with the individual, and suggesting "call me by name," and soon, repeating if necessary.)
4. If you were physically attacked (supposedly as a joke), what would your response be? (Review dealing with difficult, verbally hostile people: stand up for yourself, don't engage in further argument; physically hostile: secure your safety, stand up for yourself, report to personnel director.)
5. What advantages do you see to joining a union? Professional organization?

REFERENCES

1. Anderson, P., & Pulich, M. (2000). Recruiting good employees in tough times. *Health Care Manager, 18*(3), 32–40.
2. Haimann, T. (1994). *Supervisory management,* 5th ed. Dubuque, IA: W. C. Brown.
3. Title VII of the Civil Rights Act. (1964). 42 U.S.C. 2000e.
4. Equal Employment Opportunity Commission. (1980). Guidelines on discrimination because of sex. *Federal Register, 45,* 51266–51269.
5. O'Keefe M.E., (2001). *Nursing practice and the law.* Philadelphia: F.A. Davis, p. 219.
6. Age Discrimination Act. (1976). 29 U.S.C. 621.
7. Pregnancy Discrimination Act. (1978). 49 U.S.C. 2000e(d).
8. Americans with Disabilities Act. (1990). 42 U.S.C. 12101.
9. Immigration Reform and Control Act. Retrieved from the World Wide Web: *http://www.usda.gov/oce/labor-affairs/ircasdisc.*
10. Consolidated Omnibus Budget Reconciliation Act, Retrieved from the World Wide Web: *http://www.consumerlawpage.com*
11. O'Keefe, M.E. (2001). *Nursing practice and the law.* Philadelphia: F.A. Davis, p. 447.
12. Bularzik, M, (1978). *Sexual harassment at the workplace: Historical notes.* Somerville, MA: New England Free Press.
13. Seagrave, K. (1994). *The sexual harassment of women in the workplace, 1600–1993.* Jefferson, NC: McFarland & Company.
14. Safran, C. (1976, November). What men do to women on the job: A shocking look at sexual harassment. *Redbook,* 149, 217–223.
15. Farley, L. (1978). *Sexual shakedown: The sexual harassment of women on the job.* New York: Mc-Graw-Hill.
16. U.S. Merit Systems Protection Board. (1981). *Sexual harassment in the federal workplace: Is It a problem?* Washington, D.C.: Government Printing Office.
17. Gutek, B.A. (1985). *Sex and the workplace.* San Francisco: Jossey-Bass.
18. Fiedler, A., & Hamby, E. (2000). Sexual harassment in the workplace. *Journal of Nursing Administration, 30*(10), 497–503.
19. MacKinnon, C. (1979). *Sexual harassment of working women: A case of sex discrimination.* New Haven, CT: Yale University Press.
20. Fitzgerald, L.F. (1990). Sexual harassment: The definition and measurement of a construct. In M.A. Paludi (Ed.), *Ivory power: Sexual harassment on campus* (pp. 21–44). New York: State University of New York Press.
21. Frazier, P.A., Cochran, C.C., Olson, A.M. (1995). Social science research on lay definitions of sexual harassment. *Journal of Social Issues, 51,* 21–37.
22. *Meritor Savings Bank v. Vinson.* (1986). 477 U.S. 57, 40 FEP Cases 18222.18.
23. Chan, A.A. (1994). *Women and sexual harassment: A practical guide to the legal protections of Title VII and the hostile environment claim.* New York: Harrington Park Press.
24. Center for Women in Government. (1994, Spring). Cost of sexual harassment to employers up sharply. *Women in Public Service,* 1–4, 45.
25. Equal Employment Opportunities Commission. (2000, May). *National database reporting facility.* Washington, D.C.
26. Fiedler, A., & Hamby, E. (2000). Sexual harassment in the workplace. *Journal of Nursing Administration, 30*(10), 497–503.
27. Gutek, B.A., & Koss, M.P. (1993). Changed women and changed organizations: Consequences of and coping with sexual harassment. *Journal of Social Issues, 38,* 97–115.
28. Monarch, K. (2000). Protect yourself from sexual harassment. *American Journal of Nursing,* 100(5), 71.

29. U.S. Merit Systems Protection Board (U.S.MSPB). (1987). *Sexual harassment in the federal workplace: An update.* Washington, D.C.: Government Printing Office.
30. Sclafane, S. (1998). Sex-harassment rulings may hit hospitals hard, lawyers think. *National Underwriter, 40*(3), 102.
31. Phillips, J. (2000). Hostile environment, rape, and big bucks. *Tennessee Employment Law Update,* 15(1).
32. TWA will pay $2.6 million to settle suit. *St. Louis Post-Dispatch,* May 25, 2001, B8.
33. Klein, F., & Rowe, M. (1988). *Estimating the cost of sexual harassment to the FORTUNE 500 service and manufacturing firms.* Cambridge, MA: Klein Associates.
34. Monarch, K. (2000). Protect yourself from sexual harassment. *American Journal of Nursing, 100*(5), 71.
35. Moore, H.L., Cangelosi, J.D., & Gatlin-Watts, R.W. (1998). Seven spoonfuls of preventive medicine for sexual harassment in health care. *Health Care Manager*, 17(2), 1–9.
36. Beauvais, K. (1986). Workshops to combat sexual harassment: A case study of changing attitudes. *Signs, 12,* 130–145.
37. Madison, J., & Minichiello, V. (2000). Recognizing and labeling sex-based and sexual harassment in the heath care workplace. *Journal of Nursing Scholarship,* 32(4), 405–414.
38. Gutek, B.A., & Koss, M.P. (1993). Changed women and changed organizations: Consequences of and coping with sexual harassment. *Journal of Social Issues, 38,* 97–115.
39. Monarch, K. (2000). Protect yourself from sexual harassment. *American Journal of Nursing, 100*(5), 71.
40. Fiedler, A., & Hamby, E. (2000). Sexual harassment in the workplace. *Journal of Nursing Administration, 30*(10), 497–503.
41. Family and Medical Leave Act. (1993). 29 U.S.C. 2601.ct.seq.
42. Ealey, T. (1993). What you should know about the family and medical leave act of 1993. *The Journal of Long-Term Care Administration, 21,* 35–39.
43. Ealey, T. (1993). What you should know about the family and medical leave act of 1993. *The Journal of Long-Term Care Administration, 21,* 35–39.
44. The Family Medical Leave Act. (1995). *American Association of Occupational Health Nurses Journal, 43*(10), insert 2p.
45. O'Keefe, M.E. (2001). *Nursing practice and the law*, Philadelphia: F.A. Davis, 447.
46. Flarey, D.L., Yoder, S.K., & Barabas, M.C. (1992). Collaboration in labor relations: A model for success. *Journal of Nursing Administration,* 22(9), 15–22.
47. Porter-O'Grady, T. (1992). Of rabbits and turtles: A time of change for unions. *Nursing Economics, 10,* 179.
48. Helmlinger, C. (1999). ANA creates new "house" for all nurses. *American Journal of Nursing,* 99(12), 59–60.
49. Lenehan, G. (2000). On mandatory overtime and wearing blue ribbons. *Journal of Emergency Nursing, 26*(3), 201–202.
50. Reactions to editorial on strikebreakers. (2000). *The American Nurse, 32*(6), 4.
51. Price, C. (2000). A national uprising: United actions push mandatory overtime, inadequate staffing to forefront. *American Journal of Nursing, 100*(12), 75–76.
52. Gilmore-Hall, A. (2001). All for one and one for all: Using state legislation to secure federal protections. *American Journal of Nursing, 101*(3), 59–60, 62.
53. RISNA pushes to end forced overtime. (2001). *The American Nurse, 33*(3), 5.
54. Moylan, L.B. (1988). Implications of the National Labor Relations Act. *Nursing Management, 19*(6), 80.
55. Cohen, D.M., & Wick, E.F. (1995). Healthcare in transition: Labor law impact on nurse-supervisor roles. *Journal of Nursing Administration, 25*(6), 15–18.
56. *NLRB v. Health Care & Retirement Corporation of America.* 1989. 114 Sct 1778 (1994).

57. VandeWater, J. (2001, May 30). Supreme Court ruling on nurses may affect unions. *St. Louis Post-Dispatch,* C1, C8.
58. Mahoney, M.E. (1995). Supreme Court rejects longstanding labor rule for nurses. *Health Care Supervisor, 13*(4), 13–17.
59. VandeWater, J. (2001, May 30). Supreme Court ruling on nurses may affect unions. *St. Louis Post-Dispatch,* C1, C8.
60. Court bars union membership for RN supervisors. (2001). *Nurseweek (Midwest)*, 2(5), p. 22.
61. Ketter, J. (1994). Restructuring spurs debate on staffing ratios, skill mix. *American Nurse, 26,* 26.
62. Helminger, C. (1999). ANA creates new "house" for all nurses. *American Journal of Nursing, 99*(12), 59–60.
63. Court bars union membership for RN supervisors. (2001). *Nurseweek (Midwest),* 2(5), 22.
64. VandeWater, J. (2001, May 30). Supreme Court ruling on nurses may affect unions. *St. Louis Post-Dispatch,* C1, C8.
65. Ketter, J. (1994). NLRB rules on RN supervisory status at Alaska hospital. *American Nurse, 26,* 8.
66. In brief. (2001). *American Nurse, 33*(1), 10.
67. Aiken, L.H. et al. (2000). The magnet nursing services recognition program. *American Journal of Nursing, 100*(3), 26–36.
68. Giovinco, G. (1993). When nurses strike: Ethical issues. *Nursing Management, 24*, 86–90.
69. A decision that defies logic. (2001). *American Journal of Nursing, 101*(4), 57–58.
70. Policy vs. reality: What do you do when your rights are limited by the realities of the workplace? *American Journal of Nursing, 101*(5), 87.
71. Trossman, S. (2000). Waiting for care: Too many patients, too little staff. *American Nurse, 32*(6), 1, 2, 14.
72. Califano, J.T. (1996). *Contemporary professional nursing*. Philadelphia: F.A. Davis.
73. Ketter, J. (1994). Striker replacement loses in senate again. *American Nurse*, vol. 26.
74. A decision that defies logic. (2001). *American Journal of Nursing. 101*(4), 57–58.
75. Ketter, J. (1994). Striker replacement loses in senate again. *American Nurse,* vol. 26.
76. United American nurses launches campaign to address short staffing. (2000). *American Nurse, 32*(6), 12, 24.
77. Whistle-blowers have right to sue, court rules. (2001). *Nurseweek (Midwest), 2*(5), 23.
78. Real solutions to the staffing crisis. (2001). *American Nurse, 33*(3), 14.
79. Price, C. (2000). A national uprising: United actions push mandatory overtime, inadequate staffing to the forefront. *American Journal of Nursing, 100*(12), 75–76.
80. Gilmore-Hall, A. (2001). All for one and one for all: Using state legislation to secure federal protections. *American Journal of Nursing. 101*(3), 59–60, 62.
81. Lobbying efforts gain momentum. (2001). *American Journal of Nursing, 101*(3), 24.
82. California nurses win landmark victory. (2000). *American Journal of Nursing, 100*(1), 20.
83. Gilmore-Hall, A. (2001). All for one and one for all: Using state legislation to secure federal protections. *American Journal of Nursing, 101*(3), 59–60, 62.
84. Michigan nurses win new contract. (2001). *American Nurse, 33*(3), 5.
85. Kany, K. (2001). Mandatory overtime. *American Journal of Nursing, 101*(5), 67–68, 70, 71.
86. King, C.S. (1995). Ending the silent conspiracy: Sexual harassment in nursing. *Nursing Administration Quarterly, 19*(53), 48–55.
87. King, C.S. (1995). Ending the silent conspiracy: Sexual harassment in nursing. *Nursing Administration Quarterly, 19*(53), 48–55.
88. Confronting sexual harassment. (1994). *Nursing, 24*(49).

13

Managing Change

> "Those who never walk, except in other's tracks, will make no discoveries."
>
> Author Unknown

INTRODUCTION

Brookfield describes change as a societal constant evident in relationships in all settings.[1] Lutjens describes change as inherent, natural, and continuous.[2] Throughout this chapter, the focus is on the active role of nurses as initiators or participants in changes that affect nursing. Their role as participants is viewed as a critical means to preserve nursing standards and values in the face of strong influences from other power bases in large organizations where nursing is practiced. When nurses are not included in decision making about the direction of nursing practice, the quality of patient care can be compromised, as was seen during the last decade of the 20th century, because of changes primarily made by agency administrators. There is currently ongoing evidence of some reevaluation of the changes in health care delivery that took place during the 1990s. As a result, nursing is gaining greater autonomy in the way it is practiced within the health care system. Knowing how to manage the pace and process of change within nursing, therefore, takes on new meaning and importance.

KEY CONCEPTS

Change is a dynamic process by which an alteration is brought about that makes a distinct difference.

Change Agent is someone who initiates an idea for a goal-directed change, directs stages of the change process, or does both.

Empirical-Rational Strategy of change is based upon the assumption that people are rational and will follow their own self-interests.

Moving is a term given to the second stage of the change process during which the planned change is put into action.

Nonintervention is one way in which change comes about. Essentially nothing is done, which can be planned and deliberate to accomplish some end or can be a form of neglect.

Normative-Reeducative Strategy of change is based on the assumption that people are motivated to commit to societal norms.

Planned Change is a deliberate course of action that results in a change.

Power-Coercive Strategy of change is based on the belief that power lies with the person of influence.

Radical Change is one way in which change comes about. Action taken is quick and revolutionary. It can be legitimate (out of necessity) or performed through a misuse of power and a show of force.

Refreezing is the third stage of the change process during which the new goal becomes established as the expected condition.

Risk Taking is a willingness to expose oneself to the chance of some loss as a result of making a change.

Unfreezing is the first stage of the change process during which reasons for making a change are given in a way to make the change desirable.

A THEORETICAL PERSPECTIVE

Change can be planned and managed, or it can occur haphazardly. Nursing is a profession sanctioned by society, and its survival depends, in part, on how change is managed. To influence change in nursing through the design of a professional practice model that incorporates knowledge, skill, and the latest in informatics technology is a challenge to contemporary nurse leaders. Their success will depend on the support and creativity of professional nurses at all levels and in all roles. Skill in, and understanding of, the change process will be essential in moving nursing practice into a new paradigm. Nursing is challenged to engage in a transformational process that moves individuals into more complexity and diversity in their evolving professional practice.[3]

Expanded Conceptual Framework

Recent research by Menix [4] regarding change theory as it relates to nursing has identified three concepts that affect nursing that were not formerly included in change models: (1) nonlinear change, (2) cybernetics, and (3) learning dimensions, bringing to twelve the number of categories in a conceptual framework for nursing change management. The updated list follows:

Characteristics
Innovation
Responses
Principles
Environmental Influences
Cybernetics
Change Process
Strategies
Role
Planned Change
Nonlinear Change
Learning Dimensions

Nurse managers and educators agree that the expanded conceptual framework is pertinent for baccalaureate curricula in order to provide the tools that students will need in order to progress, both as students and as new practitioners. Self-paced continuing education modules, as part of an agency's staff development program, are proposed for practicing nurses to become acquainted with, and to begin to develop, the essential competencies associated with new change management approaches. The earlier belief that environmental factors were controllable now gives way to a more dynamic, unpredictable climate that surrounds the change process. The result is greater complexity in change management.

A description of the 12 concepts for managing accelerated change in today's health care organizations follows:

The *characteristics* of change include constancy, inevitability, unpredictability, intrusiveness, variation in rate and intensity, and the need for adaptation. The change process is a natural, social phenomenon impacting individuals, groups, organizations, and society.

The ongoing efforts of **change agents** and participants when implementing and managing change is the *change process.* How the process is enacted depends on a variety of organizational factors; stage of development, past use of research findings, degree of participation by employees in change, past successes in implementing and managing the effects of change, and adherence to organizational strategic planning in applying the change process all play a role in the outcome of change efforts. Changes may be major or minor, positive or negative, permanent or temporary, and can influence the power base within the organization.

Innovation is the outcome of creativity and originality. Managing change by any group is fostered by having individuals who are receptive to new ideas and who promote innovation and flexibility within their organizations.

Strategies are techniques designed to achieve a specific purpose during the change process. Frequently used strategies that encourage participation include education, information sharing, communication, support, negotiation, active listening, and idea acceptance. Coercion, manipulation, and appointed participation can result in varying degrees of support for change. Empowerment of informal leaders actively engaged in the change process is essential to facilitating change, and the sharing of responsibility through delegation is expected.

Responses are the varied reactions of individuals, groups, systems, organizations, and society to a change. They range from acceptance to resistance and are cognitive or attitudinal in nature. Resistance should be anticipated, as change reactions frequently include grief and loss because of "ending." Tolerance for change occurs over time for some, not at all for some, and is completely accepted early on by others.

Role is the formalized, prescribed expectation to perform change agent functions. Change agents use power, credibility, communication, trust, timing, and knowledge of change effectively. Management of change involves planning, organizing, implementing, evaluating, feedback, and relationship building. Broad systems-based thinking promotes management of the many facets of change. Change agents assume different roles, including leader or follower, at different times during the process.

Principles are accepted truths which predict that applying a particular action will result in a specific outcome. Change principles associated with change ownership and anticipated benefits, negotiability, and feedback of change guide the change process.

Change that is expected and deliberately prepared for is **planned change.** It supports systematic, directional approaches to achieve desired goals. The goal of planned change (internal and external environmental stability) may not be achievable when there is chaos within the group. There are several models for planned change that must be evaluated for their appropriateness in reaching desired outcomes.

There are *environmental influences*, internal and external, that affect the course of change. Employees are members of social systems with unique cultures, beliefs, and values which, when combined with organizational interests, can facilitate, enhance, hinder, or obstruct change. All influences impact on the initiation and progress of change.

Nonlinear change is change occurring naturally from self-organizing patterns. Information, relationships, and conceptualization of the future are the context within which effective change occurs. Environmental factors can and do result in unplanned changes, that inhibit or enhance the achieving of desired outcomes. The magnitude of factors that influence the change environment produce fluctuation in times of stability, tension, and chaotic conditions. Health care leaders must be responsive to influences in the environment that can result in potentially beneficial unplanned changes, and to appreciate that the potential benefit can be limited due to an overly rigid moderating of the process. Each situation has unique features, and the conditions present at any given time are not likely to occur again in the same configuration. The increasingly rapid pace and complexity of change reduces the effectiveness of long-range planning while not compromising the value of the pursuit of visions and goals.

Cybernetics is the regulation of systems by managing communication and feedback mechanisms. Feedback signals the need to maintain or alter the course of change. Policies, rules, and quality studies function as feedback mechanisms. Social sanctions are demonstrated through interactions of individuals about the change process. Monitoring by information gathering can limit uncertainty and evaluate acceptance of a change while determining courses of action.

Continual learning is necessary for adequate responses to accelerated change. *Learning dimensions* in organizations provide for the ongoing learning of employees. Ongoing learning improves adaptation, resilience, and hardiness of employees that result in desired responses to accelerated change. Skills needed to maximize learning are systems thinking, personal proficiency, team learning, shared vision, and frequent dialogue. Peers can act as teachers and coaches. Skill in the use of information technology increases access to needed knowledge.

Change and Stress

During times of change, nurses need support from management. Jost[5] suggests ongoing assessment during periods of adapting to changes as an effective means of assisting individuals through periods of frustration and stress. To effectively assess and meet the needs of individuals during periods of change, an organized assessment and intervention strategy is needed to ensure a holistic approach. She suggests a model that focuses on concepts that make sense to the everyday practice of nursing. The five concepts are: (1) *conservation,* (2) *adaptation and change,* (3) *environment,* (4) *patient and nurse, and* (5) *health and disease.*

Intervention is structured according to four conservation areas:

1. Conservation of energy.
2. Structural integrity.
3. Personal integrity.
4. Social integrity.

Responses that cost the least to individuals in terms of their effort and demand on well-being will foster survival. Conservation is the result of adaptation. Through adaptation an individual reaches harmony with the precise environment of which he or she is a part. The nurse is in a temporary dependent state when adapting to unusual change and requires support in the same way that patients need support during periods of disease. Each individual nurse will present with unique needs during times of unusual change. Today's practice environment is marked by frequent changes previously not experienced by nurses, creating a demand for increased administrator interventions.

Expanded Rate and Scope of Change

The challenge to nurse executives to manage change within the profession is greater than ever before as influencing forces go beyond the confines of a local health care delivery system, and information technology becomes a common standard. The scope of influences extends to international, and even global, considerations. To the extent that nursing meets the challenge, professional standards, values, and interests will be affected. Nursing educators are charged with incorporating the latest informatics technology into their teaching. Students will need the new information technology to support their role as collaborators in the development and delivery of effective consumer health. Nursing practice models are being affected by informatics. Through competence in the use of health informatics, professional nurses can integrate relevant and valid health information that leads to improved client satisfaction and improved health care outcomes.[6] As improved information technology in the delivery of patient care becomes a norm, practitioners will encounter clients with more questions about their health and treatment and an increasing desire to participate in their health management decisions. Nurses are currently being presented with new challenges in how they are expected to relate to clients.

CHANGE STRATEGIES

Planned Change Theory

What is the contribution of beginning practitioners in meeting the challenge? Understanding and developing skill in applying the change process is essential. Recently

Tiffany pointed out that research on change theory and its use in nursing is limited[7] and that those who plan change must adopt a theory that should then be used by all within the nursing department.[8] The research by Menix has modified the previous knowledge base about change management in nursing; however, much of the work from the past remains pertinent to the study of change and its application to nursing. In a series of articles on evaluating change theories in use in nursing, the Bennis, Benne, and Chin theory was found to have the highest significance, agreeing with nursing's perspective, clarity, economy, and practicality.[9] The views put forth in the theory synchronize well with the interactionist approach. Three strategies of the Bennis, Benne, and Chin planned change theory are presented:

1. Empirical-rational.
2. Power-coercive.
3. Normative-reeducative.

As will be shown, not all three lend themselves well to nursing.

Empirical-rational strategy is based on the philosophy that rational human beings will follow their own self-interests. If a person perceives some personal benefit or gain from an innovation, he or she will support the change effort, and conversely will resist the change if the innovation causes a personal inconvenience or loss.[10] Some nurses welcome a change in staffing patterns, while others resist it for personal reasons.

Power-coercive strategy is an option that is adopted when there is a belief that power lies with the most influential individual. There is an assumption that the group will comply with the plans, directions, and leadership of power figures.[11] Loyalty is given to a person who occupies a position, and it shifts when a new person assumes the position. In any setting, therefore, cooperation depends on the group's perception of whoever is in the position of most authority.

Empirical-rational and power-coercive strategies are not appropriate for nursing. Neither fosters the professional purpose or perspective. A form of power-coercive strategy produced some of the current problems faced by the profession today as top-level administrators planned and implemented major changes in health care delivery without any input by nurse leaders.

Normative-reeducative strategy is based on the philosophy that humans are driven by a commitment to norms and values.[12] Nurses' primary concern for professional standards and values motivates them to either support or resist change based on the kind of consequence they believe the change will have on standards and values. Reeducation ensures opportunities to gain knowledge about the substance of the change and to formulate new values and attitudes. Normative-reeducative strategy is the most appropriate for nursing because it is the most likely to advance the profession. It is the strategy employed throughout nursing today to incorporate the latest informatics technology into everyday practice.

BASIS OF CHANGE IN NURSING

Forces internal and external to nursing form the basis for change that influences nursing practice. The need for changes is dictated internally as patient acuity levels, treatment modalities, and the use of technologies increase. Externally, social and economic factors exert ongoing influence on how nursing is practiced. From systems theory it is understood to be the ongoing interaction between internal and external forces that influence all segments of the open system, and thus the practice of nursing in organizations. The rate and intensity of significant changes that have occurred in the past three and a half decades remove the early 21st century from the mid-20th century as much as all others are removed from those that preceded them. We have arrived at a new century and are immersed in a kind of change turbulence that continues to be almost perpetual.

External Forces

Godfrey reports that unprecedented changes in health care occurred during the last two decades of the 20th century, when 828 U.S. hospitals closed.[13] Today, similar downsizing continues. Nursing is affected when patient care units with very high occupancy rates close because of overall organizational considerations. Staffing nursing units emerged as a serious problem caused by the drastic changes. As the century drew to a close, nursing departments faced unprecedented challenges to place nurses in other available positions and to help the displaced nurses work through their understandable anger and sense of betrayal.[14] With the shift of nursing positions out of hospitals, enrollment in schools of nursing dropped more than would have been the case from fluctuating population alone. The pool of available new graduates has shrunk, leaving the profession with a serious shortage. The problem developed when professional concerns for quality care were not represented during the planning for changes that directly affect the practice of nursing. Nurse leaders are engaged in efforts to curb the problem through dialogue with legislators to keep them informed of potential negative consequences to the country's health care. Health care organizations are in competition with each other for available nurses, and nurse administrators find themselves looking out of the country for nurses to staff their agencies.

Advances in computer technology continue to have an endless potential for continuing to generate change. Continual spiraling health care costs and shrinking resources prompted vigorous efforts to conserve in all departments of organizations. Nursing represents the largest group of health care providers, and therefore a sizable percentage of health care costs. There is a sense of powerlessness relative to political and international issues that influence our way of life. All of these changes have had long-lasting effects on nursing departments as well as on overall health care agencies.

Internal Forces

The utilization of technicians for patient care activities as a cost-cutting effort has been met with resistance by professional nurses. History shows that cost considerations without quality concerns frequently produce negative results. Nursing experienced an era following World War II when technically prepared caregivers (that is, nurse aides) performed many tasks but were unprepared to interpret patient responses to the care they had received. Because of the concern for quality at the bedside, nurse aides were retrained for nondirect care activities, such as looking after supplies and ordering equipment and materials. Consider that technicians were removed from direct patient care activities at a

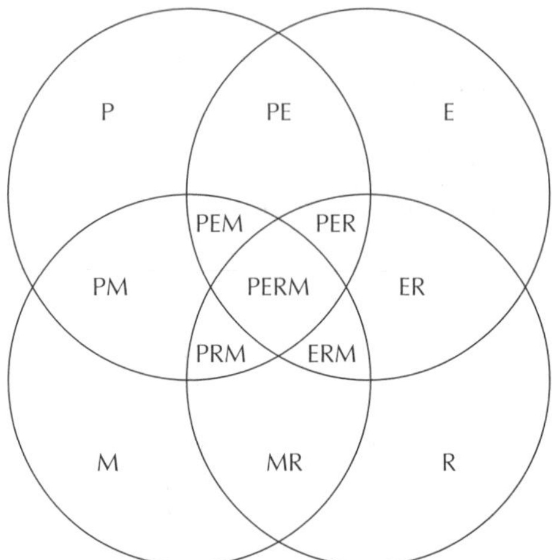

The four overlapping rings create 13 chambers:
—4 chambers with a single letter signify independent responsibilities.
—4 chambers with 2 letters each signify shared responsibilities between 2 individuals.
—4 chambers are created by the overlap of 3 rings and signify shared responsibilities among 3 individuals.
—1 chamber is created in the center and is formed by all 4 rings. It signifies responsibilities shared among all.

FIGURE 13-1. The PERM complex depicts the interaction among nurses in the four major functional roles.

time when acuity level was not as high as today and treatment modalities had fewer and less severe side effects. Through the efforts of professional nurse leaders, baccalaureate preparation was recommended as an entry level into nursing, and this practice is becoming a reality in many parts of the country. This standard is worthy of guarding and preserving. Where professional practice values are threatened, the essential task of nursing is an ongoing clarification and interpretation of professional care as cost effective. Research has demonstrated the cost effectiveness of professional care, and nurses who make use of research findings will more effectively convey the message to others.

History has shown that changes in nursing practice that are initiated and implemented by nonprofessional groups fail to represent professional norms and values. Nurses are socialized in a unique way during their education and experience in practice and are therefore prepared like no other group to monitor nursing practice. A major source of strength within nursing can be found in the collaborative efforts of nurses in the four functional roles—practitioners, educators, researchers, and managers. Together they can exert significant influence in maintaining professional practice. The four roles make up the acronym PERM. Figure 13-1 illustrates the interactional, as well as the

TABLE 13-1. The PERM Complex—Independent (I) and Shared (S) Responsibilities.

Practitioner	
I	Accurately defines changing conditions of practice.
S	Collaborates with nurse researchers in conducting studies that relate to change. Collaborates with nurse educators in providing a practice setting that supports change. Works closely with managers in identifying change ideas and supports change efforts.
Educator	
I	Prepares students for the realities of changing nursing care needs.
S	Strengthens change-agent skills in students by requiring increasingly complex use or nursing research in practice. Communicates frequently with the nursing staff about student "change" assignments. Obtains management approval for student activities that relate to change.
Researcher	
I	Conducts research studies or serves as a resource person to educators, managers, and practitioners who carry out research that relates to change.
S	Uses input from practitioners relative to changing conditions in practice and incorporates practitioners as participants in studies. Assists in the design and delivery of the research component of the curriculum. Designs research activities to conform to organizational policies and resources.
Manager	
I	Remains abreast of issues surrounding nursing care that indicate a need for change. Articulates clear expectations that non-optional changes must be supported by all personnel in the nursing department.
S	Authorizes and supports research that relates to change. Responds in a timely way to practitioners' concerns about nursing care conditions. Supports the work of joint committees of service and education representatives to explore issues of common concern relative to changing nursing care needs.

independent, nature of the work that each contributes to nursing. Table 13-1 describes the independent and the shared responsibilities of nurses in each of the roles.

Collectively, nurses have rich resources to bring to bear on time-related caregiving problems and issues. Patterns of patient care delivery undergo alterations through efforts of creative nurses to meet situational needs at various times. For example, nurses in a given hospital might handle problems associated with "float pools" in critical care or emergency units through "self-staffing"—a system that ensures caregivers are familiar with patient populations in high-acuity settings. By demonstrating a commitment to change and excellence in practice, they not only ensure quality in patient care, but also improve satisfaction, morale, autonomy, and flexibility among their staff.[15]

Regardless of the demands for change dictated from within or without, professional standards provide the stabilizing force for preserving quality and values in a volatile environment. When standards are used, what nursing is does not change, only how it is operationalized based on situational factors.

THE CHANGE PROCESS

Change occurs as a process and can be analyzed, studied, understood, and, to some extent, controlled. Lutjens says that planned change provides a way to induce structural innovations designed to make operational adjustments to meet situational demands.[16] Planned change, designed to keep the nursing department as a vital influence in the organization, is presented as the ideal form of change in this chapter. Planned change:

- Is based on empirical evidence of a need.
- Aims at improving a system of operation.
- Involves others in decisions.
- Provides time for the reeducation of those affected by the change.

The effects of change are on a continuum of minor to major, predictable to unpredictable, and positive to negative. Daloz, cited in Brookfield, refers to change as a fusion of the old and the new rather than a total abandonment.[17] Kegan, cited in Brookfield, describes change as a process of resolving old dichotomies by integrating the new with the old.[18] In fact, the success of a change effort partially depends on maintaining connections with what is valued. Usually some degree of conflict is associated with significant change. Risk and opportunity are presented simultaneously. There is a loss of the familiar and a venture into uncertainty, which is sometimes viewed as a new beginning. **Risk taking** and vision are two highly desirable qualities of participants in the change process.

What gets changed and how the change is accomplished are two major points to consider when discussing the change process. An example of a problem that came out of the turbulent times in health care during the last decade is the loss of autonomy in nursing.[19] Autonomy is a characteristic of a profession, and today nursing is fighting for greater recognition in determining the future of the profession. If business corporations continue to determine how and where nurses practice without considering input from nurses, the problems in health care delivery will compound. Ideally, what needs changing is based on careful analysis and diagnosis of existing practices with a view to future needs, and professional nurses are best equipped to provide valid data for such an analysis. If time permits, a thorough analysis to find the fundamental problem pays off in the form of finding a solution rather than treating symptoms of the problem. Symptoms are more obvious, taking the form of absenteeism, high turnover, and poor morale, while the fundamental problem might be felt as incompetency because of unfamiliar expectations. The solution for the previous problem is appropriate inservice programs, but efforts might be made in the direction of improving salaries to keep the staff happy and on the job. However, focusing on salaries is counterproductive

Problem Identification

The impetus for change has its root in some perceived conflict, which can take a variety of forms, such as not enough of something, too much of something, a practice that should be and is not, or a practice that is and should not be. It is important that whatever the perceived need, the thought process must be accompanied by a strong feeling that a change must occur. A well-thought-out problem is not sufficient for action. What is not felt, and what is not seen as improvement, will certainly produce resistance. Individuals view situations differently. What constitutes a conflict for some is not a conflict for others. These different responses can cause conflicts regarding the change itself and thereby create resistance to change efforts. It is predictable that there will be both support and resistance from individuals relative to the same event. An important part of problem identification is to envision alternatives (i.e., consider a variety of alternatives to the current practice or state of affairs). Be prepared to clarify and interpret how each alternative could improve the situation. Be realistic in acknowledging how each might produce some negative consequences, and be certain that they are only minor. Be convinced that at least one alternative is feasible and within the available resources.

Gaining Support for Change

Gaining support for change cannot be left to chance. The leadership behavior of selling is an important strategy to use when resistance threatens progress in making a needed change. Selling is done by sharing with the group all known information surrounding the changing situation so that the decision to proceed becomes a shared decision. A proposed change might be presented as a new beginning. Gaining allies early on is important if time and resources are to be used to the best advantage. Some allies might come forth from the beginning, while others have to be won. One category of potential allies consists of individuals who initially oppose your efforts, but who are open and honest about it. Such individuals are trustworthy, will listen to clarifications, and are likely to modify their positions. Other potential allies are those who are "on the fence" and who can also be characterized as honest and trustworthy when it comes to what benefits the group. Knowing the difference between true adversaries, whose agendas lie outside the overall good of the group, and potential allies is time saving. Time is wasted on trying to win support from individuals whose self-interest outweighs group interests. Beckhard and Harris recommend a technique whereby the whole group participates in problem diagnosis.[20] What is desired is stated explicitly, followed by creation of a picture of the wished-for condition. Individuals independently make "wish lists" that, if granted, would improve their work satisfaction. A group effort is more likely to result in cooperative change efforts. An example of a situation that affects staff nurses might be something like the following: A proposal has been made by nursing administration to expand the medicine room on their unit by taking space from the nurses' conference room. Sharing documented evidence that more space is needed for safe preparation of medications addresses a standard and is a convincing argument acknowledged by the nurses. The number of medication errors occurring during times of congestion in the medicine room cannot be ignored. However, space reallocation is only one possible solution to the problem.

How Changes Are Made

Administrators can use the information from the previous example about medicine errors to mandate space reallocation without giving consideration to any other possible solution. Perhaps they see their responsibility as being swift intervention. Another intervention could be to request input from the staff for other viable alternative actions, thus providing an opportunity for their active participation in arriving at the best solution. Perhaps enlarging the medicine room is not the only way to relieve congestion during medication preparation. The nurses' conference room is used for change-of-shift reports, patient care conferences, staff development programs, and periodically for social events. Reducing the size of the conference room will definitely affect the quality of the activities that take place there.

Planned Change

An alternative plan devised by staff nurses on the unit describes how better use of space in the medicine room and spreading times for medication administration could possibly reduce congestion and thus the incidence of medication errors. All stock supplies of materials used in the medicine room could be moved to a general storage area. A nurse assistant could be assigned to restock supplies according to a schedule so that the movement of the stock does not become an inconvenience or a waste of nursing hours. Schedules for standing medications could be spread out as follows:

- TID at 8 A.M., 4 P.M., and 12 midnight.
- BID at 10 A.M. and 10 P.M.
- Daily at 12 noon.

A downside of a spread-out medication schedule is that patients receiving TID, BID, and daily medications would be disturbed more frequently. The plus side of the plan is in retaining the use of the conference room for practices valued by the staff, and avoiding the expense of tearing down and reconstructing a wall. By inviting staff input, administration has two plans to consider before making a final decision.

Using the staff to generate ideas for alternative plans and then weighing all viable options that address quality standards makes the outcome a group decision. Such a move recognizes everyone who is likely to be affected by the change and addresses the need for competent professionals to be given a greater share of responsibility for the work to be done on the unit.

The example illustrates a change in which time is given to consider alternative actions and one in which input from the group is likely to produce support for the change. It is an example of planned change.

Radical Intervention

Sometimes the need for change is sudden and calls for some **radical change**. Radical intervention is an autocratic method of making changes. Sudden, drastic changes are made, usually by an individual or a select few, without any input from others. Such change can have both positive and negative consequences. When used routinely as a show of force through misuse of power, thinking, competent, professional people simply move on to other employment, while passive people who relish a dependent role support the behavior. Eventually the loss of creative group members leads to diminished-quality decision making and performance and a rigid adherence to the status quo.

Legitimate radical intervention, however, is a way to ward off or to manage a crisis. A situation can call for split-second decision making where delay would only compound or create a problem. The time required for planned change is not available during crisis situations. When it is necessary to employ radical intervention, the leadership behavior of selling is again the key to gaining support from the group. This should be done as soon as possible after the decision has been made. When rationale for the sudden action is explained to a competent group, their thinking is changed and the decision retrospectively becomes theirs, also. Sharing all relevant information surrounding the situation is usually adequate to gain support. Legitimate use of radical action considers others and strives to make them participants in decisions.

When radical action is used as a show of force, *telling* is the leadership behavior used. There is no opportunity for group members to gain the broad perspective of the situation that is needed for them to show support. Telling usually causes the loss of trust and confidence in the decision maker in future situations.

Change through Nonintervention

Nonintervention is another way in which change can come about. It can be deliberate, or it can be a form of neglect. Deliberate nonintervention is a form of planned change, whereas neglecting to intervene when intervention is warranted makes people passive recipients and sometimes victims of change.

Nonintervention as a deliberate strategy is employed to eliminate some out-of-date practice or category of worker. The unnecessary role or practice is allowed to die a natural death through attrition or depletion of materials. In some settings, not filling vacancies in the nurse aide category was the way of eliminating them as direct caregivers.

Nonintervention as a form of neglect opens the door for non-nurse groups to intervene in nursing practice issues. Although nursing was not negligent in predicting the need for baccalaureate preparation for entry into practice, forces internal to nursing caused delay in implementing the associated plan to redefine the status of workers in nursing. The move toward registered care technicians trained by non-nurse groups resulted from the long delay.

An Example of Differing Adaptations to Change

Spencer Johnson's[21] book, *Who Moved My Cheese?*, tells a story of how different individuals adapt to change. The book is a best-seller used by managers in numerous companies, large and small, to foster positive attitudes toward change in their employees. The characters in the story—two mice and two very small men the size of mice—represent different personality types and their responses as they encounter change. The mice use their instinct, as well as trial and error, to adapt to the change (moved cheese), and the two men use their ability to think and learn from past experiences in their search for the moved cheese. The lessons learned from their differing approaches in adapting to change are:

- Change happens.
- It should be anticipated and monitored.
- Early adaptation to change fosters growth.
- It can be enjoyed.
- It will occur again and again.

STAGES OF CHANGE

Once a decision has been reached to implement a change, time must be allowed for the sequence of stages designed to reduce resistance and maintain support from others. Three familiar stages in implementing change are:

1. Unfreezing.
2. Moving.
3. Refreezing.

Unfreezing

During **unfreezing**, letting go of established and familiar practices takes place. Adequate time is needed for the gradual introduction of new ideas, along with information that can serve as positive motivation for those who are going to be affected by the change. Information should include reasons why a change is needed and how the organization and individuals will benefit from it. Projecting a realistic time frame for the change to take place, giving explanations of how workers will be affected throughout the process, and being honest about temporary inconveniences to them can give workers some sense of control. Greater control can be provided by encouraging group input through a formal feedback mechanism. Objectivity of feedback review and the action taken can be ensured through representation from the group on a review committee. It also serves as testimony of flexibility in the change plan.

Commending valuable ideas submitted by the staff early on encourages wider constructive participation in feedback. Acknowledging discomfort that comes from uncertainty about a new system preserves everyone's dignity. Assurance of adequate reeducation opportunities can enable individuals to deal with their emotions over the proposed change.

Unfreezing is essentially a preparation for instituting activities to facilitate the change. During this stage, change agents have the greatest opportunity to gain allies from the staff.

Bassett says the most important element in the change process is belief in and commitment to its success.[22] Even with the best efforts to do everything right, defensive responses to being told that a system is inefficient, unnecessary, too costly, or ineffective are likely to occur. Change agents must be prepared to deal with defensiveness. All interactive processes of leadership—communication, group dynamics, decision making, and conflict management—assist change agents in overcoming obstacles to organizational change. Equally important is using systems theory and the effect of interactive parts, effective management techniques, delegation, motivation, and performance standards. At an appropriate time, a target date to begin activities of the second stage should be set to prevent nonconstructive delays. It is understood, however, that unfreezing strategies will continue to be in effect if new information surfaces that indicates a need to continue with the first stage.

Moving

The second stage of the change process is **moving**, characterized by a cognitive redefinition of how group goals can be met based on new understanding. The primary activity during moving is reeducation. Determining the specific programs needed, and for whom, gives definition to what might otherwise seem like a time vacuum when the old is gone and the new is not in place. Knowing exactly what is expected during this transitional stage and how it contributes to the new system reduces the insecurity that accompanies uncertainty. Beckhard and Harris caution that the transitional stage of change requires its own structure and strategies.[23] Ideally, the second stage does not begin until a roadmap checklist is complete.[24] The checklist implies that there is supporting evidence that the proposed change is purposeful, specific, integrated, time sequenced, adaptable, cost-effective, and has approval. The transition stage is a pilot of the larger plan and has its own temporary management structure so that there is not interference with established day-to-day operations.

Participants in the pilot project must be adequately informed as to its purpose and reeducated to be able to function proficiently. They should share the perception that the change will potentially be an improvement over current practices. A report of the pilot project should provide information on ways to avoid problems during implementation of the larger plan.

Refreezing

The third stage of the change process is **refreezing.** It occurs when there is consistent evidence that the new practice is stabilized, integrated, and internalized by the staff. Ongoing monitoring for continued quality must follow refreezing, since it provides valuable information about the ongoing effectiveness of the change. The process is only as good as its users, and follow-up findings allow for analysis to replicate success and correct errors for the future. Keeping a written record of follow-up findings on file is helpful in remembering details. More information about follow-up is discussed later under the heading of "Evaluating Change."

Knowing the ideal about the change process enables all staff to participate constructively in change efforts, either by making known their dissatisfaction through statements of their expectations or by giving their support and allegiance to change agents. Changes will continue to occur more rapidly and with higher intensity with time. Therefore, understanding change is important if nurses are to remain in control of nursing.

CHANGE AGENTS

Characteristics of Change Agents

The characteristics and qualities of change agents include experience, success, being respected, leadership skills, and management competencies. Pritchett and Pound advise that individuals who have a positive attitude about work and seize opportunities to get involved in new directions are themselves change agents.[25] They are willing to spend their time correcting problems, and they deliberately choose to be positive, optimistic, and enthusiastic. Attitude is something that is under the control of the individual, and developing a positive attitude can be fostered by anyone. Supporting more experienced change agents benefits the individual, possibly even more than the organization.

Responsibilities of Change Agents

The change agent's first responsibility is to develop a plan for action. The plan includes:

- A description of, and rationale for, the change.
- Objectives expressed in measurable terms.
- A projected timetable for each stage of implementation, leaving sufficient flexibility to accommodate new information.

Having a set deadline is a safeguard against procrastination, which can seriously compromise change efforts.

The change agent needs a keen sense of the ethical and legal elements associated with significant changes. Many people become vulnerable during change, and their rights and dignity can be unnecessarily compromised when there is insensitivity to ethical and legal factors. For example, a temporary decline in effective performance is predictable during vulnerable periods. It is therefore important that adequate time be given for personnel to assimilate all that a change incurs. Change agents must be aware of the decline in effectiveness in the early stages of change to avoid the possibility of mismanagement. He or she must know when, where, and how to intervene throughout the process.

Strategies for Change Agents

Beckhard and Harris list action strategies for change agents.[26] They are:

- Defining how much choice there is about whether to change.
- Delivering a clear message that change action is an essential, not optional, part of work.
- Developing a system of control and information flow.
- Establishing a mechanism to monitor progress.
- Planning for long-range evaluation.

Relative to developing a system of control and information flow, the temporary management structure described on page 265 under "Moving" should be established for the change plan. The regular structure in use for stable practices blurs the differences between the new and the old. Separating management of stable and changing practices permits a clearer definition of change effects. Finally, the change agent is responsible for determining the readiness for beginning the pilot project, implementing the larger plan, and determining stage progression.

Responsibilities of change agents are many and important. Selecting the best person available is an important decision. Success of a change plan is enhanced by effective change agents and informed group members who are open to new ideas and willing to take risks.

RESPONSE TO CHANGE

In field theory, described by Lewin, there are two opposing forces: driving forces and restraining forces.[27] Driving forces generate planned change, and restraining forces generate resistance to change. Planning change can be more successful when the effects of

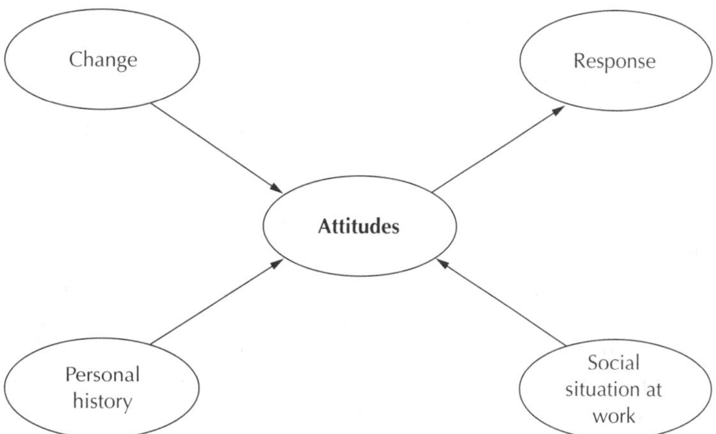

FIGURE 13-2. Formulation of attitudes toward change in work settings. Response is determined by attitude.

restraining forces are explored and managed. Force-field analysis is a technique used to determine the two opposing forces.

In this section, resistance to change and a drive toward change are explored. With an understanding of the dynamics that create both, resistance can be reduced and drive can be increased. Individuals are dynamic, growing, social beings. At any given moment, the risks involved in change can serve as a driving force, an opposing force, or even as both simultaneously. Thoughts and feelings about change and risk become modified over time with maturity and experience. Bassett says that resistance to change lies in human attitudes.[28] Lewin, the founder of the group dynamics movement in the 1930s, created the X chart to show the relationship of attitudes and response to change (see Figure 13-2).[29] Attitudes toward change are formed by a combination of the change itself, the personal history of individuals who will be affected by the change, and the social situation at work.

Resistance to Change

Being shown a better way to do things implies that current performance is not acceptable, resulting in embarrassment and insecurity. It is definitely not a good idea for a young nurse manager (e.g., in nursing for 8 years) to tell a 20-year-veteran nurse how to provide quality care. Experience is a very important qualification of change agents. Another scenario to consider is if a proposed change is a time-saving practice, what will the staff do during the saved time? Will they be given added responsibilities without additional salary? Attention must also be given to curbing rumors and speculation. When concerns such as the previous ones are apparent, the staff can be asked to list important things they would like to do but do not have the time for under the current way of doing things. Maybe there are:

- Activities they would enjoy but do not have time for.
- Developmental activities that would improve their personal potential.
- Quality problems that could be solved.

- Questions about how money released because of a better way of doing things could be used.
- Questions about what stress would be reduced because of less pressure.

This exercise could convince the staff that the change is designed to improve mission attainment and not to add to their work or reduce the staff size. The exercise is designed to reduce resistance.

When attempting to reduce resistance to change, nurses can be asked to reflect on where they learned the things they do and why they are done in just that way. Do they ever question them or consider a different routine? There is danger in allowing actions to become too routine, since they are then done out of habit rather than done thoughtfully. Frequently, a few simple questions about current practices can stir enthusiasm within the group to work toward making their practices flexible enough to fit the unique demands of a situation. Bassett presents a credo to encourage participation in change:[30]

- If you think you can't, you won't.
- If you think you can, there is a good chance you will.
- Making the effort is exhilarating.
- Reputations are made by searching for things that can't be done, and doing them.
- Aim low—boring. Aim high—soaring.

The most important element to reduce resistance is establishing trust by giving explanations, requesting input, acknowledging concerns, making changes in small doses, offering to assist, explaining benefits, and acknowledging success. Conversely, ingredients for resistance are listed as mystery, secrecy, change as punishment, pressure to speed up work, poor planning, and ignoring human nature.[31] Davis defines three types of resistance: logical–rational, psychologic–emotional, and sociologic.[32] Logical–rational objections include the time it takes to adjust, extra effort, the possibility of less-desirable outcomes, cost, and questionable feasibility. All of these points have merit, and it is wise to exercise patience with logical objectors: Show them how a delay in making truly needed changes would be destructive to the organization and that workers do help. Psychological–emotional objections include fear of the unknown, low tolerance for change, dislike of the change agent, lack of trust, and the high need for security.

Non–risk takers hold tenaciously to their objections. Diluting resistors among more adventurous peers might help them grow and overcome some of their fears. Sociologic objections include parochial and narrow views, vested interests, a wish to retain existing relationships, opposing group values, and political coalitions. Individuals who hold too strongly to self-interests at the expense of group goals need reminders of their employment responsibilities.

Some resistance will linger regardless of the correct approaches and the best efforts of competent change agents. Human behavior and interaction is far too complex to be able to gain total support for a change. Continuing to work hard toward increasing group support is productive in reducing resistance, since in the long run the strength of group influence is the most promising force in modifying resistors' behavior.

EVALUATING CHANGE

How is it known that change efforts are worthwhile, whether a change works, how much outcome is caused by chance, or whether a new practice will be maintained? How is change monitored? These are commonly asked questions. Answers can only be found during the evaluation stage of the change process. When evaluation is given low priority, the answers will be vague, subjective, or lacking altogether. When expectations are clear that evaluation is critical for effective operation, efforts are not relaxed once the change has been put into effect.

The way to arrive at answers is through the design of planned, systematic data gathering and analysis that yields the necessary information. The plan for evaluation is continuous with the overall change design, with outcomes being measured against the criteria found in statements of purpose and objectives for change. Implementation of the evaluation plan is carried out by everyone involved in the change process.

The responsibilities of each group member must be spelled out clearly, and individuals should be held accountable for their performance in this area as for any other expected behavior. Information must be explicit as to who is to receive data, on what dates, and by what collection method. It must be reinforced that completing reports is part of one's real work, not something added on to work. In other words, submitting reports is not optional. The timing of reports is important, especially when longitudinal evaluation is done. Longitudinal design requires serial collection of data at specified times to determine the effects that time, as a variable, has on outcomes. Growth grids are an example of a longitudinal design. If measurement is missed at any point, a void exists in information about the individual's progress relative to the variable time.

The method of data analysis determines whether or not the analysis will indicate how many change outcomes are due to chance. The wrong method of analysis will not provide the information, while correct methods will. Courses in statistics and research methods are requirements in nursing curricula today and orient beginning practitioners to the need for precision in determining cause-and-effect relationships. They are essential for professional monitoring of practice, in the case of change, to know whether efforts are worthwhile and cost-effective.

Stability of change is the ultimate goal. Only through systematic evaluation is the degree of stability known. Accurate information from evaluation reports permits the correction of neglect and inconsistencies. Problems are pinpointed early, and corrective action can be applied with precision. Change is costly, and justification of the cost can be found in well-documented evaluation reports. Change is incomplete without evaluation.

CASE STUDY

Planned Change Backfires

As patient acuity levels rose, nurses in a pediatric hospital looked for ways to reduce non-nurse activities. One area that was earmarked was the playroom. A play department was formed and staffed by trained workers, and a director was hired to oversee the functions and performance of the new group of workers. Meeting the play needs of hospitalized children was defined as their responsibility. Unfortunately, no distinction was made between "social play" and "therapeutic play." The latter is designed to assist children in coping with painful and, what is to them, frightening experiences that occur during the course of their treatment. The description of workers' jobs in the play department included having responsibility for the playroom, play materials, and play activities. As time went on, efforts by nurses to incorporate therapeutic play into their patients' care was viewed as interference in the domain of the play department. On one occasion, a staff nurse who was caring for a long-term 3-year-old boy requested some materials from the playroom to use for the patient's care. The response from the director of the playroom was that all play needs would be taken care of by workers in her department. The nurse explained that the patient had experienced several painful and frightening experiences and was finally showing signs of readiness to work through his feelings. The time was right for the nurse to help him gain mastery over what had happened to him by actively engaging in reenacting what had happened to him as a passive recipient. The nurse was told by the director of the playroom that using "hospital equipment for play" was scheduled for the next day at 1:00 P.M. None of the nurse's efforts were met with any success. She decided to improvise with what she had on hand and proceeded with her plan of care for her patient. A major conflict ensued when the director of the playroom discovered what the nurse had done.

- In this situation, what is at stake for patient care?
- What is at stake for play department workers?
- What was missed in the change plan?

CASE STUDY

Transition from Student to Graduate Nurse

Gretchen Hoff began her first position in nursing shortly after graduating from X University School of Nursing. She did well in school, is enthusiastic, and is hoping that she fits in on the unit she has been assigned to. The topic "Transition from Student to Graduate Nurse" is on the orientation schedule for new graduates. She had never given any thought to possible differences from the ideal world presented in school and the real world of practice. There did not seem to be any need to because she had never encountered any problems relative to patient care during her clinical experiences. She overheard a discussion about quality of care issues and that how care delivered in practice does not quite measure up to the standards she learned in school. The information is unsettling to her, and she becomes anxious about how she will be able to handle quality issues if she encounters them. For the first time, she will not have an instructor or assigned preceptor to guide her and to share responsibility for the outcomes of a conflict situation. She decides she is being overly anxious about a bridge that probably does not exist. Gretchen is about to embark on her first experience with change.

- What will be her best course of action when she does face a quality issue?
- How can she prevent being alienated from the group and still make her point about professional standards?

CASE STUDY

Parking Lot

Kathleen O'Toole, a nurse in her first year of practice, was surprised one day when she arrived, as usual, at the hospital parking lot. There was a sign at the entrance indicating that the lot would be reserved for administrators and physicians only, beginning on the first of the next month, three weeks away. A parking attendant handed her a form describing more detailed information about the change, including the lot that would be designated for staff nurses. After reviewing this information, she realized that the parking lot the nurses would have to use was located several long blocks from the hospital. The hospital's plan included a shuttle service that would transport nurses from the lot to the hospital and back again when the work period ended. Parking had been free; however, there would now be a small fee charged to cover the cost of the outside shuttle company service.

Kathleen and the other nurses were understandably upset over the change. They felt that they should have some input into a solution about the parking problems the hospital was experiencing. A major concern of theirs was the safety issue of young women waiting alone in their cars for the shuttle bus to arrive. One point that stood out in their minds was that the nursing group is the largest in the hospital, and that they are essentially the "heartbeat" of the organization.

A decision was made to organize a coalition of nurses to oppose the change and to negotiate an alternative plan to solving the ongoing parking shortage. Their focus was an approach that will be fair to nurses.

- Using the content of this chapter, prepare a written statement about the nurses' concerns that is effectively assertive. Note that the statement will be sent to top administration.

SUMMARY

In this chapter, change is described as an ongoing, societal phenomenon that can be controlled to varying degrees. Internal and external forces in the form of conflict bring about changes in nursing. Unmet professional standards generate internal nursing changes, while external forces tend to generate changes designed to solve economic problems. Planned change designed by nurses is presented as the most promising for maintaining vitality within nursing departments. Examples are given of changes that foster improved quality nursing care and those that threaten quality nursing care. Determining what should be changed depends on an analysis of the situations and predictions of decision outcomes. Only needed changes are worth the time and expense entailed in the long process. Change agents must have certain characteristics to be effective. The change plan must reduce resistance and foster support. Finally, the importance of evaluating change is stressed. The study of change is important for entry into professional practice. The reader is reminded that managing change is one aspect of a broader management system and not a discrete, isolated activity. Determining need and designing, implementing, and evaluating changes in nursing requires a collaborative effort of nurses in all categories of the PERM complex.

LEARNER EXERCISES

In 1988, the American Medical Association (AMA) proposed a new category of care workers, registered care technicians (RTCs), to alleviate the problems associated with the nurse shortage. Two years later, on June 25, 1990, the AMA House of Delegates abandoned its plan to implement pilot sites for the training of RTCs. Opposition to the RTC came from the American Nurses Association (ANA) because the duties proposed for the RTC overlapped with roles that should be performed by RNs. With the demise of the RTC proposal, the ANA resolved to work collaboratively with the AMA and other health care groups to address patient care concerns associated with nurse shortages in acute care settings.

Two issues emanate from the described situation: (1) the AMA proposal was presented because the failure of nursing to devise a workable solution to the nursing shortage, and (2) the ANA reaction demonstrates the strength of nurses' influence in monitoring standards of professional practice. Answer the following questions about the above situation:

1. Do you agree or disagree with the two issue statements? Explain your response.
2. What could have reversed the situation?
3. What are the implications for nursing practitioners, educators, researchers, and managers?
4. In your opinion, where in the PERM complex does action for effective change begin?
5. In your opinion, how effective is collaboration among nurses in the PERM complex?

REFERENCES

1. Brookfield, S. (1987). *Developing critical thinkers*. San Francisco: Jossey-Bass, p. 51.
2. Lutjens, L.R., & Tiffany, C.R. (1994, March). Evaluating planned change theories. *Nursing Management*, 25(3), 54–57.

3. Koerner, J.G., Bunkers, S.S., & Nelson, J.N. (1991). Change: A professional challenge. *Nursing Administration Quarterly*, *16*(1), 15–21.
4. Menix, K.D. (2001). Educating to manage the accelerated change environment effectively: Part 2, *Journal for Nurses in Staff Development*, *17*(1), 44–53.
5. Jost, S.H. (2000). An assessment and intervention strategy for managing staff nurse needs during change. *Journal of Nursing Administration*, *30*(1), 34–40.
6. Lewis, D. (2000). Reflections in nursing leadership. *Sigma Theta Tau International Honor Society of Nursing, Fourth Quarter*, 24–26.
7. Tiffany, C.R., Cheatham, A.B., Doornbos, D., Loudermelt, L., & Momadi, G.G. (1994, July). Planned change theory: Survey of nursing periodical literature. *Nursing Management*, *25*(7), 54–59.
8. Tiffany, C.R. (1994, February). Analysis of planned change. *Nursing Management*, *25*(2), 60–62.
9. Hageman, Z.T., & Tiffany, C.R. (1994, April). Evaluation of two planned change theories. *Nursing Management*, *25*(4), 57–62.
10. Hageman, Z.T., & Tiffany, C.R. (1994, April). Evaluation of two planned change theories. *Nursing Management*, *25*(4), 57–62.
11. Hageman, Z.T., & Tiffany, C.R. (1994, April). Evaluation of two planned change theories. *Nursing Management*, *25*(4), 57–62.
12. Hageman, Z.T., & Tiffany, C.R. (1994, April). Evaluation of two planned change theories. *Nursing Management*, *25*(4), 57–62.
13. Godfrey, C. (1994, October). Downsizing: Coping with personal pain. *Nursing Management*, *25*(10), 90–93.
14. Godfrey, C. (1994, October). Downsizing: Coping with personal pain. *Nursing Management*, *25*(10), 90–93.
15. Hausfeld, J., Gibbons, K., Holtmeier, A., Knight, M., Schulte, C., Stadtmiller, T., & Yeary, K. (1994, October). Self-staffing: Improving care and staff satisfaction. *Nursing Management*, *25*(10), 74–80.
16. Lutjens, L.R., & Tiffany, C.R. (1994, March). Evaluating planned change theories. *Nursing Management*, *25*(3), 54–57.
17. Brookfield, S. (1987). *Developing critical thinkers*. San Francisco: Jossey-Bass, p. 225.
18. Brookfield, S. (1987). *Developing critical thinkers*. San Francisco: Jossey-Bass, p. 226.
19. Anders, J.E. (1999). Doing More with Less. *American Journal of Nursing*, *99*(9), 24.
20. Beckhard, R., & Harris, R. (1977). *Organizational transitions: Managing complex change*. Reading, MA: Addison-Wesley, p. 26.
21. Johnson, S. (1998). *Who moved my cheese?* New York: G.S. Putnam's Sons, pp. 46–69.
22. Bassett, L., & Metzger, N. (1986). *Achieving excellence: A prescription for health care managers*, Rockville, MD: Aspen, p. 94.
23. Beckhard, R., & Harris, R. (1977). *Organizational transitions: Managing complex change*. Reading, MA: Addison-Wesley, p. 27.
24. Beckhard, R., & Harris, R. (1977). *Organizational transitions: Managing complex change*. Reading, MA: Addison-Wesley, p. 57.
25. Pritchett, P., & Pound, R. (1990). *The employee handbook for organizational change*. Dallas: Pritchett & Associates, p. 30.
26. Beckhard, R., & Harris, R. (1977). *Organizational transitions: Managing complex change*. Reading, MA: Addison-Wesley, p. 36.
27. England, D. (1986). *Collaboration in nursing*. Rockville, MD: Aspen, p. 213.
28. Bassett, L., & Metzger, N. (1986). *Achieving excellence: A prescription for health care managers*. Rockville, MD: Aspen, p. 104.

29. Davis, K. (1981). *Organizational behavior at work: Organizational behavior.* St. Louis: McGraw-Hill, p. 200.
30. Bassett, L., & Metzger, N. (1986). *Achieving excellence: A prescription for health care managers.* Rockville, MD: Aspen, p. 115.
31. Bassett, L., & Metzger, N. (1986). *Achieving excellence: A prescription for health care managers.* Rockville, MD: Aspen, p. 95.
32. Davis, K. (1981). *Organizational behavior at work: Organizational behavior.* St. Louis: McGraw-Hill, p. 207.

UNIT 4

Managing Resources

14

Managing Resources

The Staff

"The best executive is the one who has sense enough to pick good people to do what has to be done and self-restraint enough to keep from meddling with them while they do it."

Theodore Roosevelt

INTRODUCTION

The combination of continuing constraints on U.S. health care spending and the developing nursing shortage has increased workplace pressures on all nurses, and concern for patient safety is rising.[1] The reduced availability of resources such as personnel and assistive support services, the increasing acuity and age of the patients, expanding roles for registered nurses, and serious economic concerns (both wages and equipment cost) have raised concerns about safe staffing ratios, competency, and regulation.[2] Workplace staffing issues are dominating discussions among nurses, administrators, and government officials. Nursing continues to hold quality patient care as a value, and inadequate staffing poses a threat to this concept.

Today's nurse manager has a major responsibility to know what personnel are doing and where they spend their time. This allows the manager to justify the appropriate staff mix and ensure that nursing and support staff are being used to the greatest advantage. As decentralization of authority and responsibility continue, managers are mandated to allocate available resources. **Resources** are limited commodities that allow the work of the organization to be completed, and no resource is as important as the staff. This chapter will discuss the management of resources with specific attention to the staffing process.

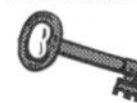

KEY CONCEPTS

Descriptive Methodology is a staffing pattern that results from variables selected by the manager.

Expert Panel Method is the staffing plan that utilizes a variety of experts to examine service- and unit-specific needs related to structure, process, and outcomes, and subsequently suggests an appropriate staffing plan.

Industrial Engineering is a staffing plan that results from techniques used by industry (i.e., time-and-motion studies).

Management Engineering is the staffing plan that results in a staffing index based on usual managerial data.

Productivity is a measure of how efficent labor resources are used in the production of a good or service.

Productivity Index is a measure of nursing hours per patient day.

Resources are commodities in limited quantities that allow the work of the organization to be performed.

Scheduling Pattern represents the actual assignment of personnel by unit or department and time.

Skill Mix refers to the type, number, and ratio of staff necessary to perform the established work; this includes the optimum ratio of professional nurses to licensed or certified support personnel for a particular unit of patient service.

Staff Plan is the actual pattern of staff distribution based on an underlying methodology.

Staffing is a complex process that determines the appropriate number of nursing resources necessary to meet the workload demand for nursing care at the unit or department level.

Workload of nursing is determined through an assessment of the patients' severity, and an estimate of the indirect and unit-based work requirements.

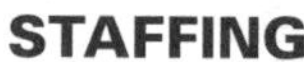

STAFFING

Process and Staffing Plan

Staffing is both a process and an outcome. Staffing may be expressed as the number of staff members required for providing care to a particular number of patients, or it can describe the way in which human resources are used in a particular setting. Staffing decisions require judgments to allocate and juggle personnel between the projects and processes (delivery of patient care) of the organization.[3] This is done by the process of staffing, or the determination of the appropriate number and the mix of nursing resources necessary to meet workload demand for nursing care at the unit or department level (see Figure 14-1).

		Week I							Week II							Week III							Week IV						
Position	**Name**	S	M	T	W	T	F	S	S	M	T	W	T	F	S	S	M	T	W	T	F	S	S	M	T	W	T	F	S
Full time	RN 1				x			x	x					x					x			x	x			x			
Full time	RN 2	x					x					x			x	x					x					x			x
Full time	RN 3			x				x	x				x					x				x	x					x	
Full time	RN 4	x				x					x				x	x				x				x					x
Full time	RN 5				x			x	x					x					x			x	x		x				
Full time	RN 6	x				x				x					x	x					x				x				x
Full time	RN 7		x					x	x				x				x					x	x			x			
Full time	RN 8	x					x					x			x	x				x					x				x
Part time	8 hrs/wk RN 9	On													On	On												On	On
Part time	8 hrs/wk RN 10							On	On													On	On						
Part time	8 hrs/wk RN 11	On													On	On												On	On
Part time	8 hrs/wk RN 12							On	On													On	On						
Total RNs on duty each day		6	7	7	6	6	6	6	6	7	7	6	6	6	6	6	7	7	6	6	6	6	6	7	6	7	8	7	6

Elements:
- Every other weekend off
- Maximum days worked: 4
- Minimum days worked: 2
- Number of split days off each period: 2
- Operates in multiples of 4, 8, 12...
- Schedule repeats itself every 4 weeks
- X: Scheduled day off

FIGURE 14-1. Master time sheet—4 week cycle.

Workload is a function of two elements: the number of patients and a measure of work. Typically, the workload of nursing is determined through the use of a patient classification system, which documents the patient severity and accompanying requirements of care (also called the direct work of nursing), as well as instruments that estimate the indirect and unit-based work requirements.[4] The purpose of using such a system is to be able to predict the correct staffing plan.

Staffing needs do vary from department to department, as well as by institutional differences. The requirements of an outpatient surgical center may vary from the staff requirement of the intensive care unit of a hospital. Today, staffing is a major complex and challenging dilemma to the entire provider community. Staffing problems occur when there is a concentration on cost savings to the detriment of quality patient care.[5] To develop an adequate staff requires taking into account a set of dynamic variables and creating a staffing plan.

The **staffing plan** is the recommended skill mix of individuals needed to provide safe and appropriate nursing care. **Skill mix** refers to the type, number, and ratio of staff necessary to perform the established work or productivity; this includes the optimum ratio of professional nurses to licensed or certified support personnel for a particular unit of patient service. A skill mix ratio may vary from department to department. However, the factors that generally predict a skill mix are as follows:

- Average daily occupancy trends and fluctuations.
- Patient classification data.
- Average length of stay.
- Staff distribution patterns for the type of health care institution.
- Type of health care being delivered.[6]

Workload Measures: Productivity Index

Because of the variety of variables necessary to determine adequate staffing, a practical method to quantify workload is a productivity measure. The emphasis on proper skill mix is aimed at using human resources efficiently, thereby increasing **productivity.** Productivity measures are estimates of how efficient labor resources are used in producing a good or service.[7] There are a variety of measures, but there are also inherent difficulties in estimating the ratio of services required (including the level of personnel required to deliver service) and hours needed to provide service. One such method, a **productivity index**, approximates the ratio of hours of nursing care needed to that which is offered. A nursing productivity measure may be estimated by comparing actual staffing hours with the staffing hours required by the patient classification system.[8] This method provides information about the adequacy of staff available to give care. The competency of the staff in delivering care is not necessarily considered. Other methods will incorporate staff level and competency.

In nursing, the criterion used most frequently is nursing hours per patient day (NHPPD). This value is a productivity standard and reflects what each unit considers a standard of nursing care. For example, the ICU may have a greater NHPPD than a general medical area, based on the acuity system of those units. The higher the acuity classification of the patient, the more nursing is required. To determine the unit specific standard NHPPD, a standard number of hours will be recommended based on the acuity system. For example, an acuity system ranging from 1 (mostly self-care) to 5 (critically ill) will necessitate the corresponding hours of nursing care. For example:

Acuity System

5 requires 20 hours/day of nursing time
4 requires 15
3 requires 10
2 requires 5
1 requires 2

The productivity formula to estimate the nursing staff productivity index is:
Patient days × unit standard = output in work hours
20 patients × 10 days each = 200 patient days
Unit standard = 10 NHPPD
200 × 10 NHPPD = 2,000 work hours (output)

8 RNs for 24 hours for 10 days = 1,920 hours worked (input)

output/input = productivity index
2,000/1,920 = 104%
This means this was a highly productive staff.[9]

Productivity, while important, is one consideration for establishing an optimum staff. Proper staffing plans require consideration of diverse and difficult-to-estimate issues, as well as nontraditional and new staffing patterns (the actual way staff is distributed throughout the organization). The American Nurses Association (ANA) suggests four questions that direct the staffing plan. These questions include:

1. How many patients can one professional nurse properly plan for, supervise, and evaluate in terms of nursing care provided?
2. How many associate nurses can one professional nurse direct, supervise, and evaluate?
3. How many patients will require the direct care of a professional nurse, and how much nursing time is involved in this care?
4. How can the autonomy of nursing practice and acceptance of accountability for results be fostered?[10]

These questions provide the structure for the database upon which the actual plan will be based. The responsibility of nursing administration, as stated by the ANA, is to develop and execute a rational program. The objective of the staffing plan is to ensure that nursing care is safe, responsive to patient needs, and scientifically and technologically sound.

STAFFING METHODOLOGIES

The emphasis on appropriate staff is guided by the development of a staffing plan or methodology. Within each plan, different criteria are involved, which allow different productivity measures to be calculated. Descriptive or consensus methodology, industrial and management engineering, and the expert panel method are various ways to begin the process of determining the correct staff configuration.[11]

Descriptive methodology refers to a staffing pattern that is based on subjective data. This means that the appropriate staffing pattern is recommended on the basis of the manager's experience and intuition. For example, using the average acuity level of patients on a unit, the manager determines that a particular ratio of staff to patient maintains quality of care, based on institutional audits. The information that is gathered to determine the staffing plan is organized around the variables selected by the manager. These variables may vary from department to department within the same institution (see Figure 14-2).

The **industrial engineering** methodology is a technique or group of techniques developed by industry to improve productivity. Typically, these techniques include task analysis, review of work distribution, and measurement of the staff work through work sampling and time-and-motion studies. Work sampling offers the possibility of an ideal staffing pattern and, even more importantly, provides empirical evidence for the establishment of a theoretical basis for staffing procedures. Work sampling combines many of the aforementioned techniques, especially time-and-motion studies. Results of these methods provide information about the time it takes to do specific work.

Nursing departments have used these techniques to develop appropriate staffing plans. The work of the unit is defined in terms of tasks to be accomplished and the level of the employee who is needed to perform the work. The problem with this precise methodology is that the complex nature of professional nursing is not entirely amenable to this type of measurement. Nursing is more than a list of tasks to be performed; rather, it involves use of the nursing process, which is analytic, instrumental, and evaluative. While aspects of this methodology are useful, relying on this exclusively would be too limiting to all that is required of the professional staff.

The **management engineering** methodology optimizes the nursing workload by developing a staffing index model. Using similar techniques of industrial engineering and a variety of other information (quality nursing care; a general description of the type and volume of patients serviced; information about institutional characteristics, such as census, bed capacity, daily visits or admission; and operating budget), a systematic analysis yields a projection for an appropriate and cost-effective staffing pattern. This methodology is as successful as the information that is provided.

This approach, referred to as the expert panel nurse staffing method, can be used to allocate resources and staff.[12] Using this model, a manager is able to examine service- and unit-specific needs related to structure, process, and outcomes. An **expert panel**, composed of nurse leaders within and related to the organization, is appointed by the chief executive nurse, and they examine the separate divisions of the organization. Data (also called minimum unit-based data set) examined by the panel differ by the mission of the organization and unit of care but usually include the patient classification system, tasks, direct and indirect costs to the delivery of care, prospective payment, availability and type of nursing and support staff, and quality-assessment findings. Following analysis of the data, staffing needs are predicted to provide coverage of the unit with calculation of a replacement factor (an estimate of the need for additional staff due to vacation, sickness, or turnover). In addition, staffing requirements are considered which allow existing staff to participate in professional and educational meetings. The outcomes of care are predicted based on increasing or decreasing the staff, and non–unit-based staff (cen-

Example of a Master Staffing Pattern								
33-bed capacity	Su	M	Tu	W	Th	F	Sa	
DAY SHIFT								
RN	4	5	5	6	6	5	4	35
LPN	1	2	2	2	2	2	1	12
AIDE	2	2	3	3	3	3	2	18
TOTAL	7	9	10	11	11	10	7	65
EVENING SHIFT								
RN	4	5	5	5	5	5	4	33
LPN	1	1	1	1	1	1	1	7
AIDE	1	1	1	1	1	1	1	7
TOTAL	6	7	7	7	7	7	6	47
NIGHT SHIFT								
RN	3	4	4	4	4	4	3	26
LPN	0	0	0	0	0	0	0	0
AIDE	1	1	1	1	1	1	1	7
TOTAL	4	5	5	5	5	5	4	33
TOTAL NURSING HRS	136	168	176	184	184	176	136	165.7 (average)
AVERAGE CENSUS	25	30.5	32	32.8	32.8	32	25	29.9 (average)
HOURS OF CARE	5.40	5.50	5.50	5.60	5.60	5.50	5.40	5.54 (average)
AVERAGE ACUITY	2.20	2.30	2.40	2.45	2.45	2.40	2.30	2.37 (average)

FIGURE 14-2. Example of a master staffing pattern.

tral staff consisting of administrators, advanced practice nurses, and staff development and support employees) are projected, which ensure all necessary nursing care is provided throughout the organization. The expert panel, in essence, recommends an ideal, professional support staff for the entire organization.

Nursing administration, with input from the lower-level managers, ultimately has the responsibility to determine which staffing methodology will be used by the department of nursing. Variables such as occupancy rate, salary scales, availability of nurses, organization of the department of nursing (structure of authority, centralized or decentralized), and type of institution influence the subsequent decision about the staffing pattern.

Scheduling Patterns

The number and type of personnel (the skill mix) needed is estimated based on the staffing methodology used. **Scheduling patterns** are proposed based on needed staff per unit. Scheduling patterns may be centralized (a member of nursing administration determines patterns for the entire organization), decentralized (scheduling occurs at the unit level), or self-scheduled (employees choose their own work schedule). Scheduling patterns are overall plans intended to provide the correct configuration of personnel for the work to be done, eliminating understaffing (not enough staff) or overstaffing (too much staff), while accommodating the individual needs of the staff.

Work Schedules

Work schedules are more specific plans by which personnel are assigned in time periods for which the organization provides service. Proper scheduling requires adequate coverage of staff for patients needing care.

Examples of work schedules include:

- **The traditional 40-hour-a-week, 8-hour shift.**
  An effective scheduling plan, this has been used for a long time and provides coverage for the work to be accomplished. Most flexible plans are in some way a deviation from this particular model. Often the manager assigns the full-time staff to the 7-day-a-week and 24-hour-a-day coverage implied by this model. In fact, this pattern of scheduling work has been the impetus for the creative and exciting changes that are occurring in staffing opportunities.

- **The 10-hour shift.**
  In this plan, a full-time employee is able to work a 4-day, 10-hour-a-shift week. This has advantages for personnel in providing a shortened work week. It also gives the added benefit of allowing enough time to ensure that the necessary work is completed for patients. The drawback to this model, besides the longer work day, has been the added expense to the personnel budget. A reduction in personnel has not been realized, and a problem of overlap exists. Fatigue has been cited as a problem for staff that needs further study. This is, however, a plan that is very attractive to many professional staff.

- **The 12-hour shift.**
  Some options within a 2-week pay period are: (1) seven 12-hour shifts, (2) seven shifts on and seven shifts off, and (3) three shifts per week in a 72-hour pay period. This plan presents many of the advantages of the 10-hour-a-week plan. It provides an intense work period and more free time while securing benefits for a full-time position. The disadvantages are also the same, particularly fatigue.

- **The Baylor plan.**
  A very interesting alternative staffing plan is the Baylor plan. In essence, it is a weekend alternative plan. The idea, originated at Baylor University Medical Center, consists of a staff for a traditional 40-hour-a-week, 8-hour-a-shift plan during the week and a second staff for weekends who work two 12-hour shifts and are paid for a 40-hour week. Its advantages include ensuring adequate weekend coverage and working fewer hours for greater pay. A problem with this method is that there is a high turnover rate because of the undesirable hours.

- **Job sharing.**
  This implies two people sharing a position, which has obvious advantages for people who desire a part-time position. This works very well at many levels of the organization and has been reported to be quite successful in the position of clinical specialist. It does require that the two individuals sharing the position be cooperative and compatible.

- **Flexible hours or part-time work.**
  Part-time work falls into any category. Professional staff are able to select working hours that are compatible with their personal needs. The hours of work may be

consistent with any of the preceding models or may be fewer working hours per day. This allows professionals with multiple responsibilities to still be part of the professional workforce. This has advantages for both the person and the organization.

- **Combination plan.**
  This plan combines part-time or full-time work with a variety of staffing schedules.

While general scheduling plans provide a structured approach to providing adequate staff, shift-to-shift variations often require staffing adjustments. Problems include the unpredictable census, variations of patients seeking care, dramatic and abrupt changes in the acuity level of critical care patients, and the competency of the staff. Flexible and innovative scheduling patterns have been proposed to induce nurses to be able to practice. The following represent some additional approaches to providing adequate staff:

- **Use of a general float pool.**
  Nurses may be hired centrally and assigned to a unit on a shift-to-shift basis. Essentially this is a unit without walls with a traditional and an administrative structure (nurse manager and assistants). The float pool staff are scheduled in 4-week blocks but are designed to address the historic census variations and staffing trends. The pool may be composed of RNs, LPNs, and paraprofessionals. The intent of this staffing model is to provide organized supplemental staff where needed.

- **Use of a unit-based float pool.**
  The same model may be used for specific highly specialized units and serve as a unit-based float pool. Instead of providing staff for the entire organization, this pool supplies staff to specific units.

- **Per diem nurses.**
  Per diem nurses are hired on a daily basis and are not guaranteed an assignment or benefits from the organization. They may be hired from outside agencies or from within the organization's staff hiring. Typically, these nurses are paid a higher hourly wage to make the position appeal more to them.

- **Float-float policy.**[13]
  Each institution should decide what will be the policy for asking nurses to float to other areas and what restriction will limit the practice. One such suggestion is to cluster the units that nurses may be expected to staff. Rather than expecting nurses to be available for the entire organization, clusters (a few related patient-care areas) may be formed to which the nurse may be asked to provide care.

Shared Staffing Help List

A shared staffing help list (SSHL) is essentially an in-house pool of various levels of staff that will serve the needs of the institution. Each unit posts their needs and a central staffing manager fills their requests with members of the SSHL.[14]

Flexibility and versatility have to be characteristics of today's staffing schedules. Providing options for professional nurses is an excellent way to prevent attrition and to enhance work satisfaction. Giving autonomy and decision making about working conditions to the staff is good management.

MANAGEMENT'S ROLE: PLANNING THE STAFFING PROGRAM

The role of administration is to determine the staffing program for the institution. The staffing program consists of phases for the selection of a staffing plan. Phases of the staffing plan include:

1. *Phase One*. A statement of the purpose of the organization and the services offered, as well as the standard of care to be provided.
2. *Phase Two*. The application of a specific method to determine the number and kind of staff to deliver care.
3. *Phase Three*. Development of an assignment pattern using policies and guidelines to steer the process.
4. *Phase Four*. Evaluation of the process through an analysis of patient outcome data, quality indicators, and personnel issues such as staff turnover, absenteeism, and attrition.[15] In addition to the overall staffing plan, the nurse manager at the unit level will implement the organization's staffing plan, as well as determine highly specific unit policies. These policies, when developed, provide adequate coverage for shifts or patients' needs, ensure stability for the nursing staff, and incorporate flexibility and fairness in work assignments. The various questions that require policy guidance include the following:

   Who determines the staffing schedule and what authority does this individual have over the staff?
   What is the type and length of the staffing cycle (Is it fixed, weekly, biweekly, monthly)?
   Is there a rotation-of-shift policy?
   Where and at what time is the staffing schedule posted?
   What is the duration of time for shifts?
   What is the weekend-off policy?
   What is the tardiness policy?
   What are the low census procedures?
   Is there a policy for trading shifts or days off?
   Is there a policy for rotation to other divisions?
   How are vacation and holiday requests handled?
   How are conflicts over requests handled?
   What is the emergency-time-off policy?[16]

To a great extent, the previous questions, when guided by organization policy and modified at the unit level, will reduce a great deal of ambiguity and conflict about staffing assignments. The more the staff knows and controls their assignments, the more satisfied they are likely to be.

Economic and Regulatory Issues

Economics dictates to what extent staff may be procured. Budgetary restrictions exist that allocate percentages of the operating budget to deal with personnel salary and benefits. In the current environment, budgets have been drastically revised to adjust to a different system of reimbursement. Every professional and nonprofessional position has to be justified as to its ability to meet the mission of the organization. Information regarding the patients and services offered are also instrumental in developing an appropriate staffing model. Type of patients, acuity levels, and prospective prediction of anticipated patients and services offered provide baseline data for predicting staff requirements.[17]

Regulatory policies from government to the variety of insurance plans direct, in part, the limits of how much and what kind of staff is economically possible. Regulations about safety, infection control, and quality-control measures also play a part in quantifying staffing plans. A certain level of environmental quality must exist for any agency to be accredited. Thus, to some extent, regulatory bodies add a dimension to "safe" staff distributions.

Professional concerns that affect policies about working conditions may also influence staffing. These concerns include mandatory overtime (as a way of providing adequate staff) and mandatory staffing ratios. The problem of requiring nurses to continue working after their allotted time has expired resulted in a federal bill. The Registered Nurses and Patient Protection Act[18] was introduced into Congress as a way of protecting patient safety. Nursing organizations galvanized support to prohibit the practice of insisting that nurses work beyond the usual shift time. This is a dangerous practice that creates the opportunity for error. There are currently state-to-state differences in what constitutes overtime. The ANA in response has placed workplace issues, especially mandatory overtime, high on its agenda to eliminate this practice.[19]

In 1999, California instituted legislation to mandate appropriate nurse-patient ratios. Currently, there is before the state legislation, rules that set, minimum staffing levels for nurses. The difficulty with this initiative is the lack of empirical data to describe adequate nurse-patient ratios. At this time, research studies are being conducted to answer the question of what constitutes appropriate staffing plans based on quality indicators and patient outcome data. The goal of these studies is to understand the association between the use of resources for patient care, their characteristics and processes (direct nursing interventions), and the effect on patients (nurse-sensitive patient care outcomes). This data will be prerequisite to the correct number and skill level of nurses and other direct care providers to provide safe and quality care.[20]

Institutional policies for recruiting, providing, maintaining, and retaining staff will involve a mutual agreement between management and personnel. Involving staff in decisions concerning their working hours can create a positive work climate. Allowing autonomy in decision making facilitates staff growth and enhances morale. The most expensive personnel costs to an organization, besides providing benefits, comes from staff turnover and absenteeism. These activities require that additional personnel be hired for temporary or permanent positions.

CASE STUDY

An Understaffed Unit

Michael Clay, a registered nurse on the 10th floor ICU, had just completed his fifth night of work and was looking forward to having the next two days off. The unit had been filled to capacity and extremely busy. As Michael was leaving, the charge nurse approached him and asked him if he would work one more night because they were really short-staffed. He paused and, looking exhausted, said, "OK, but this is it." At the same time, Stephanie, another RN, walked into the report room, and was greeted with "What are you doing here today? I thought you were off." Stephanie said, "I was called at 5 this morning to come in and help." Another nurse, Jane, joined the group and said, "I feel like quitting. I couldn't even take a break last night."

The charge nurse, who overheard the conversation, said, "You are aware of the fact that we lost three permanent staff members, and their positions have not been filled, and frankly, I am not sure if those positions will be filled by RNs or technicians." She went on, "Several proposals are being considered, including flexible hours, innovative staffing patterns, and self-scheduling. The aim is to provide autonomy and flexibility to the current and potential staff."

- What kind of staffing patterns should be offered?
- How much flexibility should be suggested?
- How would you handle financial compensation for part- and full-time staff?

SUMMARY

This chapter has dealt with the most important resource to any organization: the staff. Staffing is a highly complex process that, because of the volatility in health care today, requires management know-how. Staffing is the process that provides adequate personnel to do the work of the organization. This is based on a staffing plan that uses a particular methodology. These methodologies include descriptive or consensus, industrial engineering, management engineering, and the expert panel method.

Following the development of a staffing plan, which includes an acceptable skill mix, a scheduling plan is provided that allocates personnel to a time frame. The role of management includes the choice of a staffing plan and the evaluation of its effectiveness. Issues to keep in mind for the choice of a proper professional staff model are environmental, organizational, and professional working conditions. Staffing is the means by which the work of the organization is operationalized.

LEARNER EXERCISES

1. Plan a staffing pattern for a 30-bed, step-down, coronary care unit for 24 hours per day for 7 days. Which staffing methodology did you use? Why?
2. What would you do to recruit and retain staff?
3. What working conditions are the most important to you?
4. What should be the criteria for hiring a new staff nurse?

REFERENCES

1. American Association of Critical-Care Nurses. (2001). *Maintaining patient-focused care in an environment of nursing staff shortages & financial constraint: A statement from AACN public policy.* Retrieved from the World Wide Web in October, 2001: *http://www.aacn.org,* 1–4.
2. American Association of Critical-Care Nurses. (2001). *Maintaining patient-focused care in an environment of nursing staff shortages & financial constraint: A statement from AACN public policy.* Retrieved from the World Wide Web in October, 2001: *http://www.aacn.org,* 2.
3. Strickland, B., & Neely, S. (1995, March). Using a standard staffing index to allocate staff. *Journal of Nursing Administration,* 25(3), 15–21.
4. Dunne, M.A., Norby, R., & Cournoyer, P., et al. (1995). Expert panel method for nurse staffing and resource management. *Journal of Nursing Administration,* 25(10), 63–67.
5. Marron, S. (2001). Staffing summit: Addresses gap between patient needs and RN staffing. *The Oregon Nurse,* 65(4), 1–4.
6. Pederson, A., Hoover, C., & Kisiel, T. (1995). Redesigning a skill mix in the ICU. *Nursing Management,* 26(7), 32J–32P.
7. Managing teams for peak performance: Three in a series. *Healthcare Continuing Education,* LT.U Extension, 39–41.
8. Managing teams for peak performance: Three in a series. *Healthcare Continuing Education,* LT.U Extension, 39–41.
9. Managing teams for peak performance: Three in a series. *Healthcare Continuing Education,* LT.U Extension, 39–41.
10. American Hospital Association. (1983). *Managing under medical prospective pricing.* Chicago, IL: AHA.
11. Strickland, B., & Neely, S. (1995, March). Using a standard staffing index to allocate staff. *Journal of Nursing Administration,* 25(3), 15–21.
12. Dunne, M.A., Norby, R., & Cournoyer, P. et al. (1995). Expert panel method for nurse staffing and resource management. *Journal of Nursing Administration,* 25(10), 63–67.
13. Landergan, E. (1997). Staffing for census fluctuations. *Nursing Management,* 28(5), 77–78.
14. Bania, K. (1997). A tool for improving supplemental staffing. *Nursing Management,* 28(5), 78.
15. Cardello, D. (1995, April). Monitoring staffing variances and length of stay. *Nursing Management,* 26(4), 38–41.
16. Managing teams for peak performance: Three in a series. *Healthcare Continuing Education,* LT.U Extension, 41.
17. Taunton, R., Hope, K., Woods, C., & Bott, M. (1995). Predictors of absenteeism among hospital staff nurses. *Nursing Economics,* 13(4), 217–229.
18. Registered Nurses and Patients Protection Act (H.R. 5179). 106th U.S. Congress. September 14, 2000.
19. ANA House of Delegates. (2000, August 24). Retrieved from the World Wide Web in September, 2000: *http://www.nursingworld/org/about/summary/oohodact.htm.*
20. Bolton, L.B., Jones, C., Aydin, L.E., Donaldson, N., Brown, D.S., Lowe, M., Lenihan, P.M., & Harms, P. (2001). A response to California's mandated nursing ratios. *Journal of Nursing Scholarship, 2nd Quarter,* 179–189.

15

Managing Resources

Time

"I recommend you to take care of the minutes, for the hours will take care of themselves."

Lord Chesterfield

INTRODUCTION

Effective managers use time efficiently. In essence, taking control over time gives them control over the work. **Time** refers to the number of seconds, minutes, hours, or days available to the manager to accomplish a given task. Using time profitably has implications for both the manager as well as the professional staff. The objective of this next discussion is the process of time management.

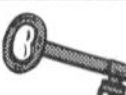

KEY CONCEPTS

Crisis Control refers to the communication and delegation of a new plan reorganized around priorities to manage an unexpected and untoward event.

Effectiveness refers to the quality of doing the right task correctly.

Efficiency refers to the resource utilization of doing the right task.

Self-Management is an individualized approach to using time best according to one's particular needs.

Stress is the sum of all the nonspecific biologic phenomena elicited by adverse, external influences. Stress may be either physical, psychological, or both.

Time is the number of seconds, minutes, hours, or days available to the manager to accomplish a given task.

Time Management is based on principles and is a variety of techniques that facilitate the best use of time.

Time Styles are the predispositions (action, idea, logic, or people) of behavioral patterns that influence how a person uses time.

TIME MANAGEMENT

Time impacts individuals in complex ways. Coordinating activities with others may cause psychological distress to some; in addition, individuals tend to be more effective at different times of the day. The ability to manage people with different concepts of time involves patience and knowledge of **time management.** Effective managers evaluate the constraints on time, as well as develop and implement methods that conserve and use time effectively. Time management is intended to foster good work habits that use time productively. The activities for organizing time should take into account a variety of principles, including:

- Communication
- Planning
- Delegating
- Prioritizing goals[1]

PRINCIPLES OF TIME MANAGEMENT

Communication

Effective communication facilitates time management. Use of the communication process is an important tool to provide complete and appropriate information. Managers need explicit and correct information to plan and direct work. Managers deal with information and make decisions based on changing and shifting information. Errors can lead to wasted time and the useless expenditure of energy. Proper information guides correct action. Communication should include clear messages and feedback in order for correct perceptions. Decisions about the work to be completed should only be made after the necessary information is known. Poor decisions and indecision are time wasters. Good communication is fundamental to the effective use of resources. Time is a resource that, when managed well, will enable the process of management.

Planning

Strategies for success begin with the planning process. Planning is the essential ingredient for the effective use of time. Managers spend a major part of their time in the planning process, which may actually exceed the time required to implement the activity. The ability to plan effectively is essential to the effective use of time. Planning charts the course of action in order of importance. Every minute spent in planning saves time in the execution of activities. The fundamental issue in "time-saving" planning is that optimal results occur with the least amount of effort and consumption of resources. Planning also involves creating objectives and goals in accord with a time frame. If the plan includes realistic deadlines (not underestimating or overestimating the time needed), there will be less stress associated with the implementation of the work. **Stress** refers to the sum total of all the nonspecific, biological, phenomena elicited by adverse, external influences. Stress may be either physical, psychological, or both. In every plan of action the possibility of unanticipated consequences should be considered. By constructing alternatives and adopting an attitude of flexibility, the manager will be able to cope with forces beyond his or her control.

The manager who uses planning properly is in a position to not only manage his or her time well but also that of others. This manager does not procrastinate because it will prevent others from doing their work. Building in alternatives facilitates the work of others in the face of barriers. A manager who routinely reviews plans on a daily, weekly, and monthly basis is using planning properly. Planning is a key ingredient to successful time management.

Delegation

Delegation is used by the manager as a way to ensure that the work of the organization is completed on schedule. The most efficient and effective use of time is when the manager manages, and the professional staff does the operative work. **Efficiency** refers to doing the right task with the least amount of resources, and **effectiveness** refers to doing the right task correctly and securing good outcomes. The manager who is results-oriented executes the plan of the organization through the appropriate use of delegation. To ensure that the delegated tasks are properly executed, the manager should maintain a delegation record. The record should include the person, the task, and the time in which it is to be completed. Delegating the work of the department to others is not only a part of management but also a strategy for time management.

Prioritizing Goals

By analyzing activities, a hierarchy of goals can be developed and a plan of time created to meet them. The manager is, then, in a position to selectively allocate varying amounts of time and energy to accomplishing the goals. Prioritizing involves ordering goals, tasks, and responsibilities from the most important to least important. This process involves knowledge about the managerial role and the nature of the work to be completed. Spending time thinking through how best to meet the goals is time well spent. It is far more efficient to spend time planning for problems than to spend time to correct them.

Matching the managerial goal with monitoring criteria to ensure appropriate progress is a useful way to map the best use of time. Take the following example: The manager has a goal of having all performance appraisals completed within a three-month period so that pay raises will be on schedule. This is an important responsibility with implications for the nursing staff. The manager plans how best to proceed by completing all performance evaluations and conducting scheduled interviews in accord with mutually established dates. The manager also knows that other activities impinge on the manager's time, and must allocate time each day to complete the evaluation forms and schedule ample time for the performance appraisal interviews.

TIME MANAGEMENT STRATEGIES

Time management strategies are practical techniques to preserve, conserve, structure, and use time well to meet goals. These strategies are, in large measure, ways to individualize the best use of time according to one's particular needs (**self-management**). How an individual best manages time can vary and is referred to as a time style.

Since managing time is a personal experience, one must know what his or her time style is, and how time is spent. **Time styles** are based on personality characteristics and habit. These styles have been categorized on dominant behavioral preferences and are named the following:

- Action
- Idea
- Logic
- People's time styles[2]

An action-oriented person tends to view time in the present and organize activities one at a time to be completed immediately. This individual is not comfortable with unexpected tasks, and tends not to prioritize, as each task is seen as important. Idea-oriented persons are creative and don't usually pay attention to time. They have a hard time meeting deadlines and estimating proper time use. Logic-oriented persons are orderly, rational, sequential planners who are comfortable with and able to use time well. Lastly, people-oriented people are most effective at team building and may not see time as a priority. These individuals are often over-committed and over-extended. They tend to underestimate the amount of time required to complete tasks. Most individuals tend to have a dominant time style.

Strategies have been devised to help managers and professional staff use their time wisely and productively, no matter their personal preference. Suggested strategies are discussed below.[3]

Time Analysis

To discover your own style, a time analysis may be used. This is a personal diary in which all activities are recorded in 15-minute blocks for approximately 1 week. This log will become the basis of analysis. It will be apparent where time is spent, wasted, and properly used. For those who wish to enhance their use of time, this method will allow them to examine their individual time style and where they might be able to use time more effectively. It has been advised that this procedure be repeated yearly to discover if bad habits remain. A typical time analysis sheet is pictured in Figure 15-1.

Daily Planning

Planning is effective when time frames correspond with the manager's responsibility. This means daily, weekly, and monthly plans. Ultimately all long- and short-range goals and activities become subject to daily planning. Prior to the implementation of a project, time lines may be applied so that activities can be broken down into daily segments.

Goals
1. Plan patient care
2. Attend inservice
3. Evaluate nursing care

Start time		Time/activity *Activity*
7:15	Receive report	
30	Give report	
45		
0		
15		
30		
45		
0		
1:15	Attend inservice	
30		
45		
0		
4:00	*Day ends*	Discuss patient care
	Evaluation	

Time savers—Planning activities
Time wasters—Unnecessary trips to Central Service

FIGURE 15-1. An example of a time-analysis worksheet.

It is recommended that the daily plans be formulated or reviewed the preceding evening by the manager. In this way, the manager is prepared to make sure certain activities are completed. This may be through the process of delegation or the manager's own effort. An example of a daily plan is pictured in Figure 15-2.

Crisis Control

No amount of planning can prevent periodic crises. In any social system, crises do occur from time to time. It is during a crisis that time-management skills are the most important. Keep in mind the principles of time management: communication, planning, delegation, and prioritizing. **Crisis control** is accomplished when communication and delegation of a new plan is reorganized around priorities to manage an unexpected and untoward event. In a crisis, certain people will be involved in its resolution. These people should be informed at once with the necessary details of the problem. Ordinarily, this group will be composed of superiors and selected subordinates.

The plan that has been established may have to be rearranged to deal with priorities. Other work may have to be delayed until a later date. Sound planning will guide the necessary day-to-day activities while effort is directed at resolution of the crisis. The manager may have to delegate tasks to the professional staff while dealing with the impending problem. The manager is in a position to communicate, reorganize, and delegate. In a crisis situation, the manager's flexibility and ability to activate alternative solutions represents good management of time.

	Morning	*Afternoon*	*Late afternoon*
Goals			
1. Begin performance appraisal evaluations.			
2. Prepare budget for next quarter.			
3. Review quality assurance records.			
Activities			
1. Review anecdotal performance records.			
2. Review budget report.			
3. Prepare a report to staff on quality scores.			

FIGURE 15-2. An example of a time-management daily planner.

Problem Analysis

Problem analysis is essential to be an effective manager as well as to use time properly. Managers must be able to distinguish a crisis from an urgent or an important event. Each type requires a different type of response. The crisis requires major reorganization of priorities. The urgent situation requires immediate action. The important event requires analysis and planning.

Another aspect of problem analysis that has implications for the manager's time is that not every problem requires an immediate solution. Some problems go away with little or no intervention. Managers, in making decisions about what to do or not to do, are also making decisions about effective or ineffective use of time.

Task Analysis

One of the most efficient ways to save time is to evaluate the tasks that are performed. By reviewing tasks, the manager may discover which tasks are of low value and therefore could be eliminated, consolidated, or delegated. Similar or related activities may be able to be grouped in such a way as to allow a more efficient performance from a manager or from personnel. This is very much like functional assignments on a nursing division. One individual takes vital signs for all patients on a postoperative step-down unit. Tasks can be more efficiently handled if all the necessary "tools" are available before beginning the activity. Assembling essential equipment prior to implementing a nursing skill saves time, energy, and frustration.

Time Control

Periodically, the manager should simply be unavailable by planning office time to think or to clear up pressing business. In this way, the manager controls interruptions except for important messages. Planned office time should be built into the manager's plans and communicated to staff.

Time Evaluation

Periodic evaluation of how time is spent is a helpful technique to assess the use of time. The ability to organize and use time effectively is the hallmark of good management.

Thus, time-analysis techniques can be helpful guides to improve both effectiveness and efficiency.

BARRIERS TO EFFECTIVE TIME MANAGEMENT

In the development of new skills, barriers may exist. Being aware of problems alerts the manager to possible pitfalls. In addition, considering problems will be helpful in the evaluation process. Some barriers to the effective management of time are discussed below.

Habit

People are creatures of habit. Habits are comfortable ways of behaving because they do not require conscious thought. It is also very difficult to change habits. Because of this, certain behaviors, while comfortable, do not use time effectively. Time analysis will show exactly where habitual behaviors take precedent over time-efficient behaviors. The manager should be mindful of negative habits, particularly procrastination, and make time more productive.

Work Expansion

Work sometimes takes on a life of its own. If 3 hours are allotted for a specific task and 1 hour is sufficient, the work may, still end up taking 3 hours. Time frames attached to work will provide realistic guidelines.

Oversupervision

The manager must be mindful of what the employee is to accomplish and how much supervision is necessary. To give too much supervision to a competent professional presents interpersonal as well as time problems. Allowing the staff to complete their work is the best use of everyone's time.

Underdelegation

The manager who does not delegate appropriately ends up with more work than is necessary. A manager has enough responsibility without assuming that of subordinates.

Losing Sight of Objectives

A manager who loses sight of the work that has to be accomplished will surely waste time. An important element of the managerial role is maintaining a course of action. Periodically reviewing what and how objectives are to be met is a productive use of time. Suggestions to help the new manager develop time-management skills are summarized below:

1. Analyze your time for an average week. Use the time-analysis tool.
2. Plan your work day the evening before.

3. Know your peak energy time. Do the most difficult work then.
4. Begin with the most important job.
5. Start the day by reviewing what you will be doing.
6. Don't waste time at work by doing too much socializing.
7. Give yourself time each day to think, plan, and create.
8. Organize the necessary "tools" to complete a task.
9. Consolidate similar tasks or work.
10. Eliminate unnecessary work.

CASE STUDY

Time Management and the Need to Prioritize

Joanne Burns is a new graduate and has begun her career in the cardiac thoracic intensive care unit (ICU). Joanne has finished her orientation and is working with experienced professional nurses.

Joanne feels relatively secure with the responsibilities of the position. She knows she has a great deal to learn and is open to suggestions. She hopes her transition period from new member of the team to experienced registered nurse (RN) will be smooth. She is pleased that her first assignment includes two fairly stable patients.

During the first day of her new position, Joanne is assigned to two postoperative patients. Everything proceeds smoothly until one patient's blood pressure drops and bleeding is suspected. Joanne is a wreck. She becomes disorganized and anxious. The other patient is neglected while she cares for the patient in crisis, who eventually returns to the operating room.

Following the episode, Joanne, who had not gone to lunch or had a break, overhears the assistant head nurse say, "I am just not sure about Joanne. She didn't have anyone take over for the other patient, and she was really shaken and disorganized." Joanne feels that the assessment of her performance was unfair, but she does not say anything.

- What would help Joanne to be more organized in the future?

CASE STUDY

Delegation and Communication Problems

Cindy Smith, a new RN, and Kim Jones, RN, were finishing work on the day shift of a postoperative surgical floor when a new patient arrived from the emergency room. Cindy stopped what she was doing (calculating Intake/Output ratios) and proceeded to admit the new patient. When Cindy got to her room, the transporter allowed the new patient, a woman, to get up off the cart and walk to her bed, which she did easily. Cindy helped her get settled, noting no acute distress, and told her she would return in 10 minutes. The patient said, "Fine, I don't need anything." Cindy went back to finish the end-of-shift duties.

Just as Cindy was about to finish her last room, Kim walked in and asked her, "Where's the admission sheet you started on the new admit?" Cindy stated she hadn't started one yet, as she wanted to finish these tasks before report, and planned on admitting the patient next. Kim abruptly walked away from Cindy and began the process of admitting the new patient. Cindy walked into the room and tried to help, but Kim said, "You should always take vital signs immediately when a new patient is admitted."

Outside the patient's room, Cindy tried to explain herself, when Kim screamed at her. "You don't do anything right! I hate to work with you! You are lazy, and you put a patient at risk!" Cindy didn't know what to say. She completed the admission, gave her report, and left the division.

- What is your analysis of what happened in this situation?
- Are new patient admissions a priority?
- What could Cindy have done differently? What could Kim have done differently?

SUMMARY

This discussion has provided an overview of time management. Using time properly involves prioritizing goals and applying time-management principles and strategies. The principles of time management include effective communication, planning, and delegation. Strategies are methods aimed at facilitating self-management of time. Barriers exist that are problematic to the effective use of time. The manager who uses time efficiently and effectively is managing a personal and group resource in an appropriate manner.

LEARNER EXERCISES

1. Keep your own record of time for an average week. Identify where you could save time.
2. Observe someone whom you believe uses time well. What is the most significant activity this individual uses?
3. In your clinical experience, try to utilize (1) time analysis, (2) daily planning, and (3) task analysis for 1 week. Is there a difference in your efficiency?
4. Consider this situation: Ms. Smith, the head nurse on a busy surgical division, notices that for the next 2 days, staffing will be slightly inadequate for the acuity of the patients on the division. This also happens to be during summer vacation. What might be done to deal with understaffing for a very short period of time and yet ensure quality of service? Since the example is general, provide a solution that deals with principles.

REFERENCES

1. Blanchard, K., & Johnson, S. (1986). *The one minute manager*. New York: Berkeley Books.
2. Tager, M.J. (1992). *Time styles, time management, personal action*. New York: Great Performances.
3. Day Timers: Retrieved from the World Wide Web: *http://www.daytimer.com*, (800) 225-5005.

SUGGESTED READINGS

Barkas, J.L. (1994). *Creative time management.* Englewood Cliffs, NJ: Prentice Hall.

Haynes, M.E. (1991). *Practical time management.* Los Altos, CA: Crisp Publications.

Matejka, J.K., & Dunsing, R.J. (1988). Time management: Changing some traditions. *Management World, 17*(2), 6–7.

Morgenstern, J. (2000). *Time management from the inside out.* New York: Henry Holt & Co.

16

Managing Resources
The Book Budget

"There are no victories at bargain prices."

Dwight D. Eisenhower

INTRODUCTION

Financial stability is a major concern in today's health care industry. It is not surprising that health care personnel at all levels of management are aware of, and are participating in, cost-saving strategies. The new nurse manager must be aware that nursing care is labor intensive and demands human resources, since personnel costs represent the largest expense for hospitals, with nursing representing the largest human resource cost. The function of all managers demands that attention be directed toward the organization's financial status. This chapter provides basic concepts of financial management with a special focus on budgeting at the unit level.

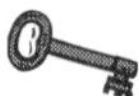

KEY CONCEPTS

Accounting is the activity that records and reports all financial transactions.

Assets are resources of the organization that have a dollar value.

Budget is a planning document used by a department or organization that forecasts both revenues and expenses.

Capital Budget is the plan for the acquisition of buildings and equipment that will be used by the organization for greater than 1 year beyond the year of acquisition.

Capital Equipment is an item with an expected life (usually greater than 3 years) beyond the date of purchase. The administrators of an organization who are responsible for financial policies usually determine a dollar threshold.

Corporation is a legal entity authorized by a state to operate under the rules of the entity's charter. Corporations are classified as either for-profit or not-for-profit, depending upon the nature of the business and the distribution of profits.

1. For-profit corporations are businesses whose mission includes earning a profit that may be distributed to its owners (shareholders).
2. Not-for-profit corporations are businesses whose mission does not include earning a profit for distribution to owners. A not-for-profit business may earn a profit, but the profit is reinvested in the organization for the replacement or expansion of services. There are no shareholders.

Cost Accounting is that activity that reports to the organization or department how much it is costing to provide specific services or products to the organization's clients.

Cost Center is a revenue- or non-revenue-producing unit or department in an organization in which the manager is assigned responsibility for costs.

Double-Entry Accounting is today's accounting method, which requires that for every amount added to one account an equal amount must be taken away from one or more other accounts.

Expenses are the costs of assets or services needed for the provision of patient care and generating revenue.

Financial Management is a major department and an activity that handles financial resources in an organization.

Financial Management System is the result of the actual plan to use and maximize the economics of the organization.

Financial Structure represents the components that are essential to managing finances and includes centralized policies, decentralized operations, and the interrelated responsibilities of those who play a part in financial management.

Fiscal Year is a 1-year period defined for financial purposes; it may start at any point during a calendar year.

Fringe Benefits are additional personnel costs other than salary. Typically, they are health insurance, life insurance, social security, and other employee benefits.

Full-Time Equivalent (FTE) represents the time of one full-time employee working for 1 year. This is calculated as 40 hours per week for 52 weeks, or a total of 2,080 paid hours per year. A FTE includes productive and non-productive time.

1. Productive time is actual hours worked, including overtime.
2. Non-productive time is paid time for nonworked hours, such as vacation, holiday, and sick time.

Gross Patient Revenues are the charges and payment for health care services provided.

Indirect Costs are costs that may be assigned to an organizational unit from elsewhere or may be unit costs that are not incurred for direct patient care.

Liabilities are the legal financial obligations an organization has to outsiders; essentially the money owed.

Long-Range Financial Plan is a document prepared by every organization to cover the next 5 to 10 years in terms of goals and dollars.

Net Patient Revenue represents the gross patient revenue minus the contractual advances, bad debt, and charity monies.

Nursing Hours per Patient Day (NHPPD) are the nursing hours provided per patient day by various levels of nursing personnel. NHPPD are determined by dividing total productive hours by the number of patients on the unit.

Operating Budget is the annual plan of revenues and expenses for the organization.

Standard Accounting refers to those procedures that prepare reports on a monthly, quarterly, or yearly basis to show financial performance.

Unit of Service is the basic measure of an item being produced by an organization (i.e., patient days, procedures, or visits).

Variable Costs are the costs that vary in relation to volume.

Variance is the difference between the planned costs (budget) and the actual costs.

MANAGING FINANCIAL RESOURCES

Preparing a department's budget is actually one of the last steps in handling a **corporation's** or organization's finances. It is part of the interrelated activities that fall within the scope of financial management. This major department in health care institutions coordinates financial operations throughout the entire organization or network. The objectives of **financial management** are as follows:

- To ensure that the organization has an efficient and effective financial management structure that supports strategic objectives, including those of individual operating units.
- To establish a uniform set of internal financial controls across the entire organization.
- To provide appropriate financial information to make timely decisions.

These objectives can only be met with the cooperation of all managers who plan and evaluate budgeted resources.

FINANCIAL STRUCTURE

The creation of a **financial structure** enables managers to know what is expected of them and, in so doing, to judge the organization's viability in today's competitive environment. A **financial management system** is a plan that uses and maximizes the economic resources of the organization. This plan consists of:

1. Centralized policies (control policies that apply to all departments).
2. Decentralized financial operations (each department has separate operating costs).
3. Establishment of interrelated responsibilities of those who play a part in financial management.

The financial system that results from the financial management plan balances **assets** (those holdings of the organization that are of value) and revenues with expenditures and **liabilities.** Financial data are integrated into the day-to-day operations, and subsequent reporting on financial conditions keeps the system functioning. The usual means of incorporating financial data is through the **budget**, or the planning document, used by a department and organization that forecasts both receipts and expenditures.

THE BUDGETING PROCESS

Budgeting is an important part of every organization's planning and control function. It requires that the manager:

- Review the financial performance during the prior budgeting time frame (month, quarter, or year).
- Formulate a new budget or financial plan for the coming period in relation to the organization's goals and financial projections.

The budgeting process can be filled with anxiety and uncertainty. Anxiety exists because the prior budget must be assessed, and **variances** (the difference between the budget numbers and the actual results) must be fully understood and explained to upper management. Uncertainty exists because translations of long-term goals and projections into detailed dollar estimates raise questions that are difficult, if not impossible, to answer precisely; yet, the process must go forward. Nevertheless, budgeting can be an exciting and challenging activity for the nurse manager to focus on for the overall plan of the organization.

Fundamental to the budgeting process is careful design and direction. This is accomplished through a general policy statement as well as through clear goals and reciprocal financial projections, which follow.

A Policy Statement

A general policy statement makes clear that: (1) budgeting is an important part of the organization's planning and control process, (2) uniform standards and definitions are used across the organization in carrying out the budgeting process, and (3) all managers are expected to provide the necessary data within a specific time frame. This policy statement is general in nature, widely publicized, and should rarely be changed, if at all.

Goals and Financial Projections

Specific goals and financial projections are prepared on a regular, set schedule (e.g., every 12 months for publication in a formal document). Goals and projections contain operating (that which affects day-to-day activities) and capital (that which affects major or unusual expenditures) plans. They convey a general sense of where the organization is headed and enough specifics so that goals can be integrated with the **capital** and **operating budget.** These statements and projections demand the attention of administrators and managers who must use them when doing their own budgeting tasks. These statements must be detailed enough to provide each department or division manager with the hard numbers needed to begin the budgeting process.

RELATED BUDGETING CONCEPTS

Budgeting is a complex process which requires specific knowledge and skill. The following section describes related concepts that are necessary to complete a budget. These concepts include: (1) accounting, (2) long-range financial plans, and (3) budget types. Accounting methods provide an accurate record of expenditures and drive the budgeting process. Long-range financial plans focus the budget. Budget types are offered to differentiate the different aspects of the budgeting process. The reader may select appropriate sections to review.

Accounting

Accounting is the activity that records and reports all financial transactions and thus generates the data for the budget. There are different types of accounting methods. This section will discuss standard accounting, cost accounting, and a method that is used by both types of accounting activities, double-entry accounting. **Standard accounting,** or general accounting, consists of activities that formulate reports of financial performance on a monthly, quarterly, or yearly basis. These reports can be prepared in many formats, but the most common formats fall into one of three categories:

Accounting Reports

1. Income statements
2. Balance sheets
3. Cash-flow statements

Category One: Income Statements

Income statements (also known as profit or loss statements) record receipts and expenditures. These statements disclose whether the organization or department made or lost money in the time period in question (month, quarter, or year). The income statement has two important sections. In the revenue section, the organization records all its receipts (or expected receipts due) from its normal operating activities. These would typically include such things as income from patient services or **net patient revenue.** The **expenses** section records: (1) the expenses directly incurred in caring for patients (labor, material, utilities, and so on); (2) the prorated portion of the cost of buildings and equipment used by the enterprise; and (3) the overhead expenses incurred in running the organization (administrators' salaries, interest expense on debts, and so on).

Category Two: The Balance Sheet

The balance sheet (also known as the position statement) records where the organization stands financially at any given point in time. These are usually prepared at the end of a period (month, quarter, or year). The balance sheet reports two types of resources:

those owned by the organization and those owed to others. Those that are owed to others are further divided into those that are owed to others as a matter of debt and those that are owed to the owners of the organization.

The balance sheet is divided into two sections. Assets make up the section for the organizations' owned resources: cash, buildings, equipment, inventory, and so on. In this section, assets are generally ranked by the speed with which they could be converted into cash. Cash is presented first, money due from others for services already rendered is second, inventory ready to be sold is third, and so on.

Liabilities and owner's equity is the section where resources owed to others are shown. In the liabilities portion, debts are shown, such as amounts due to suppliers for goods and services already received, and amounts due to bankers for loans received. Liabilities are generally ranked by urgency. Those that will have to be paid quickly are ranked first. Owner's equity is the difference between assets and liabilities. This difference is normally a positive amount and represents what the owners would receive if all the organization's assets were sold and all its debts paid.

Category Three: Cash-Flow Statements

The third form of accounting format is a cash-flow statement, which records the sources and uses of cash for a period. This statement is used to determine if the organization improved (or hurt) its cash position over a specific time period. This report is different from an income statement in that it measures the organization's ability to pay its bills. An organization can be profitable while at the same time be weak from a cash position. For example, the organization's cash may have been used to buy too many nonliquid items, such as buildings or equipment.

Cost Accounting

Another type of accounting is cost accounting. **Cost accounting** activities produce reports that tell managers how much it is costing to provide specific services. These reports are published on a monthly, quarterly, or yearly basis and contain details about the various elements of cost: labor, material, and overhead. There are two ways to approach cost accounting. Standard costing is used in an organization where all services or products fall into a manageable number of groups and where the costs to produce each item in that group are identical or so close to identical that the differences are not meaningful. The current prospective payment system uses standard costing concepts.

Actual costing (also known as job costing) is used in an organization where each product, patient, or client is unique and will have its own unique requirements. This is the actual cost system that is used by today's acute care organizations.

Cost accounting also takes into consideration the change in value through depreciation and amortization. Depreciation is the expense item that shows the drop in the value of a major asset from time period to time period. A related term is amortization, which is the drop in the value of a major, nonphysical asset from period to period. Items that are depreciated are buildings, equipment, additions, improvements, furniture, and so on. Items that are amortized are copyrights, patents, legal fees associated with organizing the organization, and so on. Although both depreciation and amortization are expense items on the income statement, they do not require any expenditure of cash and do not weaken the organization's cash position. An organization with depreciation and amortization may show losses on its income statement while actually improving its cash position.

Double-Entry Accounting

Double-entry accounting is the system used by today's accountants to record all financial transactions. This system requires that for every amount added to one account, an equal amount must be taken away from one or more other accounts. The system works because some accounts are expected to have negative balances (called credit balances), while other accounts are normally expected to have positive balances (called debit balances). Assets and expense items normally have debit (positive) balance accounts, while revenue, liabilities, and shareholder equity items normally have credit (negative) balance accounts (see Table 16-1 on pages 308–309).

Consider the following example: If the organization increases its bank debt, two things must happen. The liability account for bank debt would increase, and the asset account (cash) would also increase. The double entry must add to cash (debit) and subtract from bank debt (credit). On paper the result would be that the asset account, called cash, would increase, and the liability account, called bank debt, would also increase.

Long-Range Financial Plans

A **long-range financial plan** is a document prepared by every organization to cover the next 5 to 10 years. This plan shows how the long-range vision for the organization will take shape in terms of dollars and cents. This kind of document is also known as a projection. Typically, a goal/financial projection document will begin with a statement about the steps to be taken in the next 5 to 10 years to improve the organization. For example, the administrator of a medical clinic might include discussions about: (1) building new buildings, (2) adding a wing to modernize or increase the efficacy of certain types of care, or (3) eliminating or scaling back on underused services (e.g., obstetrics/gynecology [ob/gyn] in a clinic that serves an aging population).

The second part of the document explores the capital side of the items mentioned above. Capital expenditure plans set forth the costs for what has been planned. Where will the money come from for the new building or new wing, and when will it be finished? What disruptions will occur to the existing staff and departments? What will be necessary to accompany the improvements? Also included would be a discussion about which departments or divisions might be relocated to (or allowed to expand into) the space being vacated by the underused department.

The third part of the document discusses the operating budget of the overall clinic. An operating plan sets forth the changes that are anticipated in the organization as the long-range plan is implemented. This plan contains general and long-term language. An example of such a plan follows:

> The new building will increase our patient capacity by approximately 30 percent. This will necessitate the addition of 3 to 5 examining rooms, an "in-clinic" X-ray facility, and blood-testing machinery. Additional staff will be necessary to implement this plan.

Following the long-term discussion, a more specific, detailed discussion of the expected impact over the next 18 months would be provided.

Types of Budgets

Budgets serve different purposes. The operating budget is a planning document used by a department, a division, or the entire organization that forecasts both receipts and expenditures. The budget must be done often enough and in enough detail to allow the nurse manager to effectively address any differences that develop between the budget's numbers and the actual results. Budgets are generally prepared in one of two ways. Zero-based budgets are prepared as though all items of expense in the department, division, or organization are out and must be rejustified to be reincluded in the coming budget. This form of budgeting is time consuming. A supporting rationale must be composed for each assumption, each planned expenditure, and each planned revenue.

Flexible-based budgeting builds off the budget used in the prior period and is mostly a series of adjustments and refinements to the prior budget. Most budgeting falls into this category, mostly because zero-based budgeting is so time-consuming, and can result in major changes in direction or emphasis, and therefore may require a great deal of coordination between and among interacting departments and divisions.

Another term, variance, describes the difference between a budgeted number (or planned number) and an actual result. Some variances are positive (better than expected); some are negative (not as good as expected). All variances, both positive and negative, should be analyzed and understood. Managers are expected to classify variances as controllable and noncontrollable, simply meaning that the person responsible for the department or division had the power (or did not have the power) to control a specific variance. Although variances are classified as controllable or noncontrollable, studies of specific variances have shown that most have elements that are controllable and elements that are noncontrollable.

A more useful way to classify variances is as mix variances, volume variances, cost variances, and price variances. These classifications allow the variances to be divided into component parts and quantified by category. Each of these will be addressed below:

- A mix variance is a variance or part of a variance that is attributable to a change in the mix of work that the department or division experienced. For instance, a division whose budget for the year was devised with the expectation that most patients would be middle-aged to older patients recovering from elective gastrointestinal (GI) surgery would experience a super mix variance if suddenly it became a step-down unit for patients from a cardiac intensive care unit (ICU). The occupancy rates might be the same, but the budget numbers on staffing and supplies would never match the actual.
- A volume variance occurs when the utilization rate is higher or lower than expected. If a budget is built around a utilization rate, even a small variation from that rate will create a variance.
- A cost variance occurs when the cost of the key inputs to the process begin to change. If labor rates go up in the organization, a cost variance will result.
- A price variance occurs when the price paid for the product or service offered is different from that used in the budget.

The managerial structure needed to support a budgeting effort is substantial. Top-level decisions must be made and reinforced. Computer systems must be revised to support two parallel sets of numbers (budgeted numbers and actual accounting results) so that side-by-side comparison reports can be generated. The timing of the budgeting cycle and the

TABLE 16-1. An Example of Double Entry Accounting for St. John's Clinic from December 25 to December 31

	Dec 25, 1996		Activity for Week		Dec 31, 1996	
	DR+	*CR–*	*DR+*	*CR–*	*DR+*	*CR–*
BALANCE SHEET:						
Assets:						
Cash in clinic's account	$ 2,913				$ 2,913	
Due from patients	4,577		50[1]		4,627	
Inventories	2,588			100[4]	2,488	
Land	60,000				60,000	
Equipment	20,000				20,000	
less: depreciation	0			2,000[3]	–2,000	
Buildings + improvements	220,000				220,000	
less: depreciation	0			7,333[3]	–7,333	
Goodwill (amt paid for practice)	140,000				140,000	
less: amortization	0			14,000[3]	–14,000	
Liabilities						
Due to suppliers		$ 1,879		4,000[6]		$ 5,879
Due to doctors		11,923		3,577[5]		15,500
Due to nurses		2,884		866[6]		3,750
Due to other employees		641		192[5]		833
		673		6,500[2]		7,173
Equity						
St. John's initial capital		422,000				422,000
Profit & Loss for year		10,078				–28,440
PROFIT AND LOSS STATEMENT:						
Revenues:						
Patient fees year to date		394,338		50[1]		394,388

Expenses						
Doctors	$182,423		3,577[5]		$186,000	
Nurses	54,134		866[5]		55,000	
Other employees	9,808		192[5]		10,000	
Supplies	52,500		100[4]		52,600	
Maintenance	24,000				24,000	
Utilities and office supplies	7,155				7,155	
Rent for trailers	51,000		4,000[6]		55,000	
Uncompensated & emergency	3,240		6,500[2]		9,740	
Cash Flow (year to date)		$10,078				$ –5,107
Cash Flow (during 12/25–12/31 period)				–15,185		
Depreciation	0		9,333[3]		9,333	
Amortization	0		14,000[3]		14,000	
Profit and Loss (year to date)		10,078				–28,440
Profit and Loss (during 12/25–12/31 period)				–38,518		

Notes:

[1]The clinic's revenues are credited with $50, the usual St. John's HMO/PPO reimbursement for an expectant mother visit. (Thirty-three patients from Lobsterville visited the St. John's ER during the week. St. John's billed the insurance carriers, the patients' HMO/PPO, or these patients directly.)

[2]The clinic was charged with $6,500 emergency expense for delivering the doctors and equipment during the storm.

[3]Depreciation for the year is charged on Dec. 31. This amount is 1/30 of the value of the building & improvements ($220,000) and 1/10 of the value of the equipment ($20,000). Also, Goodwill is being amortized at the rate of 1/10 per year. (Goodwill is a term used when money is paid for a non-tangible asset, in this case the doctor's practice.)

[4]The shot given to the expectant mother came from the clinic's drug supply. It was charged as a standard $100 per dose.

[5]The doctors, nurses, and other employees of the clinic are paid on the first day of each month for the prior month's work. The liabilities section of the Dec. 25th balance sheet shows the money due employees from Dec. 1 to Dec. 25. The expense section shows the amount of accrued payroll liabilities for period Dec. 25 to Dec. 31.

[6]The $4,000 rent bill for the trailers for December is received on Dec. 31.

accounting cycle must be compatible and appropriate so that those individuals who watch over the system make sure the budget and accounting systems are coordinated. Managers must be educated to the process so that the accounting and budgeting data flow accurately and quickly into the computers.

A small group of knowledgeable health facility planners must be involved to help the administrators prepare the goal statement with financial projections. The health planners cannot provide the vision that can only come from the organization's leaders, but they can see to it that the overall document is internally consistent and realistic.

PREPARATION OF THE BUDGET

The temptation for the hard-pressed department head is to put budgeting on the back burner and then rush something out the door at the last minute. This temptation should be resisted. The budgeting process, if carried out thoroughly, demonstrates the seriousness the nurse manager exhibits in controlling finances. It gives familiarity with the dollar realities in the nurse manager's area and will inevitably trigger a series of "what if" questions. Those questions are the essential ingredients of change, and change can lead to greater productivity. Below are the several steps each manager must follow to properly prepare a budget.

Step One: Review Past Performance

Past financial performance must be reviewed and understood. This involves several steps. Placing the budgeted numbers next to the actual numbers for a given time period (month, quarter, or year) and identifying any and all significant variances is the first step. The meaning of the variance is interpreted as significant under different conditions. If the budgeted number is small, variations of less than 10 percent are generally not considered significant. If the budgeted number is large, variations of 2 percent or 3 percent may be considered significant.

The interpretation of the variances is facilitated by determining the degree of control held by the nurse manager. Each item in the budget should be identified as "beyond my control," "partly under my control," or "under my control." "Revenue per patient" and "number of patients treated" are items beyond the nurse manager's control. However, "overtime expended" items might be classified as under the nurse manager's control.

Each significant variance, whether under the manager's control or not, should be looked into, commented on, and explained. Usually the reason for a variance is a function of either a volume, mix, price, or cost variance. These generic terms can be understood with a few examples.

- If the budget had been prepared on the basis of an 80 percent average occupancy rate on a unit and the actual occupancy rate was 65 percent, there would be a volume variance of significant proportions.
- If several additional beds increased the unit's capacity, as well as the need for professional staff, registered nurse (RN) budget numbers would be below actual. In this case, the total nursing-cost budget number would be below actual and both a combination mix and cost variance would exist; different and higher cost inputs had to go into providing the service.

Step Two: Review the Organization's Goals and Projections

The organization's goals and financial projections should be studied thoroughly. The manager has to assume that the administrators and the health planners have a good grasp on future plans for the organization. Items in the major report that affect an individual department should be highlighted. An example of this is as follows:

> This division is going to lose 4 beds from February to November and then gain 12 additional beds after that. A gerontologist and clinical specialist in gerontology have been added to the staff. This division will then admit older and sicker patients. If the shortage of nurses continues, the nursing service will have to consider alternative staffing patterns to deal with this situation.

Step Three: Review the Variance

Once the goal statement is finished, it, together with the actual versus budget analysis or **variable cost** done earlier, should be reviewed with higher-level management. The departmental goals proposed should be carefully considered; the variances, their causes, and proposed corrective actions should also be reviewed. Once the final statement for the department is in place, the new budgeting process can begin in earnest.

Step Four: Actual Preparation of the Budget

The actual preparation of a new budget can be done at several degrees of depth. Types of budgets were discussed earlier, but for review, different types of budgets serve different departments more appropriately. Zero-based budgets are used when prior assumptions are rejected and all items are questioned anew. Less-rigorous budgeting or flexible budgeting uses the prior year's operation as the model for the coming year, and changes are made as needed to fit new realities. Most budgeting is flexible budgeting in which the prior year becomes the model for the current year.

To complete the budget, a budget worksheet is essential, which includes a condensed version of the department's goal statement. The actual worksheet is composed of columns. These columns should include one with historic information with the old budget and a column for actual numbers with comments explaining the variances. Another column should display revenue and **cost**, both direct and **indirect**. The items that are fully controllable within the department should be highlighted.

The manager should be able to enter an estimate of the budget numbers he or she sees growing out of the process. Next to each number should be a notation on the source of the number. Some organizations provide these budgetary worksheets with guidelines that explain what each line and column should contain.

Specific Responsibilities of the Nurse Manager

The following example will illustrate how the nurse manager applies the aforementioned concepts to the budgeting process by:

1. Accurately assessing personnel needs using predetermined standards or an established patient classification system.
2. Coordinating the monitoring of budget control.

The nurse manager oversees aspects of the operating budget consisting of the personnel budget, the supply budget, and the capital budget. Each is discussed as follows:

- **Personnel Budget**
  The personnel budget is the major component of the operating budget as it is based upon the nursing care needs of patients and the subsequent number of nursing staff to meet the patients' needs. The nurse manager who knows the historical trends and who knows the present nursing care needs is well positioned to determine the number and skill mix levels of nursing personnel on a specific unit using predetermined standards.

  With the advent of sophisticated computer programs, most organizations are providing the completed operating budget for the manager. The fiscal management department usually determines the workload forecast (**units of service**) and projected **gross patient revenue** for the next **fiscal year** based upon trends and historical data. The forecast data are provided to the unit nurse manager to confirm the personnel budget, which consists of the salary and cost of **fringe benefits.** The nurse manager must analyze the number of **Full-Time Equivalents (FTEs)** required by the predetermined standards of nursing care (see Chapter 14) and the time required to give the care (**nursing hours per patient day, or NHPPD**). Therefore, it becomes essential for the nurse manager to understand the budget components and to be able to defend necessary changes that need to be implemented. Figure 16-1 shows the personnel budget for a hospital-nursing unit.

- **Supply budget**
  The supply budget for a typical nursing unit in a hospital or long-term care facility is smaller than the personnel budget. The fiscal management department provides the supply expenses in the budget preparation packet for the nurse manager. As with the personnel budget, projected patient statistics are used as a basis for identifying supply requirements. Figure 16-2 gives the steps the nurse manager must consider in determining the supply budget.

- **Capital budget**
  The capital budget (or **capital equipment**) is the unit plan for equipment that will be used beyond 1 year and has a cost threshold. For most hospital-unit managers, the capital budget consists of the purchase of new furniture for patient rooms or selected equipment such as dopplers, wheelchairs, patient scales, and lifts. Other major equipment items are seldom purchased for a nursing unit but would be found on the capital budget of an operating room. The budget of a long-term care unit may include special beds. Figure 16-3 shows the capital budget request worksheet for a cardiac care nursing unit. The worksheet should identify the item as new, a replacement, or as an addition. Priorities for purchase are weighted, with 1 being the highest. A written justification must be attached for each item requested.

Monitoring the Budget

Managers of **cost centers** are responsible for overseeing the budget operations and determining why variances occur. The manager is then expected to compare budgeted

Personnel Budget 10-Bed Coronary Care Unit 80% Occupancy Budgeted 14 NHPPD					
Column:	**A**	**B**	**C**	**D**	**E**
Position Title	**Hours Worked**	**Total Cost before Fringes**	**Fringe Rate**	**Fringe (B × C)**	**Total Personnel Costs (B + D)**
Nurse Manager	40	$ 60,000.00	19%	$ 11,400.00	$ 71,400.00
Secretary 1FTE	40	23,880.00	19%	4,537.20	28,417.20
Secretary .4FTE	16	8,400.00	8%	672.00	9,072.00
RN(1) 1FTE	40	45,760.00	19%	8,694.40	54,454.40
RN(2) 1FTE	40	43,888.00	19%	8,338.72	52,226.72
RN(3) 1FTE	40	39,520.00	19%	7,508.80	47,028.80
RN(4) 1FTE	40	43,888.00	19%	8,338.72	52,226.72
RN(5) 1FTE	40	34,008.00	19%	6,461.52	40,469.52
RN(6) 1FTE	40	32,448.00	19%	6,165.12	38,613.12
RN(7) 1FTE	40	35,984.00	19%	6,836.96	42,820.96
RN(8) 1FTE	40	30,784.00	19%	5,848.96	36,632.96
RN(9) 1FTE	40	30,784.00	19%	5,848.96	36,632.96
RN(10) 1FTE	40	29,224.00	19%	5,552.56	34,776.56
RN(11).5FTE	20	17,472.00	8%	1,397.76	18,869.76
RN(12).5FTE	20	18,720.00	8%	1,497.60	20,217.60
RN(13).5FTE	20	17,472.00	8%	1,397.76	18,869.76
RN(14).5FTE	20	18,720.00	8%	1,497.60	20,217.60
RN(15).5FTE	20	17,680.00	8%	1,414.40	19,094.40
RN(16).5FTE	20	18,200.00	8%	1,456.00	19,656.00
RN(17).5FTE	20	20,020.00	8%	1,601.60	21,621.60
RN(18).5FTE	20	17,680.00	8%	1,414.40	19,094.40
RN(19).4FTE	16	14,976.00	0%	0.00	14,976.00
LPN(1) 1FTE	40	22,360.00	19%	4,248.40	26,608.40
LPN(2) 1FTE	40	21,890.00	19%	4,159.10	26,049.10
LPN(3) 1FTE	40	23,460.00	19%	4,457.40	27,917.40
LPN(4) 1FTE	16	9,809.00	0%	0.00	9,809.00
PCA(1) 1FTE	40	27,040.00	19%	5,137.60	32,177.60
PCA(2).4FTE	16	7,904.00	0%	0.00	7,904.00
PCA(3).4FTE	16	7,904.00	0%	0.00	7,904.00
PCA(4).4FTE	16	7,904.00	0%	0.00	7,904.00
PCA(5).4FTE	16	9,152.00	0%	0.00	9,152.00
PCA(6).4FTE	16	9,152.00	0%	0.00	9,152.00
PCA(7).4FTE	16	9,152.00	0%	0.00	9,152.00
PCA(8).2FTE	8	4,576.00	0%	0.00	4,576.00
Total		$ 779,811.00		$ 115,883.54	$895,694.54

FIGURE 16-1. Personnel budget.

A Supply Budget

1. Review supply expenses for the current fiscal year.
2. Determine changes that will affect the next fiscal year's supply budget.
   —Units of service (increased or decreased)
   —New programs
   —New procedures
   —New services
3. Determine the rate of inflation for supplies (obtained from the Fiscal Management Department).

FIGURE 16-2. Steps to be considered in determining the supply budget.

Capital Budget Request Worksheet
Fiscal Year 2002

Cost Center 3CCU

Type	Quantity	Description	Unit Cost	Extended Cost	Priority
Replacement	1	Portable Defibrillator	$2,795	$2,795	1
Addition	1	Wheelchair	$540	$540	1
Replacement	2	Cardiac ICU bed with built-in scale	$4,950	$9,900	2
Addition	1	Portable Infusor	$1,200	$1,200	3
Addition	1	Doppler	$485	$485	3
		Total		**$14,920**	

FIGURE 16-3. Capital budget request worksheet.

expectations with actual results. The Fiscal Management Department provides the manager with a monthly variance report for justification. The nurse manager must investigate each variance and make a determination as to the cause.

The monthly variance analysis is completed for several reasons: (1) providing insight for planning the next year's budget, (2) controlling the costs during the current fiscal year, and (3) evaluating the performance of the department and/or manager. Figure 16-4 shows a monthly responsibility report for the coronary care unit.

Upon review of the Responsibility Report, the manager is required to submit a written explanation of variances, either positive or negative. Many managers will involve their staff in this process. This investigative process helps the manager to understand what is occurring and to control future results.

	Coronary Care Unit June, 2002 10 Beds 14 NHPPD			
	Actual	Budget	Variance	Variance %
Statistics				
Patient Days	290	240	50	20.8%
FTEs	26.4	23.8	2.6	10.9%
Revenues				
Inpatient Revenue	$ 429,000	$ 361,900	$ 67,100	18.5%
Outpatient Revenue	0	0	0	
Total Gross Patient Revenues	$ 429,000	$ 361,900	$ 67,100	18.5%
Operating Expenses				
Salaries, Wages, & Benefits	$ 124,280	$ 82,150	$ (42,130)	–51.3%
Contract Employees	1,240	0	(1,240)	—
Overtime	3,856	4,320	464	10.7%
Supplies	8,600	7,350	(1,250)	–17.0%
Repairs	480	240	(240)	–100.0%
Other Fees and Services	650	550	(100)	–18.2%
Total Expenses	$ 139,106	$ 94,610	$ (44,496)	–47.0%
Gross Margin	$ 289,894	$ 267,290	$ 22,604	8.5%

FIGURE 16-4. Responsibility report.

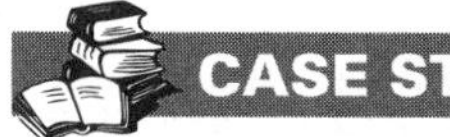

CASE STUDY

Variance Analysis

Jennifer Smith was appointed nurse manager of the coronary care unit 5 months ago. It is a 10-bed unit that was budgeted at 80 percent occupancy. Her recent responsibility report indicates some positive and negative variances. She has been asked to give a verbal report at the next hospital budget review committee meeting. Among the issues Jennifer needs to consider are:

- What are the reasons for the increase in revenue?
- What expense lines are over budget?
- Although a contribution to the gross margin was made, an explanation of the negative variances needs to be given with a corrective action plan identified.

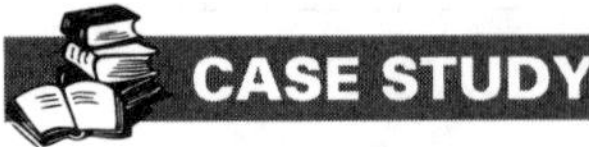

The Budget

Brenda Smith has been a head nurse on Division 6 West for 3 years. She has been a competent and thoughtful manager, and has been wanting to expand her role. She spoke to her director of nursing about her thoughts. Brenda explained that she needed to know more about the organization's plans so that she could feel she was keeping pace.

The director, Mr. Brown, suggested that Brenda think about the financial component of her division. He suggested that she consider becoming involved with the creation of the budget for her division rather than allowing financial management to dictate the budget for 6 West.

Brenda considered this possibility and felt that this would enhance her ability to plan for and control the division. However, she also considered that new technical knowledge had to be gained if she were to feel confident with this task. She devised a plan and a timetable that included what she needed to know.

She gave herself 1 year and scheduled meetings with financial management directors. She asked for and received the previous budgets for Division 6 West.

- What information and new knowledge does Brenda need?
- In what real way will this new responsibility enhance productivity on the division?

SUMMARY

This chapter has discussed the management of financial resources with special attention to the budgetary process. The major department in an organization that handles finances is the office of financial management. However, managers may be called upon to give input into decisions about finances as well as to manage a budgeted amount of money for specific divisions or departments.

It is with this responsibility in mind that a discussion concerning the budgetary process was offered. The major financial management office dictates to what degree the individual managers engage in financial management, which may include preparation of a budget.

The activity of preparing a budget requires some fundamental orientation to related budgetary concepts. Accounting is important to the process. There are different types of reports and formats, but today double-entry accounting is the most useful. Long-range financial plans for the organization dictate to what degree financial resources will be allocated for the present and the distant future. Budgetary terms are also fundamental to understanding what is involved with budgeting. Finally, the actual steps necessary to complete a budget are provided.

The manager's role may vary in relation to finances, but knowledge of the process is critical to the planning and control functions of the manager. The more information available to the manager, the better the decisions and the better the input into the long-range plans for the organization.

LEARNER EXERCISES

1. What do you think the nurse manager's role should be concerning the finances of the organization?
2. Do you think the nursing staff has a responsibility to understand the unit's budget? What role do they play in controlling it?
3. During your next clinical rotation, identify at least two cost-saving measures that the unit could implement.
4. Do some double-entry accounting of the money you began the week with and how you spent your funds. Was your spending what you anticipated?
5. On your next clinical rotation, observe the pattern of staff, use of drugs and equipment, and anything that is unusual. Determine a simple budget for the division. Use a category for salaries, drugs and equipment, and housekeeping expenses. Then observe to see if there will be a deviation from your plan. For instance, observe if extra patients are admitted, if a disaster occurs, or if too few staff require the use of nurses from an outside float pool.

SUGGESTED READINGS

Berman, H., Kukla, S.F., & Weeks, L.E. (1994). *The financial management of hospitals,* 8th ed. Ann Arbor, MI: Health Administration Press.

Finkler, S.A., & Kovner, C.T. (2000). *Financial management for nurse managers and executives,* 2nd ed. Philadelphia: Saunders.

Holder, W., & Williams, J. (1979). Better cost control with flexible budget and variance analysis. In E. Schied (Editor), *Maintaining cost effectiveness.* Chicago: Nursing Resources.

Marquis, B.L., & Huston, C.J. (1996). *Leadership roles and management functions in nursing,* 2nd ed. Philadelphia: Lippincott.

Wellever, A. (1982). Variance analysis: A tool for cost control. *Journal of Nursing Administration,* 12(7–8), 23–26.

West, D.J. (1994). Involving physicians in cost reduction strategies. *Healthcare Financial Management,* 48(4), 46–47.

Wilburn, D. (1992). Budget response to volume variability. *Nursing Management,* 23(2), 42–44.

17

Informatics in Nursing

"Progress results from persistence with purpose."

Frank Tyger

INTRODUCTION

Information technology is changing the world. Today, individuals are able to communicate on an international level, sharing information in new and exciting ways. Nursing, like other disciplines, has been greatly affected by technological advances in communication and information sciences. Nurses have benefited from the achievements made in information management, by using information systems in hospitals, clinics, and managed care settings. Organized information facilitates updating practice standards, adapting computer-based materials for clinical and patient teaching, testing computer systems for effectiveness, and structuring classification schemes for documenting the nursing process and quality patient care.[1] This chapter will discuss the role of informatics and the nursing profession.

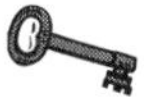

KEY CONCEPTS

Computers are machines composed of hardware and software that are used to process, manage, and store data, information, and knowledge.

Data are facts reported without interpretation.

Evidence-Based Care is nursing care that is delivered based on knowledge established through research.

Informatics combine computer and information sciences in order to manage and process data, information, and knowledge.

Information is the processing of data into relevant and meaningful statements.

Knowledge involves developing interrelationships among informational statements to create a meaningful whole.

Nursing Informatics are anything that assists nurses in the management of data in the direct care of clients (patients).

Patient Care Outcomes are the direct and measurable effects of nursing care.

Quality of Care is the degree to which the nursing care provided achieves its standards of practice.

DEFINITION OF INFORMATICS

Technological advances and concurrent changes in health care have changed every aspect of nursing.[2, 3, 4] **Informatics**, a major part of the technological revolution, has contributed to many of the changes health care is now experiencing. Informatics, by definition, is the process of combining computer and information sciences in order to manage and process data, information, and knowledge. It is through the use of this organized information that goals are set and existing information is revised. Nursing must use the best available information to forge future directions in this rapidly changing health care environment.[5, 6, 7, 8]

All practicing nurses are data gatherers. They do so by assessing and monitoring patients, communicating with patients and their families, and reviewing the patient's medical records. In turn, nurses interpret this data in a way that allows them to synthesize the knowledge needed to properly care for the patient. Subsequently, nurses rely on extensive knowledge and information to adequately make decisions and evaluate patient care. Competency requires access and the use of up-to-date information. Nursing information systems can assist in this process by identifying service demands providing data to assist in care and determining the **quality of the care** provided.[9]

The combination of informatics and information science creates an economical and efficient means of enhancing the acquisition, use, and manipulation of data. Thus, informatics is a powerful tool for knowledge development. In addition, informatics provides an effective means by which nursing science can organize and communicate its data, information, and knowledge within and outside the profession.

COMPUTERS

Future nursing practice will depend on the computer to manage data for meaningful practice and to further develop nursing informatics.[10, 11, 12] **Computers** organize data by collecting, storing, processing, retrieving, displaying, and communicating information.[13] These functions support the delivery of patient care by demonstrating effective nursing and medical regimes. For example, obstetrical patients have been discharged earlier from the hospital since a review of inpatient obstetrical patients' records indicated it is safe for them to go home earlier.

Computers also locate, transform, and provide information.[14, 15] When computer users go "online" to seek the answer to clinical questions, information can be found quickly and easily. This activity combines the requests of the user with the information available through the information network. Information can also be moved from one source to another and can be transformed or analyzed to reveal additional information. Consider the example of the public health service, which rapidly provided information about threats to health such as the 2001 anthrax scare. Providing health care providers and the general public with appropriate and scientific information as to prevention and treatment strategies can be implemented to minimize the effects of a potential lethal threat. In addition, computers can rapidly perform computations, supporting knowledge development, organization, and dissemination. Assessment of the current workforce in health care and nursing can be accomplished because of the capability of stored labor statistics, which experts are able to analyze and report.

Components of Computers: Hardware and Software

Hardware

Computers are composed of hardware and software. Computer hardware consists of the physical elements of the machine (the screen, keypad, and inner or mechanical workings). There are various ways in which this hardware is arranged, such as in supercomputers, mainframes, and personal computers.

Supercomputers are designed to compute millions of pieces of information simultaneously and carry out one task at a time. They are developed for use in meteorology, nuclear energy, and highly integrated information systems. Mainframes are designed to serve many users concurrently and are also able to run a number of programs at the same time. Personal computers are designed for individual users for word processing, accounting, database management, and communication on the Internet.

In the past, health care organizations used a central computer that was housed in the data processing division of the organization. Today, centralized computer systems have given way to distributed workstations and personal computers, which allows communication and interaction between individuals and organizations. Most divisions or units of the hospital, clinic, and offices have individual computers for the purposes of data entry, such as charting, medication administration, and laboratory reports. Pertinent patient data is entered and stored at the patient's bedside or other appropriate locations. Today, personal computers, such as laptops, personal digital assistants, and notebooks, are convenient and allow the user to have computer access almost anywhere.

The system components of a computer are a keyboard to enter data, a display screen (with personal computers), and a central processing unit (CPU), which controls the functioning of the computer. Other system components include "disk drives, hard drives, connectors, and slots for special purpose cards."[16] The motherboard (or system board) provides the connections between the system components of the computer.

The computer must be able to store data in order to process it. Random access memory (RAM) is the primary working memory of the computer.[17] RAM is a temporary form of memory. Information stored in RAM will be lost when the document is closed or the power is shut down. Read only memory (ROM) is a permanent form of storage and is used to store the programs needed when the computer is started.[18] CACHE is a special memory mechanism that allows the CPU very rapid access to information.[19]

Software

Computer software, however, directs computer functions.[20] Software tells the computer what to do and in what format. The computer operates through two basic types of software: systems and application. Systems software enables the computer to operate in a particular fashion. The operating system provides a foundation for application programs. It is the operating system that coordinates input from the keyboard with output on the screen, responds to mouse clicks, heeds commands to save a file, and transmits commands to printers and other peripheral devices.

Application programs perform specific functions for typical everyday use. The five basic types of application programs are "word processing, spreadsheets, database management, presentation software, and programs that enable computer-to-computer communication."[21] Word processing programs allow personal computer users to create and edit their written documents. Spreadsheets allow users to categorize, manage, and perform calculations on numerical information. Presentation software allows nurses to present their data, information, and knowledge in an orderly, visually appealing manner. Computer-to-computer communication manages information synthesis and exchange.

NURSING INFORMATICS

Nursing informatics is rapidly being recognized as a priority for the nursing profession. Nurses may spend up to 50 percent of their time documenting patient information, and computer assistance is mandatory. An outgrowth of hospital information systems, nursing informatics is viewed as a cost-effective application to meet nursing information requirements. **Nursing informatics** combines computer and information sciences with nursing science for the management and processing of data, information, and knowledge in support of the delivery of quality nursing care.[22, 23, 24] In addition, Turley[25] suggested including cognitive science to the model of nursing informatics. Cognitive science takes into account thinking, perceiving, understanding, and remembering. This proposed model creates a multidisciplinary framework for nursing informatics. An encompassing definition of nursing informatics is anything that assists nurses in the management of data in the direct care of clients.

Data, information, and knowledge are the building blocks of nursing informatics. **Data** are the facts that are reported without interpretation. **Information** is data that have been interpreted to create relevance and meaning. **Knowledge** is informational statements that have been synthesized into an integrated, meaningful whole. For example, the number 4 is raw data that is presented without interpretation, relevance, or particular meaning. Information is the interpretation of the raw data, or in this case, the number 4. When the data is put into a context or added to other data, relevance and meaning can be found. When the number 4 is put into the context of obstetrical nursing, it can reflect the parity of a patient. Knowledge involves critical thinking processes, taking interpretation one step further. The original data are placed into context with additional data to make decisions and create new knowledge. In our example, the nurse would provide patient education based on knowledge of the present status of the patient, the history of the

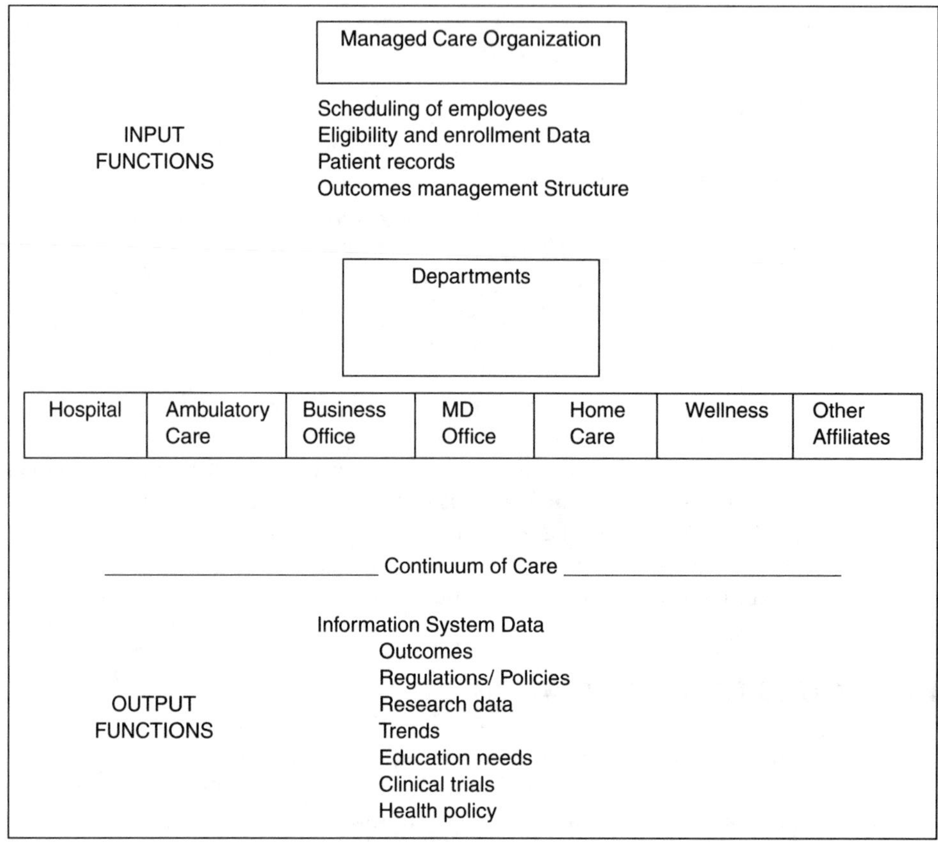

FIGURE 17-1. Health care enterprise information technology model showing inputs and outputs.

Adapted from Computers in Nursing, *17(6), November/December 1999, 278–285.*

patient, and obstetrical nursing. With nursing informatics, nurses can process, manage, and store nursing data, information, and knowledge (see Figure 17-1).

Nursing informatics allows nurses to record and evaluate their care activities. Because informatics needs a standard language, communication with other nurses, physicians, and administrators is more effective. Nursing informatics enables nurses to clarify treatments and physicians' orders expediently and with increased accuracy. Nursing informatics has been designed "to fully understand the structure of nursing knowledge, redefine nursing language so that it can properly describe this structure, and to make this new lexicon an integral component of a potential computerized model of the process of nursing information management."[26]

Significance of Nursing Informatics

Nursing informatics is essential for all nurses.[27, 28, 29, 30] Informatics allows nurses to organize and manage nursing information through various technologies. The knowledge which results from information processing leads to new questions, informed decisions to improve patient care, and provide the basis for **evidence based care**. The specific value of nursing informatics is as follows:

- **Nursing informatics facilitates communication.**
  Since Nursing informatics requires the use of standardized language for the documentation and communication of data, communication will be facilitated for interdisciplinary health care delivery and research.[31, 32, 33, 34, 35] This standardized terminology is imperative for the meaningful extraction and analysis of data. Nurses are the health care professionals who spend the most time in direct contact with patients and must be in a position to communicate clearly and effectively with respect to the delivery of nursing care.

- **Nursing informatics allows articulation of organized information.**
  A lack of consistent records and standards in the reporting process has made it difficult for researchers to determine how and why nursing care affects **patient care outcomes**. Informatics allows the articulation of patient care records, selected data, and the delivery of nursing care. Data analysis and thoughtful interpretation will provide valuable knowledge about the important role nurses play in patient outcomes.

- **Nursing informatics leads to credibility.**
  The nurse's role in successful patient outcomes is well known by the millions of patient testimonials, but a computer database designed around the recording of nursing practices could be used to quantify the exact contribution of nursing to positive patient outcomes. Nursing has developed various classification systems to document and quantify nursing practice to substantiate the contribution of professional nursing practice.

Nursing Informatics: Special Applications

Nursing education, practice, research, and administration have all benefited from the development of nursing informatics. The value of nursing informatics in each area is as follows:

- **Nursing education**
  Computers and nursing informatics have changed the face of education.[36, 37] Distance learning eliminates the barriers to accessing educational programs. Time, travel, and cost may no longer be problematic when nursing students are completing their educational programs. Educational programs have also incorporated multimedia applications into their curriculum, enhancing the learning process for nursing students at all levels of education. To be able to identify and use vital health care resources, nursing graduates must be sophisticated in the use of information technologies and must understand how these technologies interface with various health care systems. For example, schools of nursing can provide informatics education in their curricula, adapting to the different needs of the students.

- **Nursing practice**
  Nursing informatics is essential to organizing the vast amount of knowledge available to all nurses. The primary benefit from the use of nursing informatics is the increased amount of time available for patient care as a result of providing the proper information for care.

- **Patient education**
  Nursing informatics can be used for symptom management and patient education. The nurse can access the information for the patient or teach the patient where to find appropriate and helpful information. For example, on an oncology unit, nursing informatics can be used to teach patients effective symptom management of the treatment modalities which often cause pain, fatigue, and poor nutritional status. Nursing informatics can also aid in other nursing interventions of the oncology nurse, such as analgesic administration and stress-reduction techniques.

- **Clinical alert system**
  The computerized clinical alert system can be used in conjunction with the hospital pharmacy. A system design is created to alert both pharmacy and health staff when two or more drug prescriptions are incompatible.

- **Patient data**
  Nursing informatics can also be useful in a physician's office or clinic. In a managed care environment, information systems make administrative management more efficient. The private practitioner, program, or facility to manage every aspect of patient care can use one data management system (see Figure 17-2). In each of these health care settings, data management systems can be applied to treatments, diagnostics, documentation, practice management, insurance claims and referrals, and protocols, as well as treatment and diagnostics results.

- **Telehealth**
  Telehealth includes the use of telephones and sophisticated image transmission systems like EKG, faxes, and remote camera imaging. Telehealth places the ambulance

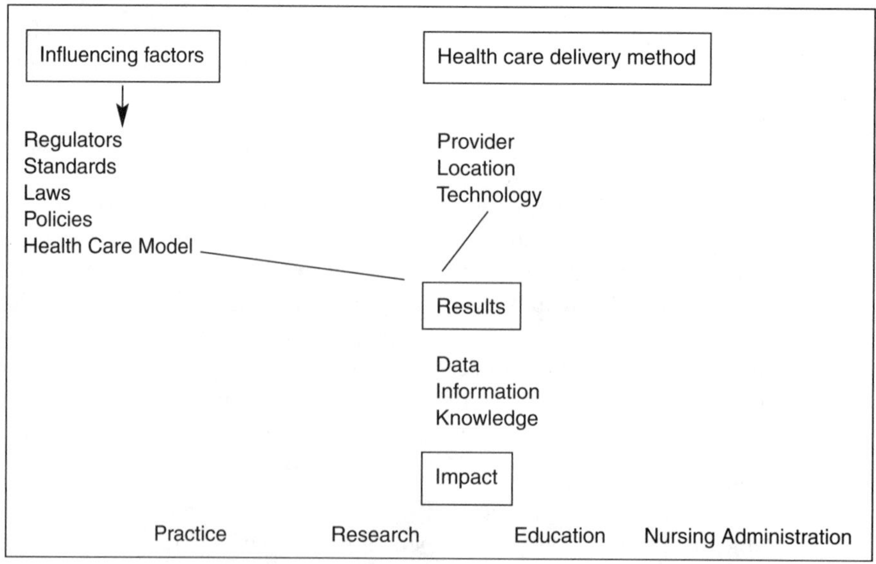

FIGURE 17-2. Patient-centered information model.

personnel in touch with the Emergency Department, and it also operates to put the generalist "nurses and doctors" at the ED in touch with specialists. Telehealth is used to evaluate stroke victims while they are in transit so appropriate therapy can be initiated quickly upon arrival at the ED. In similar fashion, a nurse practitioner in a remote ED might be guided via telephone in the proper procedure for inserting chest tubes so a man with a collapsed lung could be stabilized for subsequent transport to a major hospital. Finally, nursing informatics can be useful for interdepartmental communication. For example, ordering supplies from central supply, diagnostics, lab work, or even extra meal trays can easily be accomplished with the computer.

- **Clinical information**
  In order for the nurse to ensure the patient is receiving the most up-to-date care for a variety of chronic conditions, the National Institutes of Health (NIH) have an agency designed to offer such guidance. Clinical practice guidelines can be found at **http://www.nhlbi.nih.gov/guidelines/index.htm.** The practice guidelines found at this site provide management information for asthma, cholesterol, hypertension, and obesity.

  Clinical practice guidelines for the management of diabetes mellitus and menopause can be found at **http://www.aace.com/clinguideindex.htm.** Further information can be found through the Medscape Nurses site, and the National Institutes of Health—**http://www.nih.gov**

- **Nursing research**
  Nursing informatics is useful for nursing research. In research, nursing informatics provides a variety of ways to gather, organize, and analyze information. A researcher can easily gather specific data in order to identify specific trends in a health care population. For example, if a researcher was conducting a study on the predisposing factors of breast cancer, he or she could use a data management system in order to isolate the information on women in a specific geographical area. Within the system, he or she could then find information, such as age, past medical history, family history, occupation, and other factors affecting the health status of the individual.

- **Nursing administration**
  Nursing informatics supports the administrative processes involved in accessing health care. Using a computer program, or informatics, can reduce and simplify the "paper trail" of billing, costs, and insurance. Nursing administration in educational programs benefit from nursing informatics through the simplification of their administrative functions. Administrative personnel can access information related to health care settings, managed care settings, clinical sites, students, and other educational facilities in support of quality education.

THE HEALTH CARE RECORD

The availability of data and the technology that supports it will continue to change the way clinicians practice.[38] The primary benefit of technology and nursing informatics is the improved organization and access to information. Through computerized charting and record keeping, the work of nursing can remain focused on bedside care.

Health records, whether paper or computerized, serve four main purposes:

1. Document client care.
2. Facilitate communication among the patient's health care team.
3. Provide a financial and legal record of the care delivered.
4. Improve the quality of health care.

Computerized Patient Record

The use of a computerized patient record (CPR) has improved the communication among health professionals, increased the speed of communication, and decreased the actual amount of time nurses spend on paperwork.[39, 40] Many health care facilities are working toward computerized patient records through integrated information systems. With regard to the advantages and disadvantages of (paper versus) electronic records, electronic systems are advantageous because they:

- Have the patient's entire history.
- Can flag drug reaction problems.
- Can eliminate redundancy in record keeping.
- Eliminate the need for taking repeated histories.
- Can, if utilized properly, reduce error.

Electronic systems have the following disadvantages in that they:

- Are very expensive to set up.
- Are less secure.
- Require standardized coding systems, which force all users to use entries that the computer can understand.

A computerized patient record for data management

This data management approach revolutionizes the abilities of the informatics specialist, creating advantages for patients and health care professionals alike. The computerized patient record allows medical personnel access to pertinent patient information, such as one's name, address, phone number, next of kin, insurance information, allergies, past medical history, primary physician, any specialty practitioners, and advanced directives. This patient information must be treated with the strictest of confidentiality.

INFORMATICS SYSTEMS

Health care facilities have hired nursing informatics specialists (NISs) to create a specialized data management system. The NIS understands the nature and management of nursing knowledge and nursing information. Nursing informatics specialists build systems to support the development of information management systems. For example, a NIS may design a nursing care critical pathway to support clinical decision making. This pathway can be incorporated into a patient chart or could be used by nurses as part of the data management system. Depending on how the program is created, alarm systems can be inserted in order to alert health care personnel when making decisions related to medical intervention.

Computer programs need to be flexible enough that a nursing informatics specialist can customize a program to the needs of any health care population. For example, a program can be created in conjunction with the pharmacy department in a hospital in order to alert hospital staff when incompatible medications are prescribed to a patient.

Challenge of Nursing Informatics

Unfortunately, the substantial benefits from the use of informatics remain unrealized as evidenced through the high rate of implementation failures. Partially integrated systems that lack informational support create an extensive problem. Once a program has been installed, without the proper education or assistance, health care personnel are unable to use the system effectively. Success can only be reinforced when the system meets the needs of its users, matches the way information is processed in an organization, and the users are properly trained. One of the largest problems in informatics and data management is the lack of computer skills among those who are intended to use it. Many of the organizations that install programs, such as those used in nursing informatics, do not provide support to their customers after the product is installed. In addition, most of the "training" that is provided is inadequate and becomes more like a "quick tutoring session." Proper training and skill development are essential for the proper utilization of information systems.

Ethical Considerations

Nurses encounter ethical dilemmas every day. The advances made in technology and communication make ethical considerations an imperative in every nursing situation. As the health care marketplace changes with the growth in managed care, integrated delivery systems, and computer use, protecting the privacy, confidentiality, and security of health information has never been more critical for ethical/legal reasons.[41]

Security

Security concerns affect individuals as well as society as a whole. The safety and welfare of patients relies upon the ethical practices of all health care professionals. Information must remain secure to protect the health and lives of every patient. The subject of security could lead to an entire book; only a few problems are listed here. Security lapses have led to:

- Criminals getting the home addresses of vulnerable patients.
- Life insurance companies getting data which led to the denial of an application for insurance.
- Unauthorized people at both health insurance companies and patient employees getting patient data.

Confidentiality

The data, information, and knowledge developed in health care settings is primarily intimate in nature, requiring all health care professionals to adhere to ethical principles when communicating such information. Confidentiality involves the protection of patients in any health care setting. The identities of patients must not be connected to the information they provide and will never be made public. Patients and their families must have a sense of security and must know that their health information will remain confidential. Only those health care professionals directly dealing with the patient's health care will have access to their health information.

Privacy

The respect for privacy entails that nurses consider and protect the intimate information revealed in health care situations. Nurses must strive to protect the privacy of patients, keeping information in the strictest of confidence. Information will be accessible only to those individuals directly involved with the care and health of the patient.

A central question when considering the ethical ramifications of advances in technology is, "Who owns the client's health care data?"[42] Some experts advocate a patient-focused approach with individuals possessing ownership of their health care data. Others advocate a social approach to health care data, stating that society as a whole benefits from information gained from health care.

Legal protection has been implemented to protect health care information. Federal law protects individual's rights to privacy. Federal laws intend to appropriately balance the public's right to access and control information gathered by the government against the individual's right to protect personal information from misuse.

THE INTERNET: A RESOURCE FOR NURSING

In the past, when faced with a difficult situation, nurses referred to the standard of care set out in their nursing school textbook or asked a fellow nurse. These approaches are a poor substitute for computerized access to the latest information directly from the workplace. The World Wide Web (www) is one source that contains data, information, and knowledge. However, care must be taken to evaluate this information carefully as it may be accurate or inaccurate, complete or incomplete, and updated or outdated. However, the most recent information is often available on the web before it appears in peer-reviewed articles. Some websites are consumer- and patient-oriented, while others contain greater detail and are oriented to health care professionals.

Another source of interesting information comes from large health maintenance organizations (HMOs). These sites often provide the latest information on common diseases, as well as health promotion strategies.

Other helpful websites for obtaining nursing information include: the American Journal of Nursing (**http://www.nursingcenter.com/journals**), the Cumulative Index of Nursing and Allied Health Literature (CINAHL) (**http://www.conahl.com/**), the National Institute of Nursing Research (**http://www.nih.gov/ninr/**), and a nursing site on the World Wide Web (**http://ublib.buffalo.edu/libraries/units/hsl/internet/ nsgsites.html**).

The Internet provides a means by which nurses can communicate with one another, other health care professionals, and professional organizations. Used with understanding of its benefits and its limitations, nurses have an invaluable resource for accessing and building nursing knowledge. Valuable nursing informatics websites include the American Nursing Informatics Association (**http://www.ania.org/**), the Virtual Nursing College (**http://www.langara.bc.ca/vnc/index.html**), the Online Journal of Nursing

Informatics (http://cac.psu.edu/~dxm12/main.html), and the American Medical Informatics Association (http://www.amia-niwg.org/).

FUTURE DIRECTIONS

Nursing informatics holds great promise in all areas of nursing. It has had, and will continue to have a great impact on nursing practice. Communication will play an important role in nursing informatics as the data, information, knowledge, and health care itself become increasingly complex.

Nursing informatics must begin to focus on the interaction and interdependence of each member of the health care team. An integrated view of health informatics will depend upon interdisciplinary commitment and communication.[43] The function of health informatics is to model the data, information, knowledge, and wisdom needed in health care and to communicate that data, information, knowledge, and wisdom in an effective manner.[44] Nursing informatics must incorporate its own unique knowledge base into the larger realm of health care. In areas where various health disciplines share data, information, or knowledge, there will be shared areas of informatics as well.[45]

Nursing informatics will continue to impact every aspect of the profession. In nursing education, nursing curriculum must continue to expand its distance learning and online capabilities. Communication and information technology needs to be incorporated more fully into current nursing programs to support our participation in the future of health care. In nursing practice, CPRs will be integrated into more health care settings, resulting in the virtual elimination of traditional paper records. Informatics will change the way clinicians understand the information that is available to them.[46, 47] In nursing research, data, information, and knowledge will be communicated easily and quickly with the increased development of nursing informatics. Areas for future research in nursing informatics include "outcomes measurement using nursing information systems, decision support and expert systems, point-of-care documentation, interagency and interdisciplinary communication, and further work on individual and organizational factors.[48] In nursing administration, administrative processes will be simplified through electronic communication. Access to information and communication with students, faculty, schools of nursing, professional organizations, and health care organizations will be supported through nursing informatics.

CASE STUDY

Informatics

The Director of Nursing Service, Mrs. Arthur, was reviewing various reports from the network's administration. One report in particular grasped her attention. She noticed the degree of incident reports had been steadily rising in the nursing department and that patient falls have increased. She immediately called for a data analysis of this problem. She sought information about *who* was involved, *where* these falls were occurring, *what* time of day and season these incidents were occurring in, and *what* other trends were apparent from these incidents.

After reviewing the data, a plan was put in place to reduce the number of falls by identifying those at risk for a fall, a fall education program for the staff, and early treatment for any incident. Following the implementation of the plan, the number of falls were reduced, and the severity of the injuries were lessened.

- What kind of data is necessary to evaluate a problem of this nature?
- Where would this data come from?
- Are solutions available via electronic means?
- Is informatics a more efficient and accurate way of determining problems than discussing problems with supervisors or other leaders in the organization?
- Defend your position.

CASE STUDY

Data Analysis: Internet

Michelle Carlson, a senior nursing student, was given her clinical assignment for the next day. Michelle was working at her part-time job at the cafeteria that evening, and didn't take the time to study her assignment until late that evening. When she reviewed her patient's condition, she realized she was unfamiliar with many aspects of her patient's required nursing care. Michelle immediately went to her computer and began a search for answers to her questions in preparation for the next day's assignment. As she completed her search, she was able to review online nursing journals and a website that answered questions about patients' conditions.

- Did Michelle use the right resource or should she should have reviewed her clinical textbooks?
- Are there any problems associated with information gained from the Internet? Is it accurate, up-to-date, and useful for various levels of nursing care?
- Are there any concerns you should consider when using and interacting with patient websites?

SUMMARY

Nursing informatics is evolving every day. Information systems support the management and communication of the data, information, and knowledge generated through nursing science. The use of information and communication technologies must be based on thorough training, moderation, and ethical considerations. Only health care professionals can provide patient care. Nurses must rely on their own knowledge, skills, and abilities when providing quality patient care.

LEARNER EXERCISES

1. Define informatics.
2. What are the advantages of organized information? Disadvantages?

3. A major analysis performed by nurse researchers identified the potential of a very serious and looming nurse shortage. Is this use of organized information helpful to policymakers and administrators?
4. How can confidentiality be maintained in such an open system of communication, such as the Internet and patient records?
5. What future directions do you see for informatics?

REFERENCES

1. Saba, V. (2001). Historical perspectives of nursing and the computer. In V. K. Saba & K. A. McCormick (Eds.), *Essentials of computers for nurses: Informatics for the new millennium,* 3rd ed. (pp. 9–45). New York: McGraw-Hill.
2. Hannah, K., Ball, M., & Edwards, M. (1999). *Introduction to nursing informatics,* 2nd ed. New York: Springer, pp. 3–50, 79–113, 261–271.
3. Hebda, T., Czar, P., & Mascara, C. (2001). *Handbook of informatics for nurses and health care professionals,* 2nd ed. Englewood Cliffs, NJ: Prentice Hall, pp. 3–47, 81–98, 145–162.
4. Saba, V., & McCormick, K. (2001). Overview of computers and nursing. In V. K. Saba & K. A. McCormick (Eds.), *Essentials of computers for nurses: Informatics for the new millennium,* 3rd ed. (pp. 9–45). New York: McGraw-Hill.
5. Scott, G. (2001). Nursing informatics. *Journal of Community Nursing, 15*(3), pp. 4–6, 8, 10.
6. Thede, L. (1999). *Computers in nursing: Bridges to the future.* Philadelphia: Lippincott, pp. 3–78, 289–294.
7. Turley, J. (1996). Toward a model for nursing informatics. *Image: Journal of Nursing Scholarship, 28*(4), 309–313.
8. McGonigle, D., & Eggers, R. (1991). Establishing a nursing informatics program. *Computers in Nursing, 9*(5), 184–189.
9. Scott, G. (2001). Nursing informatics. *Journal of Community Nursing, 15*(3), 5.
10. Scott, G. (2001). Nursing informatics. *Journal of Community Nursing, 15*(3), 6.
11. Hunter, K. (2001). Nursing informatics theory. In V. K. Saba & K. A. McCormick (Eds.), *Essentials of computers for nurses: Informatics for the new millennium,* 3rd ed. (pp. 179–190). New York: McGraw-Hill.
12. McHugh, M. (2001). Computer hardware. In V. K. Saba & K. A. McCormick (Eds.), *Essentials of computers for nurses: Informatics for the new millennium,* 3rd ed. (pp. 49–65). New York: McGraw-Hill.
13. Thede, L. (1999). *Computers in nursing: Bridges to the future.* Philadelphia: Lippincott, p. 6.
14. Thede, L. (1999). *Computers in nursing: Bridges to the future.* Philadelphia: Lippincott, p. 6.
15. McHugh, M. (2001). Computer hardware. In V. K. Saba & K. A. McCormick (Eds.), *Essentials of computers for nurses: Informatics for the new millennium,* 3rd ed. (p. 50). New York: McGraw-Hill.
16. Thede, L. (1999). *Computers in nursing: Bridges to the future.* Philadelphia: Lippincott, p. 12.
17. Thede, L. (1999). *Computers in nursing: Bridges to the future.* Philadelphia: Lippincott, p. 14.
18. Thede, L. (1999). *Computers in nursing: Bridges to the future.* Philadelphia: Lippincott, p. 16.
19. Thede, L. (1999). *Computers in nursing: Bridges to the future.* Philadelphia: Lippincott, p. 17.
20. McHugh, M. (2001). Software. In V. K. Saba & K. A. McCormick (Eds.), *Essentials of computers for nurses: Informatics for the new millennium,* 3rd ed. (pp. 67–83). New York: McGraw-Hill.
21. Thede, L. (1999). *Computers in nursing: Bridges to the future.* Philadelphia: Lippincott, p. 30.

22. Hunter, K. (2001). Nursing informatics theory. In V. K. Saba & K. A. McCormick (Eds.), *Essentials of computers for nurses: Informatics for the new millennium,* 3rd ed. (pp. 179–190). New York: McGraw-Hill.
23. Graves, J., & Corcoran, S. (1989). The study of nursing informatics. *Image: Journal of Nursing Scholarship, 21,* 227–231.
24. Young, K. (2000). Nursing informatics. In J. Catalano (Ed.), *Nursing now!: Today's issues, tomorrow's trends,* 2nd ed. (pp. 373–396). Philadelphia: F.A. Davis.
25. Turley, J. (1996). Toward a model for nursing informatics. *Image: Journal of Nursing Scholarship,* 28(4), 313.
26. Jones, S. (2000). Nursing informatics. *Assignment—Ongoing Work of Health Care Students,* 6(4), 5–6.
27. Saba, V. (2001). Historical perspectives of nursing and the computer. In V. K. Saba & K. A. McCormick (Eds.), *Essentials of computers for nurses: Informatics for the new millennium,* 3rd ed. (p. 9). New York: McGraw-Hill.
28. Hannah, K., Ball, M., & Edwards, M. (1999). *Introduction to nursing informatics,* 2nd ed. New York: Springer, pp. 3–10.
29. Hebda, T., Czar, P., & Mascara, C. (2001). *Handbook of informatics for nurses and health care professionals,* 2nd ed. Englewood Cliffs, NJ: Prentice Hall, pp. 3–12.
30. Thede, L. (1999). *Computers in nursing: Bridges to the future.* Philadelphia: Lippincott, pp. 3–4.
31. Hunter, K. (2001). Nursing informatics theory. In V. K. Saba & K. A. McCormick (Eds.), *Essentials of computers for nurses: Informatics for the new millennium,* 3rd ed. (p. 180). New York: McGraw-Hill.
32. Adderly, D., Hyde, C., & Mauseth, P. (1997). The computer age impacts nurses. *Computers in Nursing,* 15(1), 43–46.
33. Bowles, K. (1997). The barriers and benefits of nursing information systems. *Computers in Nursing,* 15(4), 191–196.
34. Song, L., Ho, J., & Ho, S. (1997). The integrated patient information system. *Computers in Nursing,* 15(2), S14–S22.
35. Swart, J. (1997). A patient core data set and integrated health information system. *Computers in Nursing,* 15(2), S5–S6.
36. Bachman, J., & Panzarine, S. (1998). Enabling student nurses to use the information superhighway. *Journal of Nursing Education,* 37(4), 155–161.
37. Carty, B., & Rosenfeld, P. (1998). From computer technology to information technology: Findings from a national study of nursing education. *Computers in Nursing,* 16(5), 259–265.
38. Turley, J. (1996). Toward a model for nursing informatics. *Image: Journal of Nursing Scholarship,* 28(4), 313.
39. Song, L., Ho, J., & Ho, S. (1997). The integrated patient information system. *Computers in Nursing,* 15(2), S22.
40. Swart, J. (1997). A patient core data set and integrated health information system. *Computers in Nursing,* 15(2), S6.
41. Buckovich, S. (2001). Privacy, confidentiality, and security. In V. K. Saba & K. A. McCormick (Eds.), *Essentials of computers for nurses: Informatics for the new millennium,* 3rd ed. (pp. 155–166). New York: McGraw-Hill.
42. Young, K. (2000). Nursing informatics. In J. Catalano (Ed.), *Nursing now!: Today's issues, tomorrow's trends,* 2nd ed. (p. 386). Philadelphia: F.A. Davis.
43. Turley, J. (2000). Toward an integrated view of health informatics. *Information Technology in Nursing,* 12(4), 10–15.
44. Turley, J. (2000). Toward an integrated view of health informatics. *Information Technology in Nursing,* 12(4), 13.

45. Bachman, J., & Panzarine, S. (1998). Enabling student nurses to use the information superhighway. *Journal of Nursing Education*, 37(4), 155.
46. Turley, J. (2000). Toward an integrated view of health informatics. *Information Technology in Nursing*, 12(4), 15.
47. Bowles, K. (1997). The barriers and benefits of nursing information systems. *Computers in Nursing*, 15(4), 191.
48. Bowles, K. (1997). The barriers and benefits of nursing information systems. *Computers in Nursing*, 15(4), 191.

Index

D

M

T

U

V

W

X

Y